Preface

Drug therapy is the corner stone of the medical profession. As a medical student, resident, clinician, nurse, or pharmacist you are faced with a tremendous amount of information concerning drug therapy. In Canada it is often difficult to find a quick, convenient pharmaceutical reference that has relevant Canadian content.

I am proud to introduce the **Canadian Drug pocket**. This book is a pocket drug reference guide. A distinctly Canadian version of the already popular Drug pocket published in the US and Germany. The **Canadian Drug pocket** is unique among pocket reference guides. It includes information such as mechanisms of actions, effects, side effects and contraindications. As well as elimination half-lives, pregnancy risk categories and use during lactation. Most importantly it contains the active agents with their Canadian trade names and available forms, strengths, and recommended dosages.

I hope that this edition of the **Canadian Drug pocket** will be a useful clinical tool. It is a reference guide that is designed for the Canadian health professional. To assure continued improvement of the **Canadian Drug pocket**, any comments, criticisms, or additions would be greatly appreciated.

Carmine Nudo, M.D. C.M. FRCPC June 2008
nudo@media4u.com

Additional titles in this series:

Acupuncture pocket
Anatomy pocket
Differential Diagnosis pocket
Drug pocket 2008
Drug pocket plus 2008
Drug Therapy pocket 2006–2007
ECG pocket
ECG Cases pocket
EMS pocket
Homeopathy pocket
Medical Abbreviations pocket
Medical Classifications pocket
Medical Spanish pocket
Medical Spanish Dictionary pocket
Medical Spanish pocket plus
Medical Translator pocket
Normal Values pocket
Nursing Dictionary pocket
Respiratory pocket
Wards 101 pocket

Börm Bruckmeier Publishing LLC on the Internet:
www.media4u.com

Contents

Canadian Drug pocket 2009

www.media4u.com

Authors:

Carmine G. Nudo, M. D. C. M., FRCPC
Börm Bruckmeier Publishing LLC
111 1/2 Eucalyptus Drive, El Segundo,
CA 90245, USA
nudo@media4u.com

Andreas Russ, M. D.
Börm Bruckmeier Verlag GmbH
Nördliche Münchner Straße 28
82031 Grünwald, Germany
russ@media4u.com

Editor: Bettina Spengler, MD; Sarah Konert, MD
Production: Natascha Choffat, Anne Herhold
Cover Illustration: Lucie Mikyna
Publisher: Börm Bruckmeier Publishing LLC, www.media4u.com

Fourth Edition

IMPORTANT NOTICE - PLEASE READ!
This book is based on information from sources believed to be reliable, and every effort has been made to make the book as complete and accurate as possible and to describe generally accepted practices based on information available as of the printing date, but its accuracy and completeness cannot be guaranteed. Despite the best efforts of author and publisher, the book may contain errors, and the reader should use the book only as a general guide and not as the ultimate source of information about the subject matter.
This book is not intended to reprint all of the information available to the author or publisher on the subject, but rather to simplify, complement and supplement other available sources. The reader is encouraged to read all available material and to consult the package insert and other references to learn as much as possible about the subject.
This book is sold without warranties of any kind, expressed or implied, and the publisher and author disclaim any liability, loss or damage caused by the content of this book.
IF YOU DO NOT WISH TO BE BOUND BY THE FOREGOING CAUTIONS AND CONDITIONS , YOU MAY RETURN THIS BOOK TO THE PUBLISHER FOR A FULL REFUND.

Printed in China through Colorcraft Ltd., Hong Kong
ISBN 978-1-59103-247-2

July 2008

Tu	1	Canada Day
We	2	
Th	3	
Fr	4	
Sa	5	
Su	6	
Mo	7	
Tu	8	
We	9	
Th	10	
Fr	11	
Sa	12	
Su	13	
Mo	14	
Tu	15	
We	16	
Th	17	
Fr	18	
Sa	19	
Su	20	
Mo	21	
Tu	22	
We	23	
Th	24	
Fr	25	
Sa	26	
Su	27	
Mo	28	
Tu	29	
We	30	
Th	31	

August 2008

Fr	1	
Sa	2	
Su	3	
Mo	4	
Tu	5	
We	6	
Th	7	
Fr	8	
Sa	9	
Su	10	
Mo	11	
Tu	12	
We	13	
Th	14	
Fr	15	
Sa	16	
Su	17	
Mo	18	
Tu	19	
We	20	
Th	21	
Fr	22	
Sa	23	
Su	24	
Mo	25	
Tu	26	
We	27	
Th	28	
Fr	29	
Sa	30	
Su	31	

September 2008

Mo	1	Labour Day
Tu	2	
We	3	
Th	4	
Fr	5	
Sa	6	
Su	7	
Mo	8	
Tu	9	
We	10	
Th	11	
Fr	12	
Sa	13	
Su	14	
Mo	15	
Tu	16	
We	17	
Th	18	
Fr	19	
Sa	20	
Su	21	
Mo	22	
Tu	23	
We	24	
Th	25	
Fr	26	
Sa	27	
Su	28	
Mo	29	
Tu	30	

October 2008

We	1	
Th	2	
Fr	3	
Sa	4	
Su	5	
Mo	6	
Tu	7	
We	8	
Th	9	
Fr	10	
Sa	11	
Su	12	
Mo	13	Thanksgiving Day
Tu	14	
We	15	
Th	16	
Fr	17	
Sa	18	
Su	19	
Mo	20	
Tu	21	
We	22	
Th	23	
Fr	24	
Sa	25	
Su	26	
Mo	27	
Tu	28	
We	29	
Th	30	
Fr	31	Halloween

November 2008

Sa	1	
Su	2	
Mo	3	
Tu	4	
We	5	
Th	6	
Fr	7	
Sa	8	
Su	9	
Mo	10	
Tu	11	Remembrance Day
We	12	
Th	13	
Fr	14	
Sa	15	
Su	16	
Mo	17	
Tu	18	
We	19	
Th	20	
Fr	21	
Sa	22	
Su	23	
Mo	24	
Tu	25	
We	26	
Th	27	
Fr	28	
Sa	29	
Su	30	

December 2008

Mo	1	
Tu	2	
We	3	
Th	4	
Fr	5	
Sa	6	
Su	7	
Mo	8	
Tu	9	
We	10	
Th	11	
Fr	12	
Sa	13	
Su	14	
Mo	15	
Tu	16	
We	17	
Th	18	
Fr	19	
Sa	20	
Su	21	
Mo	22	
Tu	23	
We	24	Christmas Eve
Th	25	Christmas Day
Fr	26	Boxing Day
Sa	27	
Su	28	
Mo	29	
Tu	30	
We	31	New Year's Eve

January 2009

Th	1	New Year's Day
Fr	2	
Sa	3	
Su	4	
Mo	5	
Tu	6	
We	7	
Th	8	
Fr	9	
Sa	10	
Su	11	
Mo	12	
Tu	13	
We	14	
Th	15	
Fr	16	
Sa	17	
Su	18	
Mo	19	
Tu	20	
We	21	
Th	22	
Fr	23	
Sa	24	
Su	25	
Mo	26	
Tu	27	
We	28	
Th	29	
Fr	30	
Sa	31	

February 2009

Su	1	
Mo	2	
Tu	3	
We	4	
Th	5	
Fr	6	
Sa	7	
Su	8	
Mo	9	
Tu	10	
We	11	
Th	12	
Fr	13	
Sa	14	Valentine's Day
Su	15	
Mo	16	
Tu	17	
We	18	
Th	19	
Fr	20	
Sa	21	
Su	22	
Mo	23	
Tu	24	
We	25	
Th	26	
Fr	27	
Sa	28	

March 2009

Su	1	
Mo	2	
Tu	3	
We	4	
Th	5	
Fr	6	
Sa	7	
Su	8	
Mo	9	
Tu	10	
We	11	
Th	12	
Fr	13	
Sa	14	
Su	15	
Mo	16	
Tu	17	
We	18	
Th	19	
Fr	20	
Sa	21	
Su	22	
Mo	23	
Tu	24	
We	25	
Th	26	
Fr	27	
Sa	28	
Su	29	
Mo	30	
Tu	31	

April 2009

We	1	
Th	2	
Fr	3	
Sa	4	
Su	5	
Mo	6	
Tu	7	
We	8	
Th	9	
Fr	10	Good Friday
Sa	11	
Su	12	Easter Sunday
Mo	13	Easter Monday
Tu	14	
We	15	
Th	16	
Fr	17	
Sa	18	
Su	19	
Mo	20	
Tu	21	
We	22	
Th	23	
Fr	24	
Sa	25	
Su	26	
Mo	27	
Tu	28	
We	29	
Th	30	

May 2009

Fr	1	
Sa	2	
Su	3	
Mo	4	
Tu	5	
We	6	
Th	7	
Fr	8	
Sa	9	
Su	10	
Mo	11	
Tu	12	
We	13	
Th	14	
Fr	15	
Sa	16	
Su	17	
Mo	18	Victoria Day
Tu	19	
We	20	
Th	21	
Fr	22	
Sa	23	
Su	24	
Mo	25	
Tu	26	
We	27	
Th	28	
Fr	29	
Sa	30	
Su	31	

June 2009

Mo	1	
Tu	2	
We	3	
Th	4	
Fr	5	
Sa	6	
Su	7	
Mo	8	
Tu	9	
We	10	
Th	11	
Fr	12	
Sa	13	
Su	14	
Mo	15	
Tu	16	
We	17	
Th	18	
Fr	19	
Sa	20	
Su	21	
Mo	22	
Tu	23	
We	24	
Th	25	
Fr	26	
Sa	27	
Su	28	
Mo	29	
Tu	30	

July 2009

We	1	Canada Day
Th	2	
Fr	3	
Sa	4	
Su	5	
Mo	6	
Tu	7	
We	8	
Th	9	
Fr	10	
Sa	11	
Su	12	
Mo	13	
Tu	14	
We	15	
Th	16	
Fr	17	
Sa	18	
Su	19	
Mo	20	
Tu	21	
We	22	
Th	23	
Fr	24	
Sa	25	
Su	26	
Mo	27	
Tu	28	
We	29	
Th	30	
Fr	31	

August 2009

Sa	1	
Su	2	
Mo	3	
Tu	4	
We	5	
Th	6	
Fr	7	
Sa	8	
Su	9	
Mo	10	
Tu	11	
We	12	
Th	13	
Fr	14	
Sa	15	
Su	16	
Mo	17	
Tu	18	
We	19	
Th	20	
Fr	21	
Sa	22	
Su	23	
Mo	24	
Tu	25	
We	26	
Th	27	
Fr	28	
Sa	29	
Su	30	
Mo	31	

September 2009

Tu	1	
We	2	
Th	3	
Fr	4	
Sa	5	
Su	6	
Mo	7	Labour Day
Tu	8	
We	9	
Th	10	
Fr	11	
Sa	12	
Su	13	
Mo	14	
Tu	15	
We	16	
Th	17	
Fr	18	
Sa	19	
Su	20	
Mo	21	
Tu	22	
We	23	
Th	24	
Fr	25	
Sa	26	
Su	27	
Mo	28	
Tu	29	
We	30	

October 2009

Th	1	
Fr	2	
Sa	3	
Su	4	
Mo	5	
Tu	6	
We	7	
Th	8	
Fr	9	
Sa	10	
Su	11	
Mo	12	Thanksgiving Day
Tu	13	
We	14	
Th	15	
Fr	16	
Sa	17	
Su	18	
Mo	19	
Tu	20	
We	21	
Th	22	
Fr	23	
Sa	24	
Su	25	
Mo	26	
Tu	27	
We	28	
Th	29	
Fr	30	
Sa	31	Halloween

November 2009

Su	1	
Mo	2	
Tu	3	
We	4	
Th	5	
Fr	6	
Sa	7	
Su	8	
Mo	9	
Tu	10	
We	11	Remembrance Day
Th	12	
Fr	13	
Sa	14	
Su	15	
Mo	16	
Tu	17	
We	18	
Th	19	
Fr	20	
Sa	21	
Su	22	
Mo	23	
Tu	24	
We	25	
Th	26	
Fr	27	
Sa	28	
Su	29	
Mo	30	

December 2009

Tu	1	
We	2	
Th	3	
Fr	4	
Sa	5	
Su	6	
Mo	7	
Tu	8	
We	9	
Th	10	
Fr	11	
Sa	12	
Su	13	
Mo	14	
Tu	15	
We	16	
Th	17	
Fr	18	
Sa	19	
Su	20	
Mo	21	
Tu	22	
We	23	
Th	24	Christmas Eve
Fr	25	Christmas Day
Sa	26	Boxing Day
Su	27	
Mo	28	
Tu	29	
We	30	
Th	31	New Year's Eve

Januar 2010

Fr	1	New Year's Day
Sa	2	
Su	3	
Mo	4	
Tu	5	
We	6	
Th	7	
Fr	8	
Sa	9	
Su	10	
Mo	11	
Tu	12	
We	13	
Th	14	
Fr	15	
Sa	16	
Su	17	
Mo	18	
Tu	19	
We	20	
Th	21	
Fr	22	
Sa	23	
Su	24	
Mo	25	
Tu	26	
We	27	
Th	28	
Fr	29	
Sa	30	
Su	31	

Februar 2010

Mo	1	
Tu	2	
We	3	
Th	4	
Fr	5	
Sa	6	
Su	7	
Mo	8	
Tu	9	
We	10	
Th	11	
Fr	12	
Sa	13	
Su	14	Valentine's Day
Mo	15	
Tu	16	
We	17	
Th	18	
Fr	19	
Sa	20	
Su	21	
Mo	22	
Tu	23	
We	24	
Th	25	
Fr	26	
Sa	27	
Su	28	

1 Emergency

Adenosine	→59
Adenocard *Inj 3mg/ml*	**SVT** (not AF): 6mg rapidly IV, if no response, in 1–2min 12mg IV, then 12–18mg IV prn; **CH** ini 50mcg/kg IV, incr to 100mcg/kg, then to 200mcg/kg
Atropine →102	
Generics *Inj 0.1, 0.3, 0.4, 0.6, 1 mg/ml*	**Bradycardia, bradyarrhythmia:** 0.5–1.0 mg IV q3–5min, max 0.03–0.04mg/kg; **CH** 0.02mg/kg IV, minimum 0.1mg, max 0.5mg IV; **antimuscurinic:** 0.4–0.6mg IM/IV/SC q4–6h prn; **asystolic arrest:** 1mg IV, repeat q3–5min, max 0.04mg/kg; **organophosphate poisoning:** 1–2mg IM/IV q5–60min until symptoms disappear
Biperiden	→226
Akineton *Tab 2mg*	**Drug-induced extrapyramidal DO:** 2mg IM/IV q30min prn, max 8mg/24h; **CH** 0.04mg/kg/dose or 1.2mg/square meter/ dose IM, rep prn q30min, max 4 doses/d
Dextrose	→134
Generics *Inj 50mg/ml, 250mg/ml 2.5g/100ml, 5g/100ml, 10g/100ml, 20g/100ml, 30g/100ml, 40g/100ml, 50g/100ml, 60g/ 100ml, 70g/100ml*	**Hypoglycemia:** 25g (50ml of D50W) IV; **CH** >6mo: 0.5–1g/ kg (D25W 2–4ml/kg/dose) slowly IV, max 25g/dose, <6mo: 0.2–0.4g/kg (D10W 2–4ml/kg) slowly IV
Diazepam	→218 →232
Generics *Inj 1mg/ml, 5mg/ml*	**Seizures, status epilepticus:** 5–10mg IV, max rate 1mg/ min, rep prn q5min, max 30mg, or 10mg PR, rep prn; **CH** 1 mo–5 y: 0.2–0.5mg/kg slowly IV, rep prn q 5min, max 5mg, or 0.5mg/kg PR, rep prn in 4–12h, >5 y: 1mg IV, rep prn q5min, max 10mg or 0.3mg/kg PR, rep prn in 4–12h; **sedation:** 2–10mg IV/IM, rep prn in 4h; **muscle spasm:** 5–10mg IV/IM, rep prn in 4h

Digoxin	→60
Digoxin pediatric *Inj 0.05mg/ml* **Lanoxin** *Tab 0.0625, 0.125, 0.25mg, Inj 0.05, 0.25mg/ml, Ped elixir 0.05mg/ml* **Generics** *Inj 0.05, 0.25mg/ml, Tab 0.0625, 0.125, 0.25mg*	**AF, AF with tachyarrhythmia:** ini 0.5mg IV, rep in 4h, 0.25mg PO in 8h + 12h
Diltiazem	→49
Apo-Diltiaz *Inj 5mg/ml* **Generics** *Inj 5mg/ml*	**AF** (rapid): 20mg (0.25mg/kg) IV x 2min, rep in 15min prn 30mg (35mg/kg) IV, then prn inf at 5–15mg/h
Diphenhydramine	→251 →289
Generics *Inj 50mg/ml*	**Anaphylaxis:** 1mg/kg IV/IM, max 50mg single dose, rep prn q2–3h, max 400mg/d; **CH** 1.25mg/kg IV/IM qid, max 300mg/d
Dobutamine	→39
Dobutrex *Inj 12.5mg/ml* **Generics** *Inj 12.5mg/ml*	**Low-output-failure:** 1mg/ml (250mg in 250ml D5W) at 2.5–15mcg/kg/min, max 40mcg/kg/min
Dopamine	→39
Generics (dopamine + dextrose) *Inj 0.8mg/ml, 1.6mg/ml, 3.2mg/ml*	**Acute hypotension:** 400mg in 250ml D5W (1600mcg/ ml) a t 2–20mcg/kg/min IV, ini 2–5mcg/kg/min, incr by 1–4mcg/kg/min q 10–30min, max 50mcg/kg/min
Epinephrine	→39
Adrenalin *Inj 1mg/ml, Topical 1mg/ml* **Epipen** *Inj (IM) 0.3m g/delivery* **Epipen Jr.** *Inj (IM) 0.15mg/delivery* **Generics** *Inj 0.1mg/ml, 1mg/ml*	**Cardiac arrest:** 1mg (sol 1:10,000) IV/ET q3–5min prn; **CH** ini 0.01mg/kg IV, then prn 0.1mg/kg IV, max 0.2mg/kg IV (sol 1:10,000); **anaphylaxis:** 0.3–0.5mg/kg IV/IM/SC, rep q10–15min prn

Esmolol	→41
Brevibloc *Inj 10mg/ml, 250mg/ml*	**SVT:** ini 500mcg/kg IV x 1min, then 50mcg/kg/min IV x 4min, if response, do not change rate >25mcg/kg/min; if no response, rep 500mcg/kg IV x 1min, then 100mcg/kg/ min x 4min, prn rep 500mcg/kg IV x 1min, then incr inf by 50mcg/kg/min q4min, max 200mcg/kg/min
Fentanyl	→211
Generics *Inj 0.05mg/ml*	**Anaesthesia:** 50–100mcg IV/IM
Flumazenil	→318
Anexate *Inj 0.1mg/ml*	**Benzodiazepine overdose:** 0.2–0.5mg IV x 30sec, rep q 60 sec, max 3mg
Furosemide	→54
Lasix Special *Inj 10mg/ml* **Generics** *Inj 10mg/ml*	**Edema:** 20–40mg IV/IM, rep prn in 2h, then incr prn by 20mg >q2h until response; **CH** 1mg/kg/dose, prn incr by 0.25–0.5mg/dose q4–12h, max 10mg/kg/24h; **acute pulmonary edema:** ini 40mg slowly IV, prn incr in 1h by 40mg
Haloperidol	→247
Generics *Inj 50mg/ml, 100mg/ml*	**Agitation:** 2–5mg IM, rep prn q1–8h
Heparin	→69
Heparin Leo *Inj 100U/ml, 1000U/ml, 10000U/ml, 25000U/ml* **Heparin Lock Flush** *Inj 10U/ml, 100U/ml* **Hepalean** *Inj 1000U/ml, 10000U/ml, 25000U/ml* **Hepalean-LOK** *Inj 10U/ml, 100U/ml* **Generics** *Inj 2U/ml, 40U/ml, 50U/ml, 100 U/ml*	**DVT/pulmonary embolism:** ini 80U/kg IV, then 18 U/kg/ h, adjust by PTT testing; **CH** ini 50U/kg IV, then 10–25 U/ kg/h

Hyoscyamine	→109 →296
Levsin *Tab 0.125mg, Tab ext.rel. 0.125mg, Gtt 0.125mg/ml, Inj 0.5mg/ml*	**GI hypermotility/urinary spasm:** 0.25–0.5mg IV/IM/SC prn q4h, max 4 doses/d; **CH** 2–12y: 0.0625mg–0.125mg/dose PO/SL, prn q4h, max 0.75mg/24h, >12y: 0.125–0.25mg/dose PO/SL, prn q4h, max 1.5mg/24h
Ketamine	→212
Ketalar *Inj 10mg/ml, 50mg/ml*	**Sedation + analgesia:** 2–4mg/kg IM or 0.2–0.75mg/kg IV x 2–3min, then inf of 5–20 mcg/kg/min; **CH** 2–10mg/kg IM or 0.2–1mg/kg IV x 2–3min, then inf of 5–20 mcg/kg/min, 50% dose reduction in hypovolemia
Lidocaine	→61 →215
Xylocaine CO_2 *Inj 17.3mg/ml* **Xylocaine** *Inj 0.5%, 1%, 1.5%, 2.0%, 4.0%* **Xylocaine (with epinephrine)** *Inj 0.5%, 1%, 1.5%, 2.0%* **Xylocaine Spinal** *Inj 5.0%* **Generics** *Inj 1%, 2.0%, 10mg/ml, Inj (with epinephrine) 1%, 2.0%*	**VT/VF:** ini 1mg/kg IV, then prn 0.5mg/kg IV q5–10min, max 3mg/kg, maint 1–4mg/min; **CH** 1mg/kg/dose IV q5–10min, max 5 mg/kg, maint 10–50 mcg/kg/min; **local anesthesia:** 0.5–1% for infiltration, max 300mg
Lorazepam	→220
Ativan *Inj 4mg/ml* **Generics** *Inj 4mg/ml*	**Status epilepticus:** 4mg slowly IV, may rep after 10–15min, max 8mg; **CH** 0.1mg/kg IV, max 4mg/dose
Magnesium Sulfate	→118
Generics *Inj 500mg/ml*	**Ventricular arrhythmia:** 1–6g IV x 15min, then 3–20mg/min; **eclampsia:** ini 1–4g IV x 2–4min as 10–20% sol, maint 2–3g/h IV inf or 4–5g IM as 50% sol, rep prn q4h

Mepivacaine	→215
Carbocaine *Inj 1%, 2%* **Isocaine** *Inj 3%* **Isocaine (with levonordefrin)** *Inj 2%* **Scandonest** *Inj 3%* **Scandonest (with epinephrine)** *Inj 2%* **Polocaine** *Inj 3%* **Polocaine (with levonordefrin)** *Inj 2%*	**Brachial nerve block:** 50–400mg (1–2% sol.); **epidural nerve block:** 150–300mg (1–2% sol.); **local infiltration:** up to 400mg (0.5–1% sol.)
Methylprednisolone	→129
Depo-Medrol *Inj (M.-acetate) 20mg/ml, 40mg/ml, 80mg/ml* **Depo-Medrol (with Lidocaine)** *Inj 40mg (plus 10mg lidocaine)/ml* **Solu-Medrol** *Inj (M.-succinate) 40mg/vial, 125mg/vial, 500mg/vial, 1g/ vial* **Generics** *Inj 500mg/vial, 1g/vial*	**Status asthmaticus:** 1–2mg/kg IV; **anaphylaxis:** 125mg IV/IM or 2mg/kg IV/IM
Metoclopramide	→105
Generics *Inj 5mg/ml*	**Nausea:** 10mg IV q2–4h; **CH** 0.1–0.2mg/kg q6–8h
Morphine	→205
Generics *Inj 0.5mg/ml, 1mg/ml, 2mg/ml, 5mg/ml, 10mg/ml, 15mg/ml, 25mg/ml, 50mg/ml*	**Pulmonary edema:** 2–8mg IV; **pain:** 2–10mg IV, max 20mg prn q2–6h or 1–10mg/h IV inf, max 80mg/h or 5–20mg IM/SC; **CH** 0.1–0.2mg/kg IV/IM/SC q2–4h, max 15mg/dose or 0.025–2.6mg/kg/h IV inf
Naloxone	→207
Generics *Inj 0.4mg/ml, 1mg/ml*	**Opioid reversal (after anesthesia):** 0.1–0.2mg IV q2–3min prn; **CH** 0.01mg/kg IV, rep q2–3min; **opioid overdose:** 0.4–2mg IV, rep q2–3min, max 10mg; **CH** <20kg: 0.1mg/kg IV/IM/**ET** q2–3min, >20kg: 2mg IV, rep q2–3min

Nitroglycerin	→57
Gen-Nitro *Spray metered SL 0.4mg/Spray* **Nitrolingual Pumpspray** *Spray metered SL 0.4mg/Spray* **Nitrostat** *Tab (SL) 0.3mg, 0.6mg* **Rho-Nitro Pumpspray** *Spray metered SL 0.4mg/Spray* **Generic (NTG + dextrose)** *Inj 0.1, 0.2, 0.4mg/ml*	**Acute angina pectoris:** 1-2 sprays SL, rep prn q5min, max 3 sprays or 0.4mg Tab SL, rep prn q5min, max 3 doses; **acute MI/angina pectoris:** ini 5mcg/min IV as inf of 50mg in 250ml D5W (200mcg/ml), incr prn by 5mcg/ min q3-5min to 20mcg/min, then incr prn by 10mcg/min
Norepinephrine	→40
Levophed *Inj 1mg/ml* **Generics** *Inj 1mg/ml*	**Acute hypotension:** ini 8-12mcg/min IV (4mg in 500ml D5W), maint inf at 2-4mcg/min
Oxytocin	→299
Generics *Inj 10 U/ml*	**Postpartum hemorrhage:** 3-10U IM or 10U IV in 1L NS at 100-200ml/h
Pancuronium	→214
Pancuronium *Inj 1mg/ml, 2mg/ml* **Generics** *Inj 1mg/ml, 2mg/ml*	**Paralysis** (anesthesia): 0.04-0.1mg/kg IV
Phenobarbital	→221
Barbilixir *Elix 4mg/ml* **Generics** *Tab 15mg, 30mg, 60mg, 100mg,* **Elixir** *5mg/ml,* *Inj 30mg/ml, 120mg/ml*	**Status epilepticus:** 10-20mg/kg IV, max rate 60mg/min, max 20mg/kg
Phenylephrine	→40
Neo-Synephrin *Inj 10mg/ml*	**Acute hypotension** (mild-moderate): 200mcg IV, ini max 500mcg IV, rep prn q10-15min; **acute hypotension** (severe): inf 10mg in 500ml D5W, ini at 100-180mcg/min, prn decr to 40-60mcg/min

Phenytoin	→203
Dilantin *Cap 30mg, 100mg, Susp (oral) 30mg/5ml, 125mg/ml* **Dilantin Infatabs** *Tab (chew) 50mg* **Generics** *Inj 50mg/ml*	**Status epilepticus:** ini 15–18mg/kg IV, max rate 0.5 mg/ kg/min, max 30mg/kg, rep 100mg PO/IV q6–8h; **CH** 15–20mg/kg IV, max rate 1–3mg/kg/min
Procainamide	→62
Generics *Inj 100mg/ml*	**VF (refractory)/ paroxysmal SVT with wide QRS:** 20–30mg/min or 100mg IV q5min, until max 17mg/kg, BP ↓ , dysrhythmia suppressed or QRS/PR widens >50%, maint inf of 2g in 250ml D5W at 2–6 mg/min
Propranolol	→43
Inderal *Inj 1mg/ml*	**SVT/AF/Af:** 1–3mg IV, max 1mg/min, rep prn in 2min, rep third dose in >4h; **CH** 0.01–0.15mg/kg IV x 10min, rep prn q6–8h, max 1mg
Rocuronium	→214
Zemuron *Inj 10mg/ml*	**Paralysis** (anesthesia): 0.6–1.2mg/kg IV
Salbutamol	→83
Airomir *MDI 120mcg/dose* **Apo-Salvent** *Resp. soln 5mg/ml, MDI 100mcg/dose, Sterules 1mg/ml, 2mg/ml, Tab 2mg, 4mg* **Ventolin** *Sol (inhal) 1.25mg/2.5 ml, 2.5mg/ 2.5ml, 5mg/2.5ml, 5mg/ml* **Ventolin Diskus** *Inhal 200mcg/blister* **Ventolin HFA** *MDI 100mcg/dose* **Generics** *MDI 100mcg/dose* *Sol (inhal) 5mg/ml, 0.5mg/ml, 1mg/ml, 2mg/ml*	**Asthma:** 1–2puffs q4–6h prn

Sodium Bicarbonate	→99
Sodium bicarbonate *Inj 42mg/ml, 50mg/ml, 75mg/ml, 84mg/ml*	**Metabolic acidosis:** 1mEq/kg IV, rep prn 0.5mEq/kg IV q 10min; **CH** 1mEq/kg IV, then 0.5mEq/kg prn q10min
Sodium Nitroprusside	→52
Nipride *Inj 50mg/vial*	**HTN** (malignant): 0.3–10mcg/kg/min IV; max 70mg/kg within 14d; **CH** 0.3–10mcg/kg IV
Terbutaline	→84 →298
Bricanyl Tablets *Tab 2.5mg, 5mg*	**Asthma:** 0.25mg SC q20min, max 3 doses; **preterm labor:** 0.25–0.5mg SC q2h
Theophylline	→86
Generics *Inj 0.8mg/ml, 1.6mg/ml, 4mg/ml*	**Acute bronchospasm:** ini 4.6mg/kg IV x 6min, then inf at 0.5mg/kg/h
Thiopental	→210
Pentothal *Inj (Sol) 1g/vial, 2.5g/vial, 5g/vial, Inj (Powder) 250mg/syringe, 500mg/syringe, 500mg/vial, 1g/vial*	**Anesthesia induction:** 3–5mg/kg IV; **convulsions:** 75–125mg IV (3–5ml of a 2.5% sol)
Verapamil	→49
Generics *Inj 2.5mg/ml*	**SVT/AF/Af:** 5–10mg IV x 2min, rep prn 10mg IV in 30min; **CH** >2 y or >15kg (paroxysmal SVT): ini 0.1–0.3mg/kg IV x 2min, max 5mg/dose, rep prn in 30min, max 10mg

Advanced Life Support Algorithm

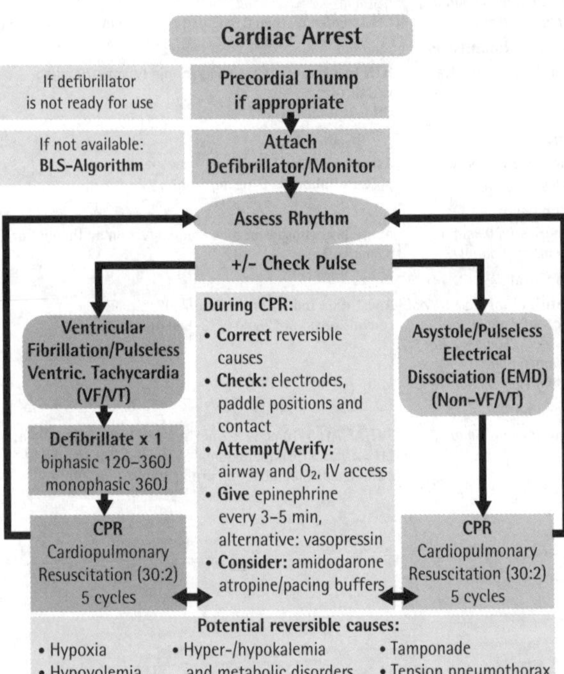
Cardiac Arrest
If defibrillator is not ready for use
Precordial Thump if appropriate
If not available: BLS-Algorithm
Attach Defibrillator/Monitor
Assess Rhythm
+/- Check Pulse
Ventricular Fibrillation/Pulseless Ventric. Tachycardia (VF/VT)
Defibrillate x 1
biphasic 120–360J
monophasic 360J
CPR
Cardiopulmonary Resuscitation (30:2)
5 cycles
During CPR:
• Correct reversible causes
• Check: electrodes, paddle positions and contact
• Attempt/Verify: airway and O_2, IV access
• Give epinephrine every 3–5 min, alternative: vasopressin
• Consider: amidodarone atropine/pacing buffers
Asystole/Pulseless Electrical Dissociation (EMD) (Non-VF/VT)
CPR
Cardiopulmonary Resuscitation (30:2)
5 cycles
Potential reversible causes:
• Hypoxia
• Hypovolemia
• Hypothermia
• Hyper-/hypokalemia and metabolic disorders
• Toxic/therapeutic disorders
• Tamponade
• Tension pneumothorax
• Thromboembolic/ mechan. obstruction

International Guidelines 2005 for CPR and ECC – a Consensus on Science, Resuscitation 2005, 67 (2–3),157–342

2 Cardiovascular System

2.1 Vasopressors

MA/EF (dobutamine): primarily beta-rec. agon., pos. inotropic, no vasoconstriction; **MA/EF** (dopamine): dose-dependent dopamine-, beta-/alpha-rec. agon, renal vasodilation, cardiac output↓, vasoconstr.
MA/EF (epinephrine): primarily beta-rec. agonist, positive inotropic, chronotropic + bathmotropic effect, syst. BP↑, diast. BP↓, bronchodilation; **MA/EF** (norepinephrine): primarily alpha-rec. agonist ⇒ syst./diast. BP↑; **MA/EF** (midodrine): alpha-adren. agonism on arteriolar + venous rec. ⇒ vascular tone↑, venous pooling↓, BP↑; **AE:** headache, anxiety, fatigue, N/V, dyspnea, angina, hypertension/hypotension, arrhythmias, parasthesia, bradycardia, palpitati., hyperglycemia; **CI** (dobutamine): pheochromocytoma, idiopathic hypertrophic subaortic stenosis, hypersensativity to the drug; **CI (dopamine):** pheochromocytoma; **CI** (epinephrine) narrow angle glaucoma, anesthesia with halogenated hydrocarbons/cyclopropane, organic brain damage, labor, cardiac dilatation, corocary insufficincy; **CI** (norepinephrine): anesthesia with halogenated hydrocarbons/cyclopropane, vascular thrombosis; **CI** (midodrine): excessive supine hypertension, severe organic heart disease, acute renal disease, urinary retention, pheochromocytoma, thyrotoxicosis, hypersensitivity to the drug

Dobutamine	EHL 2min, Dur (1x dose) 10min, PRC B, Lact ?
Dobutrex *Inj 12.5mg/ml* **Generics** *Inj 12.5mg/ml*	**Cardiac decompensation:** ini 0.5–1mcg/kg/min IV, incr to 2–20mcg/kg/min, max 40mcg/kg/min
Dopamine	EHL 2min, Dur 10min, PRC C, Lact ?
Generics (dopamine + dextrose) *Inj 0.8mg/ml, 1.6mg/ml, 3.2mg/ml*	**Hypotension, heart failure:** ini 1–5mcg/kg/min IV, incr prn by 5–10 mcg/kg/min increments, max 50mcg/kg/ min
Epinephrine	Dur 2min, PRC C, Lact ?
Adrenalin *Inj 1mg/ml, Topical 1mg/ml* **Epipen Jr.** *Inj (IM) 0.15mg/delivery* **Epipen** *Inj (IM) 0.3mg/delivery* **Generics** *Inj 0.1mg/ml, 1mg/ml*	**Cardiac arrest:** 0.5–1mg IV/ET, rep prn q 3–5min; **anaphylaxis**: 0.3–0.5 mg SC/IM, rep prn q10–15min; **CH**: 0.01mg/kg IV; 0.1mg/kg ET rep prn with 0.1mg/kg IV/ET q3–5min; **anaphylaxis:** 0.01mg/kg SC/IM (use 1: 1000 Sol), then 0.1mg/kg IV prn (IV: use 1:10.000)
Midodrine	EHL 0.5h, PRC C, Lact ?
Amatine *Tab 2.5mg, 5mg* **Generics** *Tab 2.5mg, 5mg*	**Orthostatic hypotension:** ini 2.5mg PO tid, incr prn to max 40 mg/d; **DARF:** ini 2.5mgtid

Norepinephrine	Dur 1–2min, PRC C, Lact ?
Levophed *Inj 1mg/ml* **Generics** *Inj 1mg/ml*	**Acute hypotensive states:** ini 8–12 mcg/min IV, maint 2–4 mcg/min
Phenylephrine	PRC C, Lact ?
Neo-Synephrine *Inj 10mg/ml*	**Acute hypotension:** 2–5mg SC/IM, max ini 5mg IV, rep prn q1–2h; 0.2–0.5mg slowly IV, max ini 0.5mg IV
Systemic Beta Adrenergic Agonists →63, α-β-Adrenergic Agonists →65	

2.2 Beta Blockers

MA: competitive blockage of beta-receptors;
EF: neg. inotropic + chronotropic ⇒ cardiac output↓, myocardial O_2 consumption↓, renin secretion↓, high-dose nonspecific membrane-stabilizing effect (quinidine-like);
AE: (acebutalol) congestive heart failure, bradycardia, bronchospasm, fatigue, dyspnea, nausea, dizziness, hypotension, rash (atenolol) congestive heart failure, AV block, bradycardia, bronchospasm, dizziness, vertigo, fatigue, diarrhea, nausea, dry mouth, (bisoprolol) arthralgia, dizziness, headache, insomnia, diarrhea, nausea, coughing, fatigue, edema, (carvedilol) congestive heart failure, syncope, bradycardia, hypotension, fatigue, dizziness, dyspnea (esmolo) hypotension, bradycardia, bronchospasm (labetalol) hypotension, jaundice, bronchospasm, dizziness, fatigue, headache, angina, nausea (metoprolol/nadalol) hypotension, bradycardia, congestive heart failure (AV block, bradycardia, hypotension, congestive heart failure, peripheral vasoconstriction bronchospasm, N/V, constipat., diarrhea, sexual ability↓, insulin secretion↓, glycogenolysis↓, fatigue, insomnia, dizziness, drowsiness, weakness, nervousness, anxiety, mental depression (propranolol) chf, bronchospasm, anorexia, nausea, vomiting, diarrhea, abdominal pain;
CI (betablockers): bronchospasm, congestive heart failure, sinus bradycardia, second and third degree AV block, RV failure secondary pulmonary hypertension, cardiogenic shock, hypersensativity to drug;
CI (acebutalol/bisoprolol) anesthesia that produces cardiac depression;
CI (atenolol): sick sinus syndrome, severe PVD, pheochromocytoma without alpha-blockade, metabolic acidosis ;
CI (carvedilol): severe hypotens., hepatic impairment, mental incapacity,
CI (metoprolol): severe PVD, anesthesia that produces cardiac depress.,
CI (nadalol): allergic rhinitis,
CI (oxprenolol): alleric rhinitis, anesthesia producing cardiac depression,
CI (pindolol): anesthesia produc. cardiac depression
CI (propranolol): allergic. rhinitis

Acebutolol	EHL 3-4h, PRC B, Lact ?	β_1	ISA
Sectral *Tap 100mg, 200mg, 400mg* **Rhotral** *Tap 100mg, 200mg,400mg* **Generics** *Tab 100mg, 200mg, 400mg*	**HTN:** ini 100mg PO bid, max 800mg/d PO qd or div bid; **Angina pectoris**: ini 200mg PO bid, maint 200-600mg PO div bid; DARF: GFR (ml/min) <50: 50%; <25: 25%	+	+
Atenolol	EHL 6-7h, PRC D, Lact ?	+	-
Apo, Novo, Nu-Atenol *Tab 50mg, 100mg* **Tenormin** *Tab 50mg, 100mg* **Generics** *Tab 50mg, 100mg*	**HTN:** ini 50mg PO qd, maint 50-100mg PO qd; **Angina pectoris**: ini 50 PO qd, maint 50-200mg/d PO qd or div bid; DARF: GFR (ml/ min) 15-35: max 50mg/d; <15: max 50mg/od PO		
Bisoprolol	EHL 10v12.4h, PRC C, Lact ?	+	-
Monocor *Tab 5mg, 10mg*	**HTN:** ini 5mg PO qd, max 20mg/d; **DARF/DAHF**: ini 5mg PO qd, caution with dose-titration		
Carvedilol	EHL 6-10h, PRC C, Lact ?	-	-
Generics *Tab 3.125mg, 6.25mg, 12.5mg, 25mg*	**Heart failure**: ini 3.125mg PO bid incr dose q2 wk as tolerated to max 25mg bid; DARF: not req; DAHF: contraindicated		
Esmolol	EHL 9min, PRC C, Lact ?	+	-
Brevibloc *Inj 10mg/ml, 250mg/ml*	**Periperative tachycardia/hypertension:** 1.5mg/kg (max 100mg) IV over 30sec then 0.15mg/kg/min , max 0.3mg/kg/min, **Atrial fibrillation/flutter:** ini 0.5mg/kg/min IV for 1min, then 0.05mg/kg/min IV for 4min; DARF: not req		
Labetalol	EHL 5-8h, PRC C, Lact +	-	(+)
Trandate *Tab 100mg, 200mg* **Generics** *Tab 100mg, 200mg, Inj 5mg/ml*	**Hypertensive emergency:** 20mg slow IV, then 40-80mg IV q10min prn, max 300mg total; **HTN:** ini 100mg PO bid, maint 200-400mg bid, max 1200mg/d; DARF: not req		

Metoprolol	EHL 3-7h, PRC C, Lact ?	β_1	ISA
Betaloc *Tab 50mg, 100mg, Inj 1mg/ml* **Betaloc Durules** *Tab ext.rel 200mg* **Lopresor** *Tab 50mg, 100mg, Inj 1mg/ml* **Lopresor SR** *Tab ext.rel 100mg, 200mg* **Novo-Metoprol** *Tab 50mg, 100mg* **Nu-Metop** *Tab 50mg, 100mg* **Generics** *Tab 25mg, 50mg, 100mg* *Tab ext. rel. 100mg, 200mg*	**HTN, Angina pectoris:** ini 50mg PO bid or 50-100mg PO qd (ext.rel), incr prn max 400mg/d; **acute MI:** ini 5mg IV q2min up to 15mg, if tolerated give 50mg PO q6h for 48h, then 100mg PO bid; DARF: not req	+	-
Nadolol	EHL 20-24h, PRC C, Lact ?	-	-
Corgard *Tab 40mg, 80mg,160mg* **Apo-Nadol** *Tab 40mg, 80mg, 160mg* **Generics** *Tab 40mg, 80mg,160mg*	**HTN:** ini 80mg PO qd, maint 40-80mg/d, max 320 mg/d; **Angina pectoris:** ini 80mg PO qd, maint 40-80mg/d, max 240mg/ d; DARF: GFR (ml/min): >50: q24h, 31-50: q24-36h, 10-30: q 24-48h, <10: q40-60h		
Oxprenolol	EHL 1.3-1.5h, PRC + Lact not rec	-	+
Trasicor *Tab 40mg, 80mg*	**HTN:** ini 20mg PO tid, maint 120-320mg/d, max 480mg/d	-	+
Pindolol	EHL 3-4h, PRC B, Lact ?	-	+
Apo, Novo, Nu-Pindol *Tab 5mg, 10mg, 15mg* **Visken** *Tab 5mg, 10mg, 15mg* **Generics** *Tab 5mg, 10mg, 15mg*	**Angina pectoris:** ini 5mg PO tid, maint 15-40mg/d div tid; **HTN:** ini 5mg PO bid, maint 15-45mg/d, max 45 mg/d; DARF: not req		

Propranolol	EHL 3–4h, PRC C, Lact ?	β1	ISA
Inderal LA *Cap ext.rel 60mg, 80mg, 120mg, 160mg* **Novo-Pranol** *Tab 10mg, 20mg, 40mg, 80mg* **Generics** *Tab 10mg, 20mg, 40mg, 80mg, 120mg, Inj 1mg/ml*	**HTN:** ini 40mg PO bid, maint 120–240mg/d, max 640mg/ d; ext.rel: ini 60–80mg PO qd, maint 120–160mg/d, max 640mg/d; **angina:** ini 10–20mg PO tid–qid, maint 160–240mg/d; **arrhythmias:** 1–3mg IV, rep after 2min prn; 10–30mg PO tid–qid; **MI:** 180–240mg/d PO div bid–qid; **migraine:** ini 80mg/d PO, maint 160–240mg/d; **essential tremor:** ini 40mg PO bid, maint 120mg/d; **pheochromocytoma:** preop. for 3 days 60 mg/d PO in div doses bid–tid in combination with an alpha blocking agent; **hypertrophic subaortic stenosis:** 20–40mg PO tid–qid; **CH** 2–4mg/kg/d PO div bid; DARF: not req	-	-
Timolol	EHL 2–4h, PRC C, Lact ?	-	-
Apo, Novo-Timol *Tab 5mg, 10mg, 20mg* **Generics** *Tab 5mg, 10mg, 20mg*	**HTN:** ini 10mg PO bid, maint 20–40mg/d, max 60mg/d; **MI**: 10mg PO bid; **migraine:** ini 10mg PO bid, maint 20mg/d qd; max 30mg/d; DARF: not req		

β1: selective blockage of β1-receptors;
ISA: intrinsic sympathomimetic activity = partial agonistic and antagonist activity

2.3 ACE Inhibitors

2.3.1 ACE Inhibitors - Single Ingredient Drugs

MA: competitive blockage of angiotensin converting enzyme ⇒ angiotensin II ↓, bradykinin ↑
EF: vasodilation ⇒ BP ↓, renal blood flow ↑, aldosterone ↓, catecholamines ↓, reversal of myocardial and blood vessel wall hypertrophy, protective in diabetic nephropathy
AE: acute RF, rash, dry cough, hair loss, angioedema, dizziness, fatigue, headache, hyperkalemia, hyponatremia, complete blood count changes, urticaria, hypotension
CI: angiodema, hypersensativity to drug CI (cilazapril): ascites

Benazepril	EHL 0.6 h, PRC C(1), D(2nd, 3rd trim.), Lact +
Lotensin *Tab 5mg, 10mg, 20mg* **Generics** *Tab 5mg, 10mg, 20mg*	**HTN:** ini 10mg PO qd, maint 20–40mg PO qd or div bid, max 80mg/d; DARF: GFR (ml/min) <30: ini 5mg PO qd, max 10mg/d

Captopril	EHL 1.9h, PRC C(1), D(2nd, 3rd trim.), Lact +
Apo, Nu-Capto *Tab 6.25mg, 12.5mg, 25mg, 50mg, 100mg* **Capoten** *Tab 12.5mg, 25mg, 50mg, 100mg* **Generics** *Tab 6.25mg, 12.5mg, 25mg, 50mg, 100mg*	**HTN:** ini 25mg PO bid–tid, max 450 mg/d; **heart failure:** ini 12.5–25mg PO tid, incr to 150–300mg/d div tid, max 450mg/d; **LV dysfunction after MI**: ini 6.25mg po x 1, then 12.5mg PO tid, maint. 50mg PO tid; **Diabetic nephropathy:** maint 25mg PO tid; DARF: GFR (ml/min/1.73m2) 35–75: q12–24h; 20–34: q24–48h; 8–19: q48–72h; 5–7: q72–108h
Cilazapril	EHL 8.9h, PRC contraindicated, Lact +
Inhibace *Tab 1mg, 2.5mg, 5mg* **Generics** *Tab1mg, 2.5mg, 5mg*	**HTN:** ini 2.5mg PO qd, maint 2.5–5mg qd, max 10mg/d; **heart failure:** ini 0.5mg PO qd, maint 1–2.5mg qd, max 2.5mg/d; DARF: GFR (ml/min) 10–40ml/min: ini 0.25–0.5mg qd max 2.5mg qd; <10ml/min 0.25–0.5mg qwk–biw
Enalapril/Enalaprilat	EHL 1.3h, PRC C(1st), D(2nd, 3rd trim.), Lact +
Vasotec *Tab 2.5mg, 5mg, 10mg, 20mg, Inj 1.25mg/ml*	**HTN:** ini 5mg PO qd, maint 10–40mg PO qd or div bid, max 40mg/d; 1.25mg IV q6h, max 5mg IV q6h; **heart failure:** ini 2.5 mg PO qd, maint 5–20mg/d PO div qd–bid, max 40mg/d; **CH** heart failure: 0.08mg/kg/d PO qd or div bid; DARF: GFR (ml/min) <30: ini 2.5mg PO qd, titrate prn, max 40mg/d; <30: 0.625mg IV q6h
Fosinopril	EHL 11.5h, PRC C(1st), D(2nd, 3rd trim.), Lact +
Monopril *Tab 10mg, 20mg*	**HTN:** ini 10mg PO qd, maint 20mg PO qd, max 40mg/ d; **heart failure:** ini 10mg PO qd, maint 20–40mg PO qd, max 40mg/d; DARF: not req

Lisinopril	EHL 12h, PRC C(1st), D(2nd, 3rd trim.), Lact +
Prinivil *Tab 2.5mg, 5mg, 10mg, 20mg* **Zestril** *Tab 5mg, 10mg, 20mg* **Generic** *Tab 5mg*	**HTN:** ini 10mg PO qd, maint 10–40mg PO qd, max 80mg/ d; **heart failure:** ini 2.5mg PO qd, maint 5–20mg PO qd, max 80mg/d; **acute MI:** 5mg PO then 5mg PO after 24h, then 10mg after 48h, then 10mg PO qd; DARF: GFR (ml/min) 10–30: ini 2.5–5mg PO, <10: ini 2.5mg PO, titrate dosage prn, max 40mg/d
Perindopril	EHL 0.9 h, PRC C(1st), D(2nd, 3rd trim.), Lact +
Coversyl *Tab 2mg, 4mg, 8mg* **Generic** *Tab 8mg*	**HTN:** ini 4mg PO qd, maint 4–8mg PO qd, max 8mg/d; **heart failure:** ini 2mg PO qd, maint 4mg PO qd; DARF: GFR (ml/min) 30–60: 2mg/d, 15–30: 2mg PO qod, <15: 2.5mg PO on dialysis day
Quinapril	EHL 0.8h, PRC C(1st), D(2nd, 3rd trim.), Lact +
Accupril *Tab 5mg, 10mg, 20mg, 40mg*	**HTN:** ini 10mg PO qd, max 40mg/d; **heart failure:** ini 5 mg PO qd, maint 20–40mg/d div bid; **DARF:** GFR (ml/min) >60: ini 10mg PO; 30–60: ini 5mg PO; 10–30: ini 2.5mg PO, then titrate to the optimal response
Ramipril	EHL 1–5h, PRC C(1st), D(2nd, 3rd trim.), Lact +
Altace *Cap 1.25mg, 2.5mg, 5mg, 10mg* **Generics** *Cap 1.25mg, 2.5mg, 5mg, 10mg*	**HTN:** ini 2.5mg PO qd, maint 2.5–20mg PO qd or div bid, max 20mg/d; **acute MI**: ini 2.5mg PO bid, maint 2.5–5mg bid, max 10mg/d; DARF: GFR (ml/min) <40: ini 1.25mg PO qd
Trandolapril	EHL 0.6–1.3h, PRC C(1), D(2nd,3rd trim), Lact +
Mavik *Cap 0.5mg, 1mg, 2mg, 4mg*	**HTN:** ini 1mg PO qd, maint 1–2mg PO qd, max 4mg/d; DARF: GFR (ml/min) <30: ini 0.5mg, max 1mg/d DALF: ini 0.5mg

2.3.2 ACE Inhibitors - Combinations

Cilazapril + HCTZ	PRC X, Lact +
Inhibace Plus *Tab 5 + 12.5mg* **Generics** *Tab 5 + 12.5mg*	**HTN:** 5+12.5–10+25mg PO qd; DARF: GFR (ml/min) 10–40ml/min: ini 0.5mg qd, max 2.5mg qd; <10ml/min 0.25–0.5mg qwk or biw
Enalapril + HCTZ	PRC C(1st trim.), D(2nd, 3rd trim.), Lact -
Vaseretic *Tab 5 +12.5mg, 10 + 25mg*	**HTN:** 5+12.5–10+25mg PO qd, max 20+50mg PO qd or div bid; DARF: GFR (ml/min) >30: 100%, <30: not rec
Lisinopril + HCTZ	PRC C(1st trim.), D(2nd, 3rd trim.), Lact -
Prinzide *Tab 10 + 12.5mg, 20 + 12.5mg, 20 + 25mg* **Zestoretic** *Tab 10 + 12.5mg, 20 + 12.5mg, 20 + 25mg*	**HTN:** 10+12.5 - 20+25mg PO qd; DARF: GFR (ml/min) >30: 100%, <30: not rec
Perindopril + Indapamide	PRC C(1st), D(2nd, 3rd trim.), Lact +
Coversyl Plus *Tab 4 + 1.25mg*	**HTN:** ini 4 + 1.25mg PO qd, maint 4 + 1.25mg–8 + 2.5mg PO qd; DARF (perindopril): GFR (ml/min) 30–60: 2mg/d, 15–30: 2mg PO qod, <15: 2.5mg PO on dialysis day
Ramipril + HCTZ	PRC C(1st), D(2nd, 3rd trim.), Lact +
Altace-HCT *Tab 2.5 + 12.5mg, 5 + 12.5mg, 10 + 12.5mg, 5 + 25mg, 10 + 25mg*	**HTN:** ini 2.5 + 12.5mg, maint 2.5 + 12.5mg–10 + 25mg/d
Quinapril + HCTZ	PRC C(1st trim.), D(2nd, 3rd trim.), Lact -
Accuretic *Tab 10 + 12.5mg, 20 + 12.5mg, 20 + 25mg*	**HTN:** 10+12.5–20+25mg PO, max 40+25mg PO qd; DARF: GFR (ml/min) >30: 100%, <30: not rec
Trandolapril + Verapamil SR	PRC C(1), D(2nd,3rd trim), Lact +
Tarka *Tab 2 + 180mg, 1 + 240mg, 2 + 240mg, 4 + 240mg*	**HTN:** 1+180–4+240mg PO qd, max 8+480mg/d; DARF: GFR (ml/min) <30: ini 0.5mg (trandolapril), titrate to opt. response

2.4 Angiotensin II Receptor Blockers

2.4.1 Angiotensin II Receptor Blockers - Single Ingredient Drugs

MA (ARBs): inhibition of type 1 angiotensin II receptor
EF: selective blockage of angiotensin II-effects without action on bradykinin breakdown
AE: headache, dizziness, nausea, abdominal pain
CI: hypersensativity to drug

Candesartan	PRC C(1st), D(2nd, 3rd trim.), Lact ?
Atacand *Tab 8mg, 16mg*	**HTN:** ini 16mg PO qd, max 32mg/d
Eprosartan	EHL 6h, PRC C(1st), D(2nd, 3rd trim.), Lact -
Teveten *Tab 400mg, 600mg*	**HTN:** ini 400-600mg PO qd, max 800mg qd or div bid
Irbesartan	EHL 11–15h, PRC C(1), D(2nd, 3rd trim.), Lact ?
Avapro *Tab 75mg, 150mg, 300mg*	**HTN:** ini 150mg PO qd, max 300mg/d; DARF: not req
Losartan	EHL 1.5–2h, PRC C(1.), D(2nd, 3rd trim.), Lact ?
Cozaar *Tab 25mg, 50mg, 100mg*	**HTN:** ini 50mg PO qd, max 100mg qd or div bid; DAHF: ini 25mg PO qd
Telmisartan	EHL 24h, PRC C(1st), D(2nd, 3rd trim.), Lact ?
Micardis *Tab 40mg, 80mg*	**HTN:** ini 40mg PO qd, max 80mg/d
Valsartan	EHL 6–9h, PRC C(1st), D(2nd, 3rd trim.), Lact ?
Diovan *Cap 80mg, 160mg*	**HTN:** ini 80mg PO qd, max 160mg/d; DARF: GFR (ml/min) >10: not req

2.4.2 Angiotensin II Receptor Blockers - Combinations

Candesartan + HCTZ	PRC C(1st), D(2nd, 3rd trim.), Lact ?
Atacand Plus *Tab 16 + 12.5mg*	**HTN**: 16+12.5mg–32+25mg PO qd
Eprosartan + HCTZ	PRC C(1st), D(2nd, 3rd trim.), Lact -
Teventen Plus *Tab 600 + 12.5mg*	**HTN:** 600+12.5 PO qd
Irbesartan + HCTZ	PRC C(1st trim.), D(2nd, 3rd trim.), Lact -
Avalide *Tab 150 + 12.5mg, 300 + 12.5mg, 300 + 25mg*	**HTN:** 150+12.5–300+25mg PO qd; DARF: GFR (ml/min) >30: 100%, <30: not rec
Losartan + HCTZ	PRC C(1st trim.), D(2nd, 3rd trim.), Lact -
Hyzaar *Tab 50 + 12.5mg* **Hyzaar DS** *Tab 100 + 25mg*	**HTN:** 50+12.5–100+25mg PO qd; DARF: GFR (ml/min) >30: 100%, <30: not rec

Telmisartan + HCTZ	PRC C(1st trim.), D(2nd, 3rd trim.), Lact -
Micardis Plus *Tab 80 + 12.5mg*	**HTN:** 80+12.5–160+25mg PO qd

Valsartan + HCTZ	PRC C(1st trim.), D(2nd, 3rd trim.), Lact -
Diovan-HCT *Tab 80 + 12.5mg, 160 + 12.5mg, 160 + 25mg*	**HTN:** 80+12.5–160+25mg PO qd; DARF: GFR (ml/min) >30: 100%, <30: not rec

2.5 Calcium Channel Blockers

2.5.1 CCBs - Dihydropyridines

MA: blockage of inflow of calcium ions ⇒ neg. inotropic effect, myocardial O_2 consumption ↓, predominantly arterial vasodilation ⇒ afterload ↓, preload unchanged!
AE: hypotension, flush, reflex tachycardia, peripheral edema, headache, complete blood count changes, gingival hyperplasia;
CI: hypersensativity to drug, severe hypotension
CI (flunarizine): depression, pre-existing extrapyramidal disorders

Amlodipine	EHL 35–50h, PRC C, Lact ?
Norvasc *Tab 5mg, 10mg*	**HTN, angina pectoris:** ini 5mg PO qd, max 10mg qd; DARF: not req; DAHF: ini 2.5mg PO qd

Felodipine	EHL 10–16h, PRC C, Lact ?
Plendil *Tab ext.rel 2.5mg, 5mg, 10mg* **Renedil** *Tab ext.rel 2.5mg, 5mg, 10mg* **Generics** *Tab ext.rel 5mg, 10mg*	**HTN:** ini 5mg PO qd, maint 5–10mg/d; DARF: not req

Flunarizine	EHL 19d, PRC ?, Lact +
Sibelium *Cap 5mg*	**Migraine Prophylaxis:** 10mg/d

Nifedipine	EHL 2–5h, 10h (ext. rel.), PRC C, Lact +
Adalat XL *Tab ext.rel 20mg, 30mg, 60mg* **Apo-Nifed** *Cap 5mg, 10mg* **Apo-Nifed PA** *Tab ext. rel. 10mg, 20mg* **Novo-Nifedin** *Cap 5mg, 10mg* **Nu-Nifed** *Cap 10mg* **Generics** *Tab ext.rel 10mg, 20mg*	**HTN:** ext.rel: ini 20–30mg PO qd, max 90mg/d; **angina pectoris:** ini 10mg PO tid, maint 10–20mg tid; ext.rel: ini 30mg PO qd, max 90mg/d; DARF: not req

2.5.2 CCBs - Non-Dihydropyridines

MA: blockage of inflow of calcium ions; **EF:** neg. inotropic and chronotropic effect, myocardial O_2 consumption ↓, vasodilation (afterload ↓, preload unchanged!), AV conduction time ↑, AV refractory period ↑; **AE:** allergic reactions/dermatitis, bradycardia, AV block, cardiac arrest, congestive heart failure, N/V, constipation, diarrhea, dizziness, headache, fatigue, peripheral edema, pulmonary edema
CI: AV block II°-III°, SA block, sick sinus syndrome, cardiogenic shock, hypotension, severe congestive heart failure, bradycardia, hypersensitivity to drug

Diltiazem	EHL 3-6.6h, PRC C, Lact -
Apo-Diltiaz *Tab 30mg, 60mg, Inj 5mg/ml* **Apo-Diltiaz CD** *Cap cont. del. 120mg, 180mg, 240mg, 300mg* **Apo-Diltiaz SR** *Cap sust. rel. 60mg, 90mg, 120mg* **Cardizem** *Tab 30mg, 60mg* **Cardizem CD** *Cap cont. del. 120mg, 180mg, 240mg, 300mg* **Cardizem SR** *Cap sust. rel. 60mg, 90mg, 120mg* **Nu-Diltiaz** *Tab 30mg, 60mg* **Tiazac** *Cap ext. rel. 120mg, 180mg, 240mg, 300mg, 360mg* **Tiazac XC** *Tab ext. rel. 120mg, 180mg, 240mg, 300mg, 360mg* **Generics** *Tab 30mg, 60mg, Cap ext.rel 60mg, 90mg, 120mg, 180mg, 240mg, 300mg, 360mg, Inj 5mg/ml*	**Chronic stable and vasospastic angina pectoris:** ini 30mg PO qid, max 360mg/d; ext.rel: 120-360mg qd; HTN: cont. del.: ini 180-240mg PO qd; sust. rel.: 120-360mg/d div bid, max 360mg/d; **AF:** ini 0.25mg/kg IV over 2min, rep prn after 15min with 0.35mg/kg; continous inf: 5-15mg/h; DARF: not req
Verapamil	EHL 4-12h, PRC C, Lact +
Apo, Nu-Verap *Tab 80mg, 120mg* **Covera-HS** *Tab ext. rel. 180mg, 240mg* **Isoptin SR** *Tab ext.rel 120mg, 180mg, 240mg* **Novo-Veramil SR** *Tab sust. rel. 240mg* **Generics** *Tab 80mg, 120mg, Tab ext.rel 120mg, 180mg, 240mg, Inj 2.5mg/ml*	**HTN:** ini 80mg PO tid, ext.rel: 180-240mg PO qd-bid, max 480mg/d; **chronic stable angina:** ini 80mg PO tid-qid, max 480mg/d; **obstructive hypertrophic cardiomyopathy:** ini 80-120mg PO tid-qid; **SVT:** 5-10mg IV over 2min, rep after 15-30min prn; continuous inf: 5mg/h IV; **AF:** 240-480mg/d PO div tid-qid; **CH** 1-15 y: **arrhythmias:** 0.1-0.3mg/kg IV; DARF: not req

2.6 Adrenergic Inhibitors

2.6.1 Central Acting Alpha Agonists

MA (clonidine, methyldopa): stimulation of central alpha-2 receptors (presynaptic effect) ⇒ release of noradrenaline ↓, postsynaptic effect ⇒ peripheral sympathetic tone ↓, release of renin ↓, (⇒ inhibition of renin-angiotensin-aldosterone-system); additional agonistic effect on imidazole-receptor;
EF (clonidine, methyldopa): BP ↓ due to reduction of peripheral resistance, stroke volume and cardiac output **AE** (clonidine,): AV block, bradycardia, drowsiness, dry mouth

AE (clonidine): AV block, bradycardia, drowsiness, oral dryness
CI (clonidine): bradycardia, **CI** (methydopa): active liver disease, therapy with MAO inhibitors

Clonidine	EHL 12–16h, PRC C, Lact ?
Catapres *Tab 0.1mg, 0.2mg* **Dixarit** *Tab 0.025mg* **Generics** *Tab 0.1mg, 0.2mg*	**HTN:** ini 0.1 mg PO bid, maint 0.2–0.6mg/d div; **menopausal flushing:** 0.05mg PO bid; **CH HTN:** ini 5–10mcg/kg/d PO div bid–tid, max 0.9mg/d; DARF: not req

Methyldopa	EHL 1.7h, PRC B, Lact +
Nu-Medopa *Tab 250mg, 500mg* **Generics** *Tab 125mg, 250mg, 500mg*	**HTN:** ini 250mg PO bid–tid, maint 500–2000mg/d div bid–qid; **CH HTN:** 10mg/kg/d PO div bid–qid, max 65 mg/kg/d; DARF: GFR (ml/min) >50: q8h; 10–50: q8–12h; <10: q12–24h

2.6.2 Alpha Adrenergic Blockers

MA: reversible blockage of α_1-receptor; **MA** (phenoxybenzamine): irreversible blockage of α_1/ α_2-receptor; **EF:** vasodilation, pre- and afterload ↓ ; **AE:** reflex tachycardia (not prazosin), arrhythmia, postural hypotension, fatigue, nausea, dyspepsia, diarrhea; "adverse epinephrine effect": epinephrine → vasodilation and BP ↓ when receptors are blocked due to β-mimetic effect; **AE** (Prazosin): "first-dose phenomenon": postural hypotension after first dose ⇒ slow incr in dosage!; **CI:** hypersensativity to drug CI (doxazosin, prazosin) hypersensativity to quinazolines ; **CI** (phentolamine) myocardial infarction or history of, coronary insufficiency, angina, hypotension, hypersensativity to sulfites

Doxazosin	EHL 8.8-22h, PRC C, Lact ?
Cardura *Tab 1mg, 2mg, 4mg* **Generics** *Tab 1mg, 2mg, 4mg*	**HTN (not first line):** ini 1mg PO qd, max 16mg/d; **benign prostatic hypertrophy:** ini 1mg PO qd, max 8mg/d
Phentolamine	EHL 19min., PRC C, Lact +
Rogitine *Inj 10mg/ml* **Generics** *Inj 5mg/ml*	**Treatment of alpha-adren. drugextravas.:** Infiltrate area SC with small amount of 5–10 mg in 10 ml NS solution within 12h; max 0.1–0.2 mg/kg or 5 mg total; **diagnosis of pheochromocytoma**: 5 mg IM/IV; **CH**: 0.05–0.1 mg/kg/dose; max single dose 5 mg; **surgery for pheochromocytoma/HTN**: 2–5 mg IM/IV 1–2 h before procedure then q2–4 h PRN; **CH**: 0.05–0.1 mg/kg/dose 1–2 h before proce. then q2–4 h PRN; max single dose: 5 mg; **hypertens. crisis**: 5–20 mg IM/IV
Prazosin	EHL 2–4h, PRC C, Lact ?
Apo,Nu-Prazo *Tab 1mg, 2mg, 5mg* **Minipress** *Tab 1mg, 2mg, 5mg* **Novo-Prazin** *Tab 1mg, 2mg, 5mg* **Generics** *Tab 1mg, 2mg, 5mg*	**HTN:** ini 0.5mg PO qd, increase to 0.5mg PO bid–tid then 1mg PO bid–tid, max 20 mg/ d; **CH HTN:** ini 5mcg/kg PO as 1x dose; maint 25–150mcg/ kg/d div q6h, max 0.4 mg/kg/d, DARF: not req
Terazosin	EHL 9–12h, PRC C, Lact ?
Hytrin *Tab 1mg, 2mg, 5mg, 10mg* **Generics** *Tab 1mg, 2mg, 5mg, 10mg*	**HTN:** ini 1mg PO hs, maint 1–5mg PO qd or div bid, max 20mg/d; **benign prostatic hypertrophy:** ini 1mg PO qd, maint 5–10mg PO qd; DARF: not req

2.6.3 Peripheral Acting Adrenergic Blockers

MA: inhibition of vesicular storage of catecholamines; **EF:** peripheral resistance ↓ (afterload) ⇒ BP ↓, HR ↓, cardiac output ↓; **AE:** depression, gut motility ↑, bradycardia, postural hypotension, stuffy nose; **CI**: Hypersensitivity to drug, depression or history of, active peptic ulcer disease, ulcerative colitis, patients receiving electroconculsive therapy

Reserpine	EHL 50–100h, PRC C, Lact -
Generics *Tab 0.25mg*	**HTN:** ini 0.5mg/d PO for 1–2 wk, then reduce to 0.1– 0.25mg/d PO qd; DARF: GFR (ml/min) >10: 100%; <10: not rated

2.7 Direct Vasodilators

MA/EF: direct effect on the smooth muscles of the small arteries and arterioles ⇒ peripheral resistance ↓ (afterload) ⇒ BP ↓
AE (direct vasodilators): hypotension, Na^+, H_2O retention, tachycardia, dizziness, headache;
AE (nitroprusside): cyanide poisoning;
AE (minoxidil): hypertrichosis, pericardial effusion, changes in T-wave
AE (hydralazine): Gi disturbance, blood dyscasias
CI (diazoxide): hypersensativity to drug or thiazide
CI (epoprostenol) congestive heart failure due to LV systolic dysfunction, hypersensativity to drug
CI (nitroprusside): compensated HTN (aortic coarctation, AV shunt), high output failure, metabolic acidosis, congenital optic atrophy, tobacco amblyopia
CI (minoxidil): pheochromocytoma, pulmonary HTN with mitral stenosis, hypersensitivy to drug

Epoprostenol	EHL 3–5min, PRC B, Lact ?
Flolan *Inj 0.5mg/vial, 1.5mg/vial*	**Primary pulmonary HTN:** 2ng/kg/min IV, incr by 2ng/kg/ min q15min
Hydralazine	EHL 3–5h, PRC C, Lact +
Apresoline *Inj 20mg/ml* **Novo-Hylazin** *Tab 10mg, 25mg, 50mg* **Nu-Hydral** *Tab 10mg, 25mg, 50mg* **Generics** *Tab 10mg, 25mg, 50mg*	**HTN emergencies:** 5–10mg IV, rep q20–40min prn; IV infusion: ini 200–300mcg/min, maint 50–150mcg/min; **HTN:** ini 10mg PO qid, incr by 10–25mg/dose every 2–5d, max 300mg/d; **CH HTN emergency:** 0.1–0.5mg/kg IM/IV ; **CH HTN:** 0.75–1mg/kg/d PO div q4–6h
Minoxidil	EHL 2.3–28.9h, PRC C, Lact +
Loniten *Tab 2.5mg, 10mg*	**Severe HTN:** ini 2.5mg PO bid, incr to 10–40mg/d div bid, max 100mg/d; **CH** <12y:ini 0.2mg/kg/d PO div bid, incr q3d, max 50mg
Nitroprusside Sodium	EHL 3–4min
Nipride *Inj 50mg/vial*	**HTN emergencies:** ini 0.3–0.5mcg/kg/min IV, incr by 0.5mcg/kg/min, max 10mcg/kg/min; DARF: not req

2.8 Endothelin Receptor Antagonists

MA/EF (bosentan): specific and competitive antagonist at endothelin receptor types ETA and ETB ⇒ inhibition of endothelin-1 effects ⇒ pulmonary artery pressure ↓
AE (bosentan): headache, nasopharyngitis, hypotension, flushing, edema, liver injury
CI (bosentan): pregnancy, coadmin. with cyclosporine A, glyburide, moderate to severe liver impairment, known hypersensitivity

Bosentan	EHL 5h, PRC X, Lact -
Tracleer *Tab 62.5mg, 125mg*	**Pulmon. arteri. HTN** (WHO III–IV): ini 62.5mg PO bid for 4wk, then 125mg bid; DARF: not req

2.9 Diuretics

2.9.1 Thiazide Diuretics

MA: inhibition of the reabsorption of Na^+, Cl^- and H_2O in the distal convoluted tubule, secretion of K^+ ↑; **EF:** elimination of Na^+, Cl^-, H_2O and K^+ ↑, excretion of Ca^{2+} and PO_4^{3-} ↓
AE: hypokalemia, hypercalcemia, hyperuricemia, thrombosis, anemia, hyperglycemia
CI: anuria, renal insuff., sulphonamide hypersensitivity, hepatic coma

Chlorthalidone	EHL 40–89h, PRC B, Lact ?
Generics *Tab 50mg, 100mg*	**HTN:** ini 12.5mg PO qd, maint 12.5–50mg/d, max 50mg/d; **edema**: ini 25–100mg PO/d div tid–qid, max 200mg/d
Hydrochlorothiazide	EHL 10–12h, PRC B, Lact +
Apo-Hydro *Tab 25mg, 50mg, 100mg* **Novo-Hydrazide** *Tab 25mg, 50mg* **Generics** *Tab 12.5mg, 25mg, 50mg*	**Edema:** 25–100mg PO/d div qd–tid, max 200mg/d; **HTN:** ini 12.5mg PO qd, maint 12.5–50mg/d, max 50mg/d; **CH:** 1–2mg/kg/d PO qd or div bid
Indapamide	EHL 14–15h, PRC B, Lact ?
Lozide *Tab 1.25mg, 2.5mg* **Generics** *Tab 1.25mg, 2.5mg*	**HTN:** ini 1.25mg PO qd, incr prn, max 5mg/d; **edema**: ini 2.5mg PO qd, max 5mg/d
Metolazone	EHL 8–14h, PRC B, Lact +
Zaroxolyn *Tab 2.5mg*	**Edema:** 5–10mg PO qd, max 20mg/d; **HTN:** ini 2.5mg PO qd, max 10mg/d

2.9.2 Loop Diuretics

MA/EF: inhibition of the reabsorption of Na^+, Cl^-, K^+ and H_2O, primarily in the ascending limb of the loop of Henle ⇒ increased elimination of Na^+, Cl^-, K^+, H_2O, Ca^{2+} and Mg^{2+}
AE: orthostatic hypotension, hypotension, thrombosis, appetite loss, diarrhea/constipation, N/V, headache, dizziness, hypokalemia, hypocalcemia, hyperuricemia, blurred vision, reversible hearing loss, skin photosensitivity; **CI:** severe electrolyte depletion, hypovolemia, oliguria/anuria, hepatic coma, hypersensitivity to the drug

Bumetanide	EHL 1-1.5h, PRC C, Lact ?
Burinex *Tab 1mg, 5mg*	**Edema:** 0.5-2mg PO qd, rep prn doses at 4-5h intervals, max 10mg/d; 0.5-1mg IV/IM, rep prn at 2-3h intervals, max 10mg/d; DARF: not req
Ethacrynic Acid	EHL 1-4h, PRC B, Lact -
Edecrin *Tab 50mg, Inj 50mg/vial*	**Edema:** 50-200mg/d PO div bid; 0.5-1mg/kg IV, max 100mg/d; **CH:** ini 25mg PO, incr prn q2-3d by 25mg, max 2-3mg/kg/ d;
Furosemide	EHL 30-120min, PRC C, Lact ?
Lasix *Tab 20mg, 40mg, Sol (oral) 10mg/ml* **Lasix Special** *Tab 500mg, Inj 10mg/ml* **Novo-Semide** *Tab 20mg, 40mg, 80mg* **Generics** *Tab 20mg, 40mg, 80mg, Inj 10mg/ml*	**Edema:** ini 20-80mg PO, max 200mg/d or 20-40mg IV, incr by 20-40mg q6-8h prn, max 600mg/d; **HTN:** ini 20-40mg PO bid, incr prn; **CH:** ini 1-2mg/kg IV/IM/PO, incr by 1-2mg q6-8h until desired effect is achieved, max 6mg/kg/dose

2.9.3 Potassium-Sparing Diuretics

MA (amiloride, triamterene): inhibition of the reabsorption of Na^+, Cl^- and H_2O as well as inhibition of the K^+-secretion in the distal convoluted tubule
MA (spironolactone): competitive blockage of aldosterone receptor in late-distal tubule
EF: elimination of Na^+, Cl^- and H_2O ↑, K^+ elimination ↓
AE (amiloride): hyperkalemia, metabolic acidosis, megaloblastic anemia
AE (spironolactone): hyperkalemia, gynecomastia, impotence, amenorrhea, hirsutism, voice DO, skin DO
CI (amiloride): hyperkalemia, renal insufficiency, anuria, use of other antikaliuretics/K-salts
CI (spironolactone): renal insufficiency, hyperkalemia, anuria

Amiloride	EHL 6-9h, PRC B, Lact ?
Generics *Tab 5mg*	**cirrhosis ascites, edema:** ini 5mg PO qd in combination with another diuretic or monotherapy ini 10mg PO qd or div bid, max 20mg/d, **cardiac edema/HTN:** ini 5-10mg PO qd, max 20mg/d
Spironolactone	EHL 1.3-1.4h, PRC D, Lact +
Aldactone *Tab 25mg, 100mg* **Novo-Spiroton** *Tab 25mg, 100mg*	**Edema with heart failure, cirrhosis, nephrotic syndrome:** ini 100mg PO qd or div bid, incr prn until diuretic effect is achieved, max 200mg/d; **HTN:** 50-100mg PO qd or div bid; **CH:** 1-3mg/kg/d PO

2.9.4 Potassium-Sparing Diuretics - Combinations

Amiloride + HCTZ	PRC B, Lact -
Apo, Nu-Amilzide *Tab 5 + 50mg* **Novamilor** *Tab 5 + 50mg* **Generic** *Tab 5 + 50mg*	**HTN, edema:** 50+5-100+10mg PO qd or div bid, max 4 tab/d
Spironolactone + HCTZ	PRC C, Lact ?
Aldactazide *Tab 25 + 25mg, 50 + 50mg* **Novo-Spirozine** *Tab 25 + 25mg, 50 + 50mg*	**Edema:** 25+25-200+200mg PO qd or div bid; **HTN:** 50+50-100+100mg PO qd or div bid
Triamterene + HCTZ	PRC D, Lact -
Apo, Nu-Triazide *Tab 50 + 25mg* **Novo-Triamzide** *Tab 50 + 25mg*	**HTN, edema:** 50+25mg PO qd

2.9.5 Diuretics - Carbonic Anhydrase Inhibitors

MA/EF: noncompetitive inhibition of the enzyme carbonic anhydrase ⇒ urine volume ↑, urinary excretion of bicarbonate and sodium ↑ ⇒ metabolic acidosis
AE: taste disturbances, paresthesia, metabolic acidosis, tinnitus; **CI**: hypersensitivity to drug, hyponatremia, hypokalemia, severe liver or renal impairment, hyperchloremic acidosis, suprarenal gland failure **CI** (methazolamide): severe pulmonary obstruction

Acetazolamide	EHL 4–8h, PRC C, Lact ?
Novo-Zolamide *Tab 250mg* **Generics** *Tab 250mg*	**Acute angle closure glaucoma and pre-op:** 500mg IV q2–4h prn; 250mg PO q4h; **CH:** 8–30mg/kg/d PO div tid; **Edema:** 250–375mg PO qd; **mountain sickness**: 0.5–1g PO div bid–tid, ini 48h before ascent, continue prn; DARF: 10–50ml/min: 250mg PO q12h
Methazolamide	EHL 14h, PRC C, Lact ?
Generics *Tab 50mg*	**Acute angle closure glaucoma:** ini 50–100mg PO bid–tid; **Chronic open angle:** 250mg/d in div doses, max 1g/d

2.10 Antihypertensive Combinations

Atenolol + Chlorthalidone	PRC D, Lact -
Tenoretic *Tab 50 + 25mg, 100 + 25mg*	**HTN:** 50+25–100+25mg PO qd; DARF: GFR (ml/min) 15–35: 50mg qd, <15: 50mg qod
Pindolol + HCTZ	EHL 3.5h,PRC D, Lact +
Viskazide *Tab 10 + 25mg, 10 + 50mg*	**HTN:** 10+25–20+100mg PO qd

2.11 Nitrates

MA: NO relaxes vascular smooth muscles
EF: dilates both arterial and venous vessels, preload ↓, afterload ↓, coronary spasmolysis
AE: facial flushing, N/V, hypotension, tachycardia, headache, dizziness, tachyphylaxis
CI: hypotension (monitor BP), shock, severe anemia, early MI, constrictive pericarditis, pericardial tamponade, head trauma/cerebral hemorrhage, hypovolemia

Isosorbide Dinitrate	EHL 4h, PRC C, Lact ?
Apo-ISDN *Tab (SL) 5mg, Tab10mg, 30mg* **Cedocard SR** *Tab sust. rel. 20mg, 40mg* **Coronex** *Tab (SL) 5mg, Tab10mg, 30mg* **Novo-Sorbide** *Tab10mg, 30mg* **Generics** *Tab (SL) 5mg, Tab 10mg, 30mg*	**Angina Tx:** 5–10 mg PO/SL, rep prn q5–10min up to 3 doses in 30min; **angina PRO:** ini 10–30mg PO tid; ext.rel: ini 20–40mg PO bid, a daily dose-free interval of 10–12h is advisable to avoid nitrate tolerance; DARF: not req
Isosorbide-5-Mononitrate	EHL 6.2 and 6.6h, PRC C, Lact ?
Apo-ISMN *Tab ext.rel 60mg* **Imdur** *Tab ext.rel 60mg*	**Angina PRO:** ext.rel: ini 30mg PO qd, incr prn to 120mg/d

Nitroglycerin IV	EHL 19–33min, PRC C, Lact ?
Generic (NTG + dextrose) *Inj 0.1, 0.2, 0.4mg/ml*	**Acute angina, heart failure:** ini 5mcg/min IV, incr by 5mcg/min q3–5min to 20mcg/min, if no response incr by 10mcg/min q3–5min, max 200mcg/min; **hypertensive emergency:** ini 10–20mcg/min IV, incr to max 100mcg/min
Nitroglycerin Spray	EHL 2–33min, PRC C, Lact ?
Gen-Nitro *Spray metered SL 0.4mg/Spray* **Nitrolingual Pumpspray** *Spray metered SL 0.4mg/Spray* **Rho-Nitro Pumpspray** *Spray metered SL 0.4mg/Spray*	**Acute angina:** 0.4–0.8mg SL, rep prn, max 1.2mg in 15min
Nitroglycerin Sublingual	EHL 2–33min, PRC C, Lact ?
Nitrostat *Tab (SL) 0.3mg, 0.6mg*	**Acute angina:** 0.3–0.6mg SL or in the buccal pouch, rep prn q5min up to 3 doses in 15min; **angina PRO:** 0.3–0.6mg 5–10min before activities which might precipitate an acute attack; DARF: not req
Nitroglycerin Transdermal	EHL 2–33min, PRC C, Lact ?
Minitran *Film (ext.rel, TD) 0.2, 0.4, 0.6mg/h* **Nitrol** *Oint. 2%* **Nitro-Dur** *Film (ext.rel, TD) 0.2, 0.3, 0.4, 0.6, 0.8mg/h* **Transderm-Nitro** *Film (ext.rel, TD) 0.2, 0.4, 0.6mg/h* **Trinipatch** *Film (ext.rel, TD) 0.2, 0.4, 0.6mg/h*	**Angina PRO:** 0.2–0.8mg/h; patch should remain for 12–14h and then be removed, oint: ini 1.25cm to skin q6–8h and wipe off at bedtime, maint 2.5–5cm

2.12 Antiarrhythmics

Class IA antiarrhythmics (quinidine, disopyramide, procainamide)

MA/EF: inflow of Na^+ blocked ⇒ delayed depolarization, conduction velocity ↓ (neg. dromotropic), threshold potential of the AV node ↑ (excitability ↓), neg. inotropic, K^+-outflow blocked ⇒ action potential length ↑, refractory time ↑
AE: GI impairment, dizziness, confusion, dysopias, BP ↓, AV block, tachycardia
AE (disopyramide): urinary retention, constipation, accommodation impaired, dry mouth
AE (procainamide): appetite loss, diarrhea, allergic reactions/dermatitis, itching, dizziness, systemic lupus, hypotension, QT interval prolongation
CI: AV block II°–III°;
CI (quinidine): myasthenia gravis, history of drug induced Torsades, uncompensated heart failure, junctional or intraventricular conduction delay, prolonged QT interval, digitalis overdose;
CI (disopyramide): shock, extensive myocardial disease, glaucoma, urinary retension, renal failure, intraventricular conduction delay;
CI (procainamide): history of Torsades de Pointes, SLE, myasthenia gravis

Class IB antiarrhythmics (lidocaine, mexiletine)

MA: Na^+ inflow ↓, K^+ outflow ↑, slowed phase 4 depolarization
EF: excitability ↓, especially in the ventricles, action potential duration and refractory time in Purkinje fibers ↓, in atria and ventricles ↑; high-frequency excitations are filtered out (premature contractions), possible AV conduction time ↑, negative inotropic effect smaller than class Ia, in high concentrations neg. dromotropic, neg. inotropic
AE (lidocaine): anxiety, drowsiness, dizziness, nervousness, convulsions, pain at injection site, paresthesia, allergic reaction, N/V
AE (mexiletine): dizziness, heartburn, lightheadedness, N/V, nervousness, tremors
CI: AV block II°–III°;
CI (lidocaine): Adam-Stokes syndrome, SA or intraventricular conduction delay;
CI (mexiletine): cardiogenic shock

Class IC antiarrhythmics (flecainide, propafenone)

MA: conduction and refractory time ↑ (AV node and ventricle), no vagolysis
AE: hypotension, AV block, nausea, pro-arrhythmias, cholestatic hepatitis
CI (flecainide): AV block II°–III°, shock, bi- or trifascicular block;
CI (propafanone): sinus or AV dysfunction, bradycardia, severe cardiac insufficiancy, bronchospastic disease, severe electrolyte imbalance or hepatic failure

Class II antiarrhythmics (Isoproterenol), see Beta Blockers →40

Class III antiarrhythmics (amiodarone, sotalol)
MA/EF: blockage of K^+ channels ⇒ action potential length ↑ **AE** (amiodarone): corneal microdeposits, pulmonary fibrosis, hepatic damage, photosensitivity, dysopias, erythema nodosum, hypo- and hyperthyroidism; **AE** (sotalol): see Beta Blockers **CI** (amiodarone): AV block II° -III°, bradycardia, thyroid diseases, iodine allergy, acute hepatitis, thyroid dysfunction, pulmonary interstitial abnormalities **CI** (sotalol): see Beta Blockers
Class IV antiarrhythmics see Calcium Channel Blockers - Non-Dihydropyridines
Other antiarrhythmics (adenosine, atropine, digoxin , epinephrine)
MA/EF (adenosine): brief blockage of the AV node ⇒ termination of re-entry tachycardias, neg. chronotropic at the sinus node **MA** (atropine): competitive antagonism at muscarinic receptors **EF** (atropine): tachycardia, antispasmodic, tear production ↓; sputum, sweat and bronchial secretion ↓, mydriasis, blurred vision **AE** (adenosine): flush, dyspnea, bronchospasm, nausea; **AE** (atropine): decrease of sweat production, urinary retention, restlessness, hallucinations, oral dryness, acute glaucoma **CI** (adenosine): AV block II°-III°, sick-sinus, bradycardia **CI** (atropine): narrow angle glaucoma, micturition disturbance, prostatic hypertrophy, tachyarrhythmias, pyloric stenosis, thyrotoxicosis, GI obsruction, paralytic ileus, severe ulcerative colitis, toxic megacolon, myasthenia gravis

Adenosine	Group IA, EHL < 10s, PRC C, Lact:?
Adenocard *Inj 3mg/ml*	**SVT:** 6mg IV as rapid bolus; if tachycardia persists after 1-2min then 12mg IV; **CH** : **SV arrhythmias conversion:** ini 0.05mg/kg IV as rapid bolus, then 0.05-0.1mg/kg IV, max 12mg/dose; DARF: not req
Amiodarone	Group III, EHL 28-107d, PRC D, Lact -
Cordarone *Tab 200mg, Inj 50mg/ml* **Generics** *Tab 200mg, Inj 50 mg/ml*	**Ventricular arrhythmias:** ini 150mg IV over 10min, then 360mg over 6h (1mg/min), hen 540mg IV over 18h (0.5mg/min); or 800-1600mg/d div qd-bid for 1-3 wk, then 600-800mg/d div qd-bid for 1 mo, then maint 200-400mg/d; DARF: not req

Atropine	EHL 4h, PRC C, Lact ?
Generics *Inj 0.1, 0.3, 0.4, 0.6, 1 mg/ml*	**Bradycardia, bradyarrhythmia:** 0.5–1.0 mg IV q3–5min, max 0.03–0.04mg/kg; **CH:** 0.02mg/kg IV, minimum 0.1mg, max 0.5mg IV; **antimuscurinic:** 0.4–0.6mg IM/IV/SC q4–6h prn; **asystolic arrest:** 1mg IV, repeat q3–5min, max 0.04mg/kg; **organophosphate poisoning:** 1–2mg IM/IV q5–60min until symptoms disappear
Bretylium	EHL 7–11h, PRC C, Lact +
Generics *Inj 50mg/ml*	**Ventricular arrhythmias.**: ini 5 mg/kg IV over 1 min, if arrhythmia persists, 10 mg/kg IV over 1 min, and repeat PRN, max 30–35 mg/kg; maint 5–10 mg/kg q6–8 h IV/IM; **CH:** ini 5 mg/kg IV, attempt electrical defibrillation; if persists repeat PRN with 10 mg/kg, max 30 mg/kg; maint 5 mg/kg IM/IV q6 hours; DARF: CrCl 10–50 mL/min 25%–50% , ClCr <10 mL/min: 25% .
Digoxin	EHL 1.3–2.2d, PRC C, Lact +
Digoxin pediatric *Inj 0.05mg/ml* **Lanoxin** *Tab 0.0625, 0.125, 0.25mg, Ped elixir 0.05mg/ml* **Generics** *Inj 0.05, 0.25mg/ml, Tab 0.0625, 0.125, 0.25mg*	**AF, heart failure:** ini 0.5mg IV, then 0.25mg q6h for 2 doses or ini 0.5–0.75mg PO then 0.125mg–0.375mg PO q6–8h until effect, maint 0.125–0.375mg PO/IV qd; **CH** 5–10 y: ini 20–35mcg/kg PO div q6–8h, maint 25–35% of loading dose; DARF: GFR (ml/min) 10–50: 25–75% or q36h, <10: 10–25% or q48h
Disopyramide	Group IA, EHL 4–10h, PRC C, Lact +
Rythmodan *Cap. 100mg, 150mg* **Rythmodan LA** *Tab 250mg*	**Ventricular arrhythmias:** 400–800mg/d div qid; can change to ext. rel. bid once stable; for rapid control: loading 300mg PO then 100mg PO q6h, incr to 150–200mg PO q6h prn; DARF: GFR (ml/min) 30–40: 100mg q8h; 15–30: 100mg bid; <15: 100mg qd

Epinephrine	EHL no data, PRC C, Lact ?
Adrenalin *Inj 1mg/ml, Topical sol. 1mg/ml* **Epipen** *Inj (IM) 0.3mg/delivery* **Epipen Jr.** *Inj (IM) 0.15mg/delivery* **Generics** *Inj 1mg/ml*	**Cardiac arrest:** 0.5–1mg IV/ET, rep.ed prn q3–5min; **anaphylaxis**: 0.3–0.5 mg SC/IM, rep.ed prn q10–15min; **CH cardiac arrest:** 0.01mg/kg IV; 0.1mg/kg ET rep.ed prn with 0.1mg/kg IV/ET q3–5min; **anaphylaxis:** 0.01mg/kg SC/IM; 0.1mg/kg IV if response is inadequate; IV: use 1:10.000 Sol; SC/IM: use 1: 1000 sol
Flecainide	Group IC, EHL 14h, PRC C, Lact +
Tambocor *Tab 50mg, 100mg* **Generics** *Tab 50mg, 100mg*	**ventricular arrhythmias:** ini 100mg PO q12h, max 400/d; **SV arrythmia:** ini 50mg PO q12h, max 300mg/d; **CH** >6 mo: 100–200mg/m²/d PO; DARF: GFR (ml/min) <35: 50mg PO bid
Isoproterenol	Group II, EHL 2.5–5min, PRC C, Lact ?
Generics *Inj 0.2mg/ml*	**Cardiac arrhythmias**: ini 2 mcg/minute IV; titrate to patient response, maint 2–10 mcg/min; **CH**: ini 0.1mcg/kg/min IV; maint 0.2–2 mcg/kg/minute
Lidocaine	Group IB, EHL 1.5–2h, PRC B, Lact +
Generics (lidocaine + dextrose) *Inj 0.2, 0.4, 0.8, 2%*	**Ventricular arrhythmia:** ini 1–1.5mg/kg IV over 2–3 min, repeat doses of 0.5–0.75mg/kg in 5–10min prn, max 3mg/kg; continuous infusion: 1–4mg/min; **CH ventricular arrhythmia**: ini 1mg/kg IV, may repeat dose q10–15 min prn x 2 doses, then 20–50mcg/kg/min as continuous inf
Mexiletine	Group IB, EHL 6–17h, PRC C, Lact +
Generics *Cap 100mg, 200mg*	**Ventricular arrhythmia:** ini 200mg PO q8h or 400mg PO x 1, maint 200–300mg PO q8h, max 1.2g/d; Hepatic impair: 25–30%

Procainamide	Group IA, EHL 2.5–8h, PRC C, Lact ?
Procan SR *Tab sust. rel. 250, 500, 750mg* **Generics** *Cap 250mg, 375mg, 500mg, Inj 100mg/ml*	**Recurrant VF/pulseless VT:** ini 20–30mg/min until arryth. resolved or widened QRS, max 17mg/kg; **Ventricular arrhythmias:** IV: ini 100–200mg or 15–18mg/kg IV q5min prn, max 1g, then 1–4mg/min; PO: 250–500mg PO q3–6h (imm. rel.) or 500mg–1g PO q6h (sust. rel.); max 4g/d; A.fib/PAT: ini 1.25g PO, then 0.75g in 1h, then 0.5–1g q2h until resolved
Propafenone	Group IC, EHL 5–8h, PRC C, Lact ?
Rythmol *Tab 150mg, 300mg* **Generics** *Tab 150mg, 300mg*	**ventricular arrhythmias:** ini 150mg PO q8h, incr q3–4d to 300mg q12h, max 300mg q8h; DARF: not req; **Hepatic impair**: ini 150mg PO qd, then bid, then tid, max 300mg PO bid
Quinidine Bisulfate	
Biquin Durules *Tab cont. rel. 250mg*	**Ventricular arrythmias, supraventricular arrythmias:** ini 250mg PO in am, then 500mg in pm, maint 500–1.25g PO bid
Quinidine Gluconate	Group IA, EHL no data, PRC C, Lact ?
Generics *Tab 325mg*	**Maintenance after conversion of AF:** 325–975 mg PO q8–12h; DARF: not req
Quinidine Sulfate	Group IA, EHL no data, PRC C, Lact ?
Generics *Tab 200mg, Inj 190mg/ml*	**Ventricular arrythmias, PAC/PVC:** 200–400mg PO q6–8h or 12mg/kg loading then 6mg/kg PO q4–6h; **CH:** 6mg/kg PO q4–6h; DARF: not req
Sotalol	Group III, EHL 7–18h, PRC B, Lact ?
Generics *Tab 80mg, 160mg*	**AF, ventricular arrhythmia:** ini 80mg PO bid, maint 160–320mg/d div bid; DARF: CrCl 30–60: 50%, 10–30: 25%, <10: avoid

2.13 Cardiac Glycosides

MA: inhibition of active Na^+-K^+-transport into heart muscle cells ⇒ intracellular Na^+ ↑ ⇒ Na^+-Ca^{2+} exchange ⇒ intracellular Ca^{2+} ↑, vagal nerve activity ↑, sympathetic activity ↓
EF: pos. inotropic, stroke volume ↑, higher efficiency of the insufficient heart, tissue perfusion ↑, coronary perfusion ↑, neg. chronotropic and dromotropic, refractory time at S-A node ↑, at the myocardial ↓, ⇒ activation of ectopic pacemakers, pos. bathmotropic
AE: AV block, arrhythmias, extrasystoles, allergic reaction, allergic dermatitis, skin rash, N/V, diarrhea, blurred vision, visual halos, confusion
CI: AV block II°–III°, WPW-syndrome, VT, carotid sinus syndrome, hypertrophic obstructive cardiomyopathy, myocardial ischemia, acute MI, pacemakers, hypercalcemia, hypokalemia, thoracic aortic aneurysm, V. fib.

Digoxin	EHL 1.3–2.2d, PRC C, Lact +
Digoxin pediatric *Inj 0.05mg/ml* **Lanoxin** *Tab 0.0625, 0.125, 0.25mg, Ped elixir 0.05mg/ml* **Generics** *Inj 0.05, 0.25mg/ml, Tab 0.0625, 0.125, 0.25mg*	**AF, heart failure:** ini 0.5mg IV, then 0.25mg q6h for 2 doses or ini 0.5–0.75mg PO then 0.125mg–0.375mg PO q6–8h until effect, maint 0.125–0.375mg PO/IV qd; **CH** 5–10 y: ini 20–35mcg/kg PO div q6–8h, maint 25–35% of loading dose; DARF: GFR (ml/min) 10–50: 25–75% or q36h, <10: 10–25% or q48h
Digoxin-Immune Fab	EHL 15–20h, PRC C, Lact +
Digibind *Inj 38mg/vial*	**Digoxin/digitoxin-intoxication:** **average-dose:** 400mg IV; 40mg will bind 0.5–0.6mg digoxin or digitoxin

2.14 Phosphodiesterase Inhibitors

MA: inhibition of phosphodiesterase ⇒ intracellular accumulation of cAMP ⇒ intracellular Ca^{++} ↑ ⇒ myocardial contractility ↑
EF: pos. inotropic effect (stroke volume, cardiac output ↑), pos. chronotropic effect, vasodilation (preload ↓, afterload ↓), bronchodilation
AE: cholestasis, nausea, hypotension, tachyarrhythmias, thrombocytopenia, splenomegaly, vasculitis, myositis, lung infiltration
CI: hypersensitivity to drug

Milrinone	EHL 1–3h, PRC C, Lact ?
Generics *Inj 1mg/ml*	**Heart failure:** ini 50mcg/kg IV over 10min, maint 0.375–0.75mcg/kg/min; DARF: GFR (ml/min). 41–50: 0.43*, 31–40: 0.38, 21–30: 0.33*, 11–20: 0.28*, 6–10: 0.23*, <5: 0.2* (* = mcg/ kg/min)

2.15 Antilipidemics

2.15.1 Bile Acid Sequestrants

MA/EF: intestinal binding of bile acids ⇒ interruption of the biliary cycle ⇒ bile acid production from cholesterol ↑ ⇒ serum cholesterol ↓; LDL-receptor activity ↑ ⇒ LDL-resorption of the liver ↑ ⇒ serum cholesterol ↓
AE: constipation, abdominal discomfort/pain, nausea, diarrhea, resorption failure of drugs and fat-soluble vitamins
AE (colestipol): constipation, fat soluble vitamin deficiency, N/V, flatulence, abdominal distention;
AE (cholestyramine): constipation, abdominal discomfort/pain, flatulence, N/V, bleeding tendencies due to hypoprothrombinemia
CI: bile duct obstruction
CI (colestipol): hypersensitivity to colestipol products, complete biliary obstruction, phenylketonurics
CI (cholestyramine): complete biliary obstruction, hypersensitivity to bile-sequestering resins

Colestipol	EHL no data, PRC , Lact +
Colestid *Tab 1g, Granules (oral) 5g/pkt*	**Hypercholesterolemia:** Tab: ini 2g PO qd/bid, max 16g/ d; Gran: ini 5g PO qd/bid, incr by 5g increments at 1–2 mo intervals, max 30g/d; DARF: not req
Cholestyramine	EHL no data, PRC C, Lact ?
Generics *Powder (oral) 4g/packet*	**Hypercholesterolemia:** ini 4g PO qd, maint 4g 1–6 times/d, max 24g/d; DARF: not req

2.15.2 Cholesterol Absorption Inhibitors

MA/EF (ezetimib): inhibition of the intestinal absorption of cholesterol ad related phytosterols; **AE** (ezetimib): fatigue, pharyngitis, sinusitis, abd. pain, diarrhea, back pain, arthralgia, cough, viral infection; **CI** (ezetimib): hypersensitivity to e., hepatic dysfunction

Ezetimibe	EHL 22h, PRC C, Lact -
Ezetrol *Tab 10mg*	**Primary hypercholesterolemia, homozyg. fam. hyperchol., homozyg. sitosterolemia:** 10mg PO qd, may be administered with an HMG-CoA reducatse inhibitor; DARF: not req

2.15.3 HMG-CoA Reductase Inhibitors ("Statins")

MA: competitive inhibition of HMG CoA reductase; **EF:** intracellular cholesterol synthesis ↓, LDL↓, HDL ↑;
AE: skin reactions, myopathy, vasculitis, headache, abdominal pain, transaminases↑, dyssomnia; **AE** (atorvastatin): headache, liver enzymes↑, abdominal pain;
AE (fluvastatin): dyspepsia, diarrhea, abdominal pain, nausea, headache;
AE (lovastatin): headache, rhabdomyolysis, diarrhea, hepatotoxicity;
AE (pravastatin): GI disturbances, liver enzymes↑, headache, weakness, flu- like symptoms;
AE (simvastatin): headache, GI upset, rhabdomyolysis, transient hypotension, liver dysfunction
CI: hepatic diseases, pregnancy, lactation, hypersensitivity to product ingredients
CI (rosuvastatin): cyclosporine use

Atorvastatin	EHL 14h, PRC X, Lact ?
Lipitor *Tab 10mg, 20mg, 40mg, 80mg*	**Hypercholesterolemia, mixed dyslipidemia:** ini 10–20mg PO qd, maint 10–80mg PO qd, depending on lipid levels DARF: not req
Fluvastatin	EHL < 3 h, PRC X, Lact ?
Lescol *Cap 20mg, 40mg*	**Hypercholesterolemia:** ini 20–40mg PO qd, max 80mg/ d, give 80mg in div doses bid
Lovastatin	EHL no data, PRC X, Lact ?
Mevacor *Tab 20mg, 40mg* **Generic** *Tab 20mg, 40mg*	**Hypercholesterolemia:** ini 20mg PO qd, maint 10–80mg/ d PO
Pravastatin	EHL 2.6–3.2 h, PRC X, Lact ?
Pravachol *Tab 10mg, 20mg, 40mg* **Generics** *Tab 10mg, 20mg, 40mg*	**Hypercholesterolemia:** ini 10–20mg PO qd, maint 10–40 mg/d; DARF: ini 10mg PO qd

Simvastatin	EHL no data, PRC X, Lact ?
Zocor *Tab 5mg, 10mg, 20mg, 40mg, 80mg*	**Hypercholesterolemia:** ini 20–40mg PO qd, maint 10–80mg/d; DARF: ini 5mg PO qd
Rosuvastatin	EHL 19h, PRC X, Lact ?
Crestor *Tab 10mg, 20mg, 40mg*	**Hypercholesterolemia:** ini 10 PO qd, maint 10–40mg/d

2.15.4 Fibric Acids

MA/EF: lipoprotein lipase activity ↑ ⇒ triglycerides ↓, LDL ↓, HDL ↑
AE: myalgia, rhabdomyolysis, N/V, transaminases ↑, cholelithiasis, ventricular dysrhythmia, blood count changes; **AE** (clofibrate): diarrhea, flatulence, headache; **AE** (fenofibrate): rash, LFT ↑; **AE** (gemfibrozil): epigastric pain, xerostomia, diarrhea, myopathy, hepatotoxicity;
CI: primary biliary cirrhosis, great caution in children; **CI** (fenofibrate): severe hepatic or renal disease, gallbladder disease, hypersensitivity to fenofibrate;
CI (gemfibrozil): hypersensitivity to gemfibrozil, gallbladder disease/biliary cirrhosis, severe liver/kidney disease, type I hyperlipoprotenemia
CI (bezafibrate): hepatic or renal impairment, PBC, lactation, type I hyperlipoprotenemia, combination with statin in patients predisposed to myopathy

Bezafibrate	EHL 1–2h, PRC X, Lact ?
Bezalip *Tab sust. rel 400mg* **Generics** *Tab 200mg*	**Hypercholesterolemia type IIa, IIb, mixed/Hypertriglyceridemia type IV, V:** 200mg PO bid–tid or sust. rel. 400mg PO qd; CrCl 40–60ml/min 200 bid, 15–40 200 qod to qd, <15 200mg q3d
Fenofibrate	EHL 20–22h, PRC C, Lact -
Apo-Feno-Micro *Cap 67mg, 200mg* **Apo-Feno-Super** *Cap 100mg, 160mg* **Fenomax** *Cap 100mg, 160mg* **Lipidil EZ** *Tab 48mg, 145mg* **Lipidil Micro** *Cap 200mg* **Lipidil Supra** *Tab 100mg, 160mg* **Novo-Fenofibat** *Cap 67, 200mg* **Gen, PMS-Fenofibrate Micro** *Cap 200mg* **Generics** *Cap 100mg, 160mg*	**Hypertriglyceridemia:** ini 160mg PO qd, maint 100–200mg PO qd
Gemfibrozil	EHL 1.5 h, PRC C, Lact -
Lopid *Cap 300mg, Tab 600mg* **Generics** *Cap 300mg, Tab 600mg*	**Hypertriglyceridemia:** 600mg PO bid

2.15.5 Nicotinic Acid

MA/EF: blockage of the triacylglycerol lipase ⇒ lipoprotein lipase activity ↑ ⇒ triglycerides ↓, cholesterol ↓
AE: flush, a sensation of warmth in face, neck, and ears, GI disturbances, glucose tolerance ↓, fasting blood sugar ↑, pruritus, hepatotoxicity, feeling of restlessness, headache, hypotension, rash, tingling, itching, and dry skin
CI: acute CVS failure, hypersensitivity to niacin, active liver/peptic ulcer disease

Niacin	EHL 10h, PRC C, Lact ?
Niacin/Niacinamide *Tab 500mg* **Niodan** *Tab (ext rel) 500mg* **Generics** *Tab 500mg*	**Hyperlipoproteinemia/hyperlipidemia:** ini 100mg PO tid incr slowly to 3g/d, max 6g/d; ext.rel.: 375mg PO qd for 1wk, then 500mg PO qd for 1wk, then 750mg PO qd for 1wk, then 1000mg PO qd; max 2g/d

2.15.6 Combination

Niacin + Lovastatin	PRC X, Lact +
Advicor *Tab 500 (ext. rel.) + 20mg (imm. rel.), Tab 1000 (ext. rel) + 20mg (imm. rel.)*	**Hypercholesterolemia/Mixed dyslipidaemia:** 500mg + 20mg–1000mg + 20mg PO qd
Amlodipine + Atorvastatin	PRC X, Lact ?
Caduet *Tab 5 + 10mg, 5 + 20mg, 5 + 40mg, 5 + 80mg, 10 + 10mg, 10 + 20mg, 10 + 40mg, 10 + 80mg*	**HTN/angina pectoris and Hypercholesterolemia/mixed dyslipidemia:** ini 5 + 10mg PO qd, max 10 + 80mg qd; DAHF (amlodipine): ini 2.5mg PO qd; DARF: not req
Acetylsalicylic acid + Pravastatin	PRC X, Lact ?
PravASA *Tab 81mg, 162mg + Tab 10mg, 20mg, 40mg*	**Hypercholesterolemia:** (pravastatin) ini 10–20mg PO qd, maint 10–40 mg/d; DARF: ini 10mg PO qd **PRO of recurrent MI, unstable angina pectoris:** (acetylsalicylic acid) 80–325mg PO qd

3 Hematology

3.1 Plasma Expanders

MA/EF (dextran): high molecular weight polysaccharides with water-binding capability and intravascular retention ⇒ plasma volume ↑
AE (albumin): hypersensitivity (shaking, chills, urticaria)
AE (dextran): allergic to anaphylactic reactions, great amounts of low-molecular-weight dextran can be nephrotoxic
AE (pentastarch): coagulopathy
CI (blood plasma substitutes): states of hyperhydration, hypervolemia, serious cardiac insufficiency, pulmonary edema, known allergy to active ingredients
CI (dextran): hypersensitivity to dextran or corn products, hemostatic defects, cardiac decompensation
CI (albumin): hypersensitivity to albumin, severe anemia, heart failure
CI (pentastarch): hypersensitivity to pentastarch, severe RF, CHF, bleeding DO

Albumin	EHL 15–20d, PRC C
Plasbumin *Inj (5%) 50ml vial, 250ml vial, 500ml vial, (25%) 20ml vial, 50ml vial, 100ml vial*	**Hypovolemia:** 0.5–1g/kg/dose, repeat prn, max 6g/kg/d, max 5ml/min for 5% and 1–2ml/min for 25%; **hypoproteinemia:** 0.5–1g/kg/dose, repeat q1–2d bases on loses
Dextran	EHL 41min, PRC C, Lact ?
Gentran 40 *Inj 100mg dextran 40/ml* **Gentran 70** *Inj 60mg dextran 70/ml*	**Shock, hypovolemia:** Dextran 40, 10% Sol: ini 10ml/kg IV as rapid inf, max 20ml/kg on the 1st d, thereafter 10ml/ kg/d for max 4d
Pentastarch	70% elimination in 24hrs, PRC C, Lact ?
Pentaspan *Inj 10g/100ml*	**Shock, hypovolemia:** 500–2,000ml IV, max 28ml/kg/d

3.2 Anticoagulants

3.2.1 Unfractionated Heparin

MA/EF: forming complexes with antithrombin-III ⇒ inhibiting effect of antithrombin-III ↑ (by a factor of 1,000) ⇒ inhibition of thrombin, factors Xa, XIa, XIIa, and callicrein ⇒ thrombin activated conversion of fibrinogen to fibrin ↓ ; activat. of the lipoprot. lipase
AE: hemorrhage complications, allergic reactions, anaphylaxis, osteoporosis, cutaneous necrosis, hair loss, thrombocytopenia
CI: heparin allergy, heparin induced thrombocytopenia (type II), active bleeding, imminent abortion, lumbar puncture, epidural anesthesia, hemophilia, ITP, severe liver damage

Heparin Sodium	EHL 2.13h, PRC C, Lact +
Heparin Leo *Inj 100U/ml, 1,000U/ml, 10,000U/ml, 25,000U/ml* **Heparin Lock Flush** *Inj 10U/ml, 100U/ml* **Hepalean** *Inj 1,000U/ml, 10,000U/ml, 25,000U/ml* **Hepalean-LOK** *Inj 10U/ml, 100U/ml* **Generics** *Inj 2U/ml, 40U/ml, 50U/ml, 100 U/ml*	**DVT, pulmonary vembolism Tx:** ini 80 U/kg IV, maint 18 U/kg/h IV, adjust dose based on PTT; **DVT PRO:** 5,000 U SC q8–12h; **CH:** ini 50 U/kg IV, maint 10–25 U/kg/h IV, adjust dose based on PTT

3.2.2 Low-Molecular-Weight Heparins, Heparinoids

MA/EF (low-molecular-weight heparins): molecular weight ↓ ⇒ thrombin inhibition ↓, factor Xa inhibition ↑ ; effect on blood platelet function ↓, antithrombotic effect ↑, danger of hemorrhage ↓ ; neutralization ↓ through platelet factor 4; when used subcutaneously bioavailability ↑, half-life ↑ ;
MA/EF: (argatroban): specific and reversible direct thrombin inhibitor;
MA/EF: (danaparoid): = heparinoid, factor Xa inhibition;
MA/EF: (fondaparinux): selectivly binding to antithrombin III ⇒ activation of the innate neutralization of factor Xa;
MA/EF: (lepirudine): = recombined hirudin, direct inhibition of thrombin, prevention of thromboembolic diseases
AE/CI (low-molecular-weight heparins): see heparin →69
AE (argatroban): bleeding, hypotension, fever, cardiac arrest, ventricular tachycardia, diarrhea, nausea, allergic reactions;
AE (danaparoid): bleeding, tachycardia, chest pain, hyperkalemia, inj site hematoma;
AE (fondaparinux): bleeding, anemia, fever, edema, local irritation;
AE (lepirudine): bleeding, anemia, abnormal LFT, allergic reactions

CI (LMWH, dalteparin, enoxaparin, nadroparin, tinzaparin): uncontrolled active bleeding, severe HTN, hemmorhagic stoke, hypersensativity to pork, history of HIT;
CI (nadroparin): hypersensitivity to nadroparin, acute infectious endocarditis, severe hemorrhagic diathesis/states, Nadr induced thrombocytopenia
CI (argatroban): active major bleeding, hypersensitivity to argatroban
CI (danaparoid): hypersensitivity to danaparoid, severe hemorrhagic diathesis/states, IM route, bacterial endocarditis, major blood clotting disorder, active PUD, hemorrhagic CVA or retinopathy, severe HTN, surgery involving brain/spine/eyes/ears
CI (fondaparinux): severe renal impairment, endocarditis, weight <50kg, thrombocytopenia, bacterial endocarditis, active bleeding
CI (lepirudine): hypersensitivity to hirudin products

Argatroban	EHL 39-51min, PRC B, Lact ?
Argatroban *Inj 100mg/ml*	**DVT PRO and Tx in heparin-associated thrombocytopenia**: 2mcg/kg/min, adjust dose based on aPTT, max 10mcg/kg/min; DARF not req
Dalteparin	EHL 2-5h, PRC B, Lact ?
Fragmin *Prefilled syr. 2500 U/0.2ml, 5,000 U/0.2ml, 7,500U/0.3ml, 10,000U/0.4ml, 12,500U/0.5ml, 15,000U/0.6ml, 18,000U/0.72ml, Inj10,000 U/ml, 25,000U/ml*	**DVT PRO, hip replacement:** ini 5,000 U SC night preop, then 2,500 U 6h after first dose, then 5,000 U SC qd for 14d; **DVT PRO, gen. surgery:** ini 2,500 U SC 1-2h preop, then 2,500 U qd postop for 5-7d; **hip surgery:** 5,000 U SC night preop then phs for 5-7d or 2500 U SC 1-2h preop and 8-12h later, then 5,000 U qam for 5-7d; **DVT tx:** 200U/kg SC qd, max 18,000U/d; **unstable angina or NQWMI:** 120 U/kg max 10,000 U SC q12h for 5-8d; **anticoagulation, dialysis:** 5,000 U into the arterial line
Danaparoid	EHL 1h, PRC B, Lact ?
Orgaran-DVT *Inj 750U/0.6ml* **Orgaran-HIT** *Inj 750U/0.6ml*	**DVT PRO (ortho., thorac., major surg.):** ini 750 U SC 1-4h preop, then 750 U SC q12h upto 14d; **DVT PRO (stoke patient):** ini 1,000 U IV bolus then 750 U SC bid for 7-14d; **DVT/PE Tx (HIT):** 2,250-2500 IV bolus then 400 U/h for 4h, then 300 U/h for 4 h, then 150-200U/h for 5-7d; DARF req

Enoxaparin	EHL 4.5h (range 3–6h), PRC B, Lact ?
Lovenox *Inj 10mg/0.1ml, 30mg/0.3ml, 40mg/0.4ml, 60mg/0.6ml, 80mg/0.8ml, 100mg/ml, 120mg/0.8ml, 150mg/1ml*	**DVT PRO, hip/knee replacement:** 30mg SC q12h ini 12–24h postop for 7–14d; **DVT PRO abd., gyne surgery:** ini 40mg SC 2h preop, then 40mg SC qd for 7–10d; **Tx of DVT:** 1.5mg/ kg SC qd or 1mg/kg SC q12h, max 180mg/d; **unstable angina or NQWMI:** 1mg/kg SC q12h for 2–8d with ASA, max 100mg/dose; DARF req
Fondaparinux	EHL 17–21h, PRC B, Lact ?
Arixtra *Inj 2.5mg/0.5ml*	**DVT PRO, hip/knee replacement**: ini 2.5mg SC6–8h postop, then 2.5mg qd; DARF: GFR (ml/min) <30: contraind.
Lepirudine	EHL 1.3h, PRC B, Lact ?
Refludan *Inj 50mg/vial*	**Heparin-associated thrombocytopenia with VTE:** ini 0.4mg/kg bolus IV, max 44mg, maint 0.15mg/kg/h IV, max 16.5mg/ h; **ACS:** ini 0.4mg/kg IV bolus then 0.15mg/kg/h x 72h, max 40mg bolus, max 15mg/h infusion; DARF ini 0.2mg/kg bolus IV, then GFR (ml/min): 45–60: 0.075mg/kg/h; 30–44: 0.045mg/kg/h; 15–29: 0.0225mg/ kg/h; <15, dialysis: 0.1mg/kg IV qod
Nadroparin	EHL 6h, PRC B, Lact -
Fraxiparine *Inj 9,500U/ml, 1,900U/0.2ml, 2,850U/0.3ml, 3,800U/0.4ml, 5,700U/0.6ml, 7,600U/0.8ml, 9,500U/ml* **Fraxiparine Forte** *Inj 19,000U/ml, 11,400U/0.6ml, 15,200U/0.8ml*	**DVT PRO:** 2,850U SC 2–4h preop then qd for atleast 7d; **DVT PRO, hip surgery:** 38U/kg SC 12h before and 12h after surgery then qd X 3d, then 57U/kg SC qd; **DVT tx:** 171U/kg SC qd, max 17100U/d; **UA,NQWMI:** 86 U/kg IV bolus, then 86 U/kg SC q12h with ASA

Tinzaparin	EHL 3–4h, PRC B, Lact ?
Innohep *Inj 1,0000U/ml, 20,000 U/ml*	**DVT Tx with or without pulmonary embolism:** 175U/ kg SC qd; **DVT PRO, gen. surgery:** 3,500U SC 2h preop then qd for 7–10d; **hip surg:** 50U/kg SC 2h preop then SC qd for 7–10d; **knee surg.:** 75U/kg SC qd postop for 7–10d; DARF req caution

3.2.3 Heparin Antidote

MA/EF: forming of a salt-like bond with heparin ⇒ inactivation of heparin
AE: hypotension, bradycardia, hypersensitivity reactions;
CI: hypersensitivity to protamine products; Note: severe hypotension/ anaphylactoid reaction with too rapid administration; allergic reactions in fish allergy, previous exposure to protamine (including insulin); risk of allergy unclear in infertile/vasectomized men with anti-protamine antibodies

Protamine	EHL no data, PRC C, Lact ?
Generics *Inj 10mg/ml*	**Heparin overdose (usual rule):** 1mg antagonizes approx. 90 U of beef heparin or 115U porcine heparin, max rate 50mg/10min; max 1x dose 50mg

3.2.4 Oral Anticoagulants

MA/EF (warfarin): inhibition of the vitamin K negotiated carboxylation of Ca^{2+} dependant blood clotting factors (II, VII, IX, X) in the liver
MA/EF (ancrod): thrombin-like enzyme from venom of the Malayan Pit Viper, enzymatically cleaves fibrinogen
MA/EF (AT-III): inactivation of thrombin, IXa, Xa, XIa, XIIa, and plasmin.
MA/EF (nicoumalone): inhibition of the vitamin K, inhibits formation of prothrombin, VII, IX, X, protein C
AE: hemorrhage complications, skin necrosis, urticaria
CI: pregnancy, blood dyscrasias, recent CNS/eye surgery, hemmorhagic stroke, pericarditis/pericardial effusion, bacterial endocarditis, unsupervised patients, thrombocytopenia, GI ulcers, retinopathy, arterial brain aneurysms, severe HTN

Antithrombin III	EHL 2.5d, PRC B, Lact ?
Thrombate III *Inj 500U/vial, 1,000U/vial*	**AT III deficiency:** individualized dosing
Warfarin	EHL 20–60h, PRC X, Lact +
Coumadin *Tab 1mg, 2mg, 2.5mg, 3mg, 4mg, 5mg, 6mg, 10mg, Inj 5.4mg/vial* **Generics** *Tab 1mg, 2mg, 2.5mg, 3mg, 4mg, 5mg, 6mg, 7.5mg, 10mg*	**Anticoagulation:** ini 2–5mg PO qd for 2–4d, maint 2–10mg/d PO, adjust dose to PT/INR (PT: 1.2–2 times control)

3.3 Thrombolytics

MA/EF: activation of plasminogen ⇒ formation of plasmin ⇒ Plasmin proteolyses fibrin ⇒ dissolution of not yet fully organized blood clots (Streptokinase forms a streptokinase-plasminogen-complex ⇒ free plasminogen ⇒ plasmin);
AE: bleeding from wounds, gingival bleeding, hemorrhagic/thromboembolic stroke, internal bleeding, bruising, skin lesions, skin rash, hives, hypotension, fever, allergic reaction, head-/backache, arrhythmias;
Absolute CI (to fibrinolytic therapy): active internal bleeding, other thrombolytic use, CNS neoplasm, AV malformation, aneurysm, CNS procedure/trauma within 2 mo, SAH, intracranial hemmorhage, uncontrolled hypertension (over 180/110), bleeding diathesis, MI due to aortic dissection, allergy to streptokinase/anistreplase; (in acute stroke): seizure at onset of stroke, platelets <100,000/mm3, INR>1.7, PT>15 sec, heparin with 48h preceding onset;

Alteplase	EHL 26.5–46min, PRC C, Lact ?
Activase rt-PA *Inj 50mg/vial, 100mg/vial* **Cathflo** *Inj 2mg/vial*	**Acute MI:** >67kg: 15mg IV bolus, then 50mg over 30min, then 35mg over 1h; <67kg: 15mg IV bolus, then 0.75mg/ kg over 30min, then 0.5mg/kg over 1h; **acute ischemic stroke:** (within 3h of symptom onset) 0.9mg/kg, max 90mg, over 60min IV, with 10% of total dose admin as IV bolus over 1min; **thrombolysis of central venous device:** 2mg IV x 1
Anistreplase	EHL 70–120min, PRC C, Lact ?
Eminase *Inj 30 U/5ml*	**Acute MI:** 30 U IV over 2–5min
Reteplase	EHL 13–16min, PRC C, Lact ?
Retavase *Inj 10.4 U/vial*	**Acute MI:** 10 U IV over 2min, rep dose in 30min

Streptokinase	EHL 18–83min, PRC C, Lact ?
Streptase *Inj 25,0000 U/vial, 75,0000 U/vial, 150,0000 U/vial*	**Acute MI:** 1.5 million U IV over 1h; intracoronary: 20,000 U bolus, then 2,000–4,000 U/min for 30–90min; **pulmonary or arterial embolism/arterial thrombosis:** 250,000 U IV over 30min, then 100,000 U/h IV for 24h; **deep vein thrombosis:** 250,000 U IV over 30min, then 100,000 U/h IV for 72h DARF not req
Tenecteplase	EHL 17–20min, PRC C, Lact ?
TNKase *Inj 50mg vial*	**Acute MI:** single bolus IV: < 60kg: 30mg 60–69kg: 35mg; 70–79kg: 40mg; 80–89 kg: 45mg; > 90kg: 50mg
Urokinase	EHL < 20min, PRC B, Lact ?
Abbokinase *Inj 5,000U/vial, 250,000 U/vial*	**Pulmonary embolism:** 4,400 U/kg IV over 10min, then 4,400 U/kg/h for 12h; occluded IV catheter: 5,000 U instilled into catheter, remove after 5min

3.4 Antiplatelets

3.4.1 Glycoprotein IIb-IIIa Inhibitors

MA/EF: antagonist of the glycoprotein IIb-IIIa-receptor on blood platelets ⇒ inhibition of platelet aggregation
AE (abciximab, tirofiban): hemorrhage complications, thrombocytopenia, nausea, fever, headaches;
AE (eptifibatide): bleeding
CI (abciximab, tirofiban): active bleeding, cerebrovascular complications during the last 2 years, operations and traumas during the last 6 wks., intracranial neoplasm, severe HTN, use of dextran, thrombocytopenia, vasculitis, aneurysm, AV anomalies, retinopathy of hypertensive or diabetic origin;
CI (tirofibin): pericarditis, cirrhosis;
CI (eptifibatide): bleeding DO/surgery/CVA, hypersensitivity to eptifibatide products, severe renal dysfunction, platelet count < 100,000/mm(3);

Abciximab	EHL < 10min, PRC C, Lact ?
Reopro *Inj 2mg/ml*	**Percutaneous coronary intervention:** 0.25mg/kg IV over 1min 10–60min before procedure, then 0.125mcg/ kg/min, max 10mcg/min for 12h; **unstable angina not responding to conventional Tx:** 0.25mg/kg IV over 1min, then 10mcg/min for 18–24h concluding 1h after PTCA
Eptifibatide	EHL 1.13–2.5h, PRC B, Lact ?
Integrilin *Inj 0.75mg/ml, 2mg/ml*	**UA/NQWMI:** ini 180mcg/kg IV, then 2mcg/kg/min up to max 72h; **percutaneous coronary intervention:** ini 180mcg/kg IV before procedure, then 180mcg/kg bolus 10min after 1st bolus, then 2mcg/kg/min IV for 18–24h after the procedure; DARF serum-creatinine (mg/dl) <2: 100%; 2–4: ini 180mcg/kg IV, then 1mcg/kg/min
Tirofiban	EHL 90–180min, PRC B, Lact ?
Aggrastat *Inj 0.25mg/ml, 0.5mg/ml*	**Acute coronary syndrome:** ini 0.4mcg/kg/ min IV for 30min, then 0.1mcg/kg/min for upto 48h or until 12–24h after coronary intervention; DARF GFR (ml/min) <30: 50%

3.4.2 Phosphodiesterase/Platelet Aggregation-Adhesion Inhibitors

MA (aspirin): inhibition of cyclooxygenase ⇒ synthesis of thromboxane A2 ↓ (aggregation activator for blood platelets), synthesis of prostacyclin ↓ (aggregation inhibitor in endothelium);
MA (clopidogrel, ticlopidine): blockage of the ADP-receptor of blood platelets;
MA (anagrelide, cilostazol, dipyridamole): inhibition of cAMP phosphodiesterase ⇒ cAMP in platelets ↑ ⇒ inhibition of platelet aggregation
EF: inhibition of platelet aggregation
AE (anagrelide): headache, thrombocytopenia, orthostatic hypotension;
AE (aspirin): allergic reactions, gastric ulcers, skin reactions, dizziness, tinnitus, dysopias, nausea, bronchospasm, alkalosis, acidosis;
AE (clopidogrel): dyspepsia, abdominal pain, constipation, bleeding;
AE (dipyridamole): dizziness, headache, rash, abdominal distress, exacerbation of angina pectoris; **AE** (ticlopidine): agranulocytosis, pancytopenia, allergic skin reactions
CI: hypersensitivity to the drug;
CI (clopidogrel) active bleeding, significant liver impairment, cholestatic jaundice;
CI (aspirin): GI ulcers, hemorrhagic diathesis, great caution with children
CI (ticlopidine): hematopoetic or bleeding disorders, severe liver dysfunction, active bleeding; **CI** (dipyridamole): IV in shock

Acetylsalicylic acid (ASA)	EHL 4.7–9h, PRC D, Lact ?
Asaphen *Tab 80mg, 81mg* **Asaphen E.C.** *Ent. coated tab 80mg, 81mg* **Asatab** *Tab 80mg* **Aspirin** *Tab 80mg, 325mg, 500mg, Coated Tab 81mg, 325mg, 500mg Cap 325mg, 500mg, 650mg Coated Cap 325mg, 500mg, 650mg* **Bufferin** *Cap 325mg, 500mg* **Novasen** *Tab 325mg, 650mg* **Generics** *Tab 325mg*	**Ischemic stroke, TIA:** 80–325mg PO qd; **PRO of recurrent MI, unstable angina pectoris:** 80–325mg PO qd; **Acute MI:** ini 160mg chewed/crushed; **Analgesic/antipyretic:** 325–650mg PO q4h prn, **CH** <12y: 10–15mg/kg PO q6h, max 2.4g/d; **Anti-inflammatory:** 975mg PO q4–6h, **CH:** 60–125mg/kg/d div q4–6h

Anagrelide	EHL 76h, PRC C, Lact ?
Agrylin *Cap 0.5mg* **Generics** *Cap 0.5mg*	**Essential thrombocythemia:** ini 0.5mg PO qid or 1mg PO bid, after 7d incr dose prn, do not increase by more than 0.5mg/d in any 1wk, max 10mg/d or 2.5mg as single dose

Aspirin + Dipyridamole	PRC D, Lact ?
Aggrenox *Cap ext.rel 25mg + 200mg*	**Prevention of stroke/TIA:** 1 Cap PO bid

Clopidogrel	EHL 7-8h, PRC B, Lact ?
Plavix *Tab 75mg*	**PRO of recurrent stroke, MI, peripheral arterial disease:** 75mg PO qd; **ACS:** ini 300mg PO, then 75mg PO qd; DARF not req
Dipyridamole	EHL alpha: 40min, beta: 10h, PRC C, Lact ?
Apo-Dipyridamole FC *Tab 25mg, 50mg, 75mg* **Persantine** *Tab 25mg, 50mg, 75mg, Inj 5mg/ml* **Generics** *Inj 5mg/ml*	**Prevention of thromboembolism after cardiac valve replacement:** 100mg PO qid 1h before meals, max 600mg/d
Ticlopidine	EHL 12.6h, PRC B, Lact ?
Ticlid *Tab 250mg* **Generics** *Tab 250mg*	**Prevention of stroke:** 250mg PO bid

3.5 Antifibrinolytics

MA/EF (tranexamic acid): inhibition of plasminogen activation
AE (tranexamic acid): thromboembolic events, N/V, diarrhea, giddiness, hypotension;
CI (tranexamic acid): acquired defective color vision, subarachnoid hemorrhage, active intravascular clotting, SAH

Tranexamic acid	EHL 3h, PRC C, Lact +
Cyklokapron *Inj 100mg/ml, Tab 500mg* **Generics** *Inj 100mg/ml*	**Conization of cervix:** 2-3 tabs PO q8-12h, 12d postop; **Epistaxis**: 2-3 tabs PO q8-12h for 10d; **Hyphema**: 2-3 tabs PO q8-12h for 7d; **Menorrhagia**: 2-3 tabs PO tid-qid; **Hereditary angioneurotic edema**: 2-3 tabs PO bid-tid; **CH** 25mg/kg, bid-tid

3.6 Hematopoietic Drugs

MA/EF: darbepoetin/erythropoietin ↑ ⇒ production of red cells in bone marrow ↑
MA/EF: filgrastim is a granulocyte colony-stimulating factor (G-CSF) ⇒ activation of hematopoietic elements;
MA/EF (ancestrim): recombinant-methionyl human stem cell factor;
AE (darbepoetin, erythrop.): HTN, headache, arthralgias;
AE (filgrastim) bone pain, flu-like symptoms;
AE (ancestrim): injection site reaction, bone pain, rash, respiratory symptoms
CI: hypersensitivity to the drug; **CI** (darbepoetin, erythropoietin): uncontrolled HTN, children < 2; **CI** (erythropoietin): pure red cell aplasia;
CI (ancestrim, filgrastim): hypersensitivity to E. coli derived proteins, ancestrim
Note: not for immediate correction of anemia; Monitor, control BP in chronic RF, monitor hematocrit twice weekly in chronic RF, once weekly in HIV-infected and CA patients until stable. Consider iron deficiency if no response

Ancestrim	EHL 2–5h, PRC B, Lact ?
Stemgen *Inj 1875 mcg/vial*	**Mobilization of peripheral blood progenitor cells:** 20mcg/kg/d sc, use in combination with filgrastim.
Darbepoetin Alfa	EHL 21h (IV), 49h (SC), PRC C, Lact ?
Aranesp *Inj 10, 20, 30, 40, 50, 60, 80, 100, 150mcg/syringe*	**Anemia (CRF)**: ini 0.45 mcg/kg IV/SC q week; titrate to hematologic response; **anemia in chemotherapy patients**: ini 2.25 mcg/kg SC q week; titrate to hematologic response
Erythropoietin/epoetin alfa	EHL IV: 4–13h in CRF; SC: 27h, PRC C, Lact ?
Eprex *Prefilled Syr 1,000U, 2,000U, 3,000U, 4,000U, 5,000U, 8,000U, 10,000U, 40,000U, Inj 20,000 U/ml*	**Anemia (chronic RF):** ini 50–100 U/kg IV/SC 3x/wk, adjust dose to maintain target hematocrit (doses range 12.5–525U/kg 3x/wk) **anemia of zidovudine Tx:** 100 U/kg IV/SC 3x/wk x 8wk.; may be incr thereafter prn by 50–100 U/kg 3x/wk up to 300 U/kg 3x/wk; adjust dose based on AZT + hematocrit; **anemia in chemotherapy patients:** ini 150U/kg SC 3x/wk x 8wk, incr thereafter prn up to 300 U/kg 3x/wk DARF: see Prod Info

Filgrastim	EHL 2-7h, PRC C, Lact ?
Neupogen *Inj 300mcg/ml*	**Neutropenia - chemotherapy induced:** 5mcg/kg/d SC, incr prn in increments of 5mcg/kg/d for each cycle according to the duration and severity of the absolute neutrophil count (ANC) nadir; **CH** see Prod Info
Pegfilgrastim	EHL 15-80h, PCR C, Lact ?
Neulasta *Inj 6mg/syr*	**Neutropenia - chemotherapy induced:** 6mg SC per cycle of chemotherapy

3.7 Hemorheologics

MA/EF: blood viscosity↓, erythrocyte flexibility↑, microcirculatory flow↑, tissue O_2 concentrations↑; **AE:** GI disturbances, CNS depression, headaches; **CI:** hypersensitivity to pentoxifylline or xanthines, acute MI, severe CAD, PUD, bleeding diathesis

Pentoxifylline	EHL 0.4-1h, PRC C, Lact ?
Trental *Tab ext.rel 400mg* **Generics** *Tab ext.rel 400mg*	**Intermittent claudication:** ini 400mg PO bid-tid with meals

3.8 Other Hematologics

MA/EF, AE, CI (desmopressin): →119 ;
MA/EF (aprotinin): proteinase (trypsin, chymotrypsin, cathespin, plasmin, kallikrein) inhibitor;
MA/EF (dasatinib): inhibits BCR-ABL kinase, SRC family kinases (LYN, HCK), along with a number of other kinases including c-KIT, ephrin (EPH) receptor kinases, and PDGF-beta receptor;
MA/EF (drotrecogin alfa): recombinant activated protein C; inhibiting factors Va + VIIIa ⇒ antithrombotic effect; TNF-production ↓, leukocyte adhesion to selectins ↓, thrombin-induced inflammatory responses ↓ ⇒ antiinflammatory effect;
MA/EF (thrombin): clots fibrinogen of blood
MA/EF (imatinib): inhibits Philadelphia chromasome tyrosine kinase;
MA/EF (sorafenib, sunitinib): multikinase inhibitor;
AE (aprotinin): allergic reaction, renal failure;
AE (dasatinib): fluid retention, diarrhea, hemorrhage, pyrexia, headache, musculoskeletal pain, fatigue, rash, nausea, dyspnea;
AE (drotrecogin alfa): bleeding;
AE (thrombin): allergic reaction;
AE (imatinib): fluid retention, nausea, muscle cramps, diarrhea, rash, fatigue, congestive heart failure, hemmorhage;
AE (sorafenib): erythema, rash, alopecia, hand-foot syndrome, pruritus, diarrhea, fatigue, hypertension, nausea, vomiting, increased lipase, increased amylase, bleeding events, lymphopenia;
AE (sunitinib): fatigue, diarrhea, nausea, stomatitis, altered taste, skin abnormalities, hypertension, bleeding, alopecia
CI (aprotinin/thrombin): hypersensitivity to drug;
CI (drotrecogin alfa): active internal bleeding, hemor-rhagic stroke within the last 3mo, intracranial or intraspinal surgery or severe head trauma within the last 2mo, trauma with an increased risk of life-threatening bleeding, presence of an epidural catheter, intracranial neoplasm or mass lesion, or evidence of cerebral hernia-tion, known hypersensitivity,
CI (desmopressin): Type 2B vWD,
CI (factor IX): DIC, hyperfibrinolysis;
CI (imatinib): hypersensativity to drug
Note (factor VIII, IX): risk of HIV/hepatitis transmission varies by product; factor VIII: reduced response with development of factor VIII inhibitors, hemolysis with large/rep.ed doses in A, B, AB blood type; factor IX: products that contain factors II, VII, and X may cause thrombosis in at-risk patients, stop infusion if signs of DIC

Antihemophilic factor (factor VIII)	EHL 15.8h, PRC C, Lact ?
Advate *Inj 250IU/bottle, 500IU/bottle, 1,000IU/bottle, 1,500IU/bottle* **Hekixate FS** *Inj 250IU/bottle, 500IU/bottle, 1,000IU/bottle* **Kogenate FS** *Inj 250IU/bottle, 500IU/bottle, 1,000IU/bottle* **Recombinate** *Inj 250IU/bottle, 500IU/bottle, 1,000IU/bottle* **ReFacto** *Inj (moroctocog alfa) 250IU/vial, 500IU/vial, 1,000IU/vial*	**Hemophilia A:** individualize factor VIII dose; **CH:** individualize factor VIII dose
Eptacog alfa (activated factor VII)	EHL 2.3h, PRC C, Lact ?
NiaStase *Inj 1.2mg/vial, 2.4mg/vial, 4.8mg/vial*	**Hemorrhage in patients with hemophilia A or B with inhibitors to factor VIII or IX:** 70–90 mcg/kg IV q 2h until hemostasis
Aprotinin	EHL 0.7h, PRC B, Lact ?
Trasylol *Inj 10,000 KIU/ml*	**Hemorrhage due to hyperfibrinolysis:** ini 200,000 to 500,000KIU IV, up to 1,000,000 KIU/d to control bleeding
Dasatinib	EHL 5-6h, PRC C, Lact ?
Sprycel *Tab 20mg, 50mg, 70mg*	**Chronic, accelerated, or blast phase CML, Philadelphia chromosome positive (Ph+) ALL with resistance or intolerance to prior therapy:** ini 70mg PO bid, maint 90-100mg PO bid
Desmopressin	EHL IV 75.5min, PRC B, Lact ?
DDAVP *Tab 0.1, 0.2mg, Tab (dis) 60mcg, 120mcg, Spray (nasal) 10mcg/Spray, Inj 4mcg/ml* **DDAVP Rhinyle Nasal Solution** *Spray 100mcg/ml* **Minirin** *Tab 0.1mg, 0.2mg* **Octostim** *Spray (nasal) 150mcg/Spray Inj 15mcg/ml* **Generics** *Spray (nasal) 10mcg/Spray, ab 0.1mg, 0.2mg*	**Hemophilia A, Type 1 von Willebrand's disease:** 10mcg/m2 IV 20–30min, max 20mcg; **CH:** 0.3mcg/kg IV over 15–30min; **Diabetes insipidus:** 1–4mcg SC/IM/IV qd; 10v40mcg/d intranasal div qd–tid; 0.1mg PO tid, max 1.2mg/d; **Nocturnal enuresis:** 10–40mcg/d intranasal

Drotrecogin alfa	EHL no data, PRC C, Lact. ?
Xigris *Inj 5mg/vial, 20mg/vial*	**Severe sepsis**: 24mcg/kg/h IV for 96h; DARF: not req
Factor IX	EHL 12–17h, PRC B, Lact. ?
Immunine VH *Inj 160IU/vial, 240IU/vial, 480IU/vial, 720IU/vial, 960IU/vial, 1440IU/vial*	**Hemophilia B:** individualize factor IX dose, **CH:** individualize factor IX dose
Imatinib	EHL 18h, PRC D, Lact. +
Gleevec *Tab 100mg, 400mg*	**CML:** ini 400mg PO qd, incr. to 600mg PO qd to 400mg PO bid; **Gastrointestinal stromal tumor:** 600mg PO qd; Hepatic dosing: mild-mod. disease ini 400mg qd, severe disease 300mg qd; **CH:** ini 260–340mg/m^2/d PO div qd–bid, max 600mg/d
Gelatine, absorbable	EHL n/a,
Gelfoam *Powder 1g/envelope, Sponge 4cm^2, 12cm^2, 100 cm^2* **Gelfilm** *Film 12.5cm2*	**Hemostasis**: apply to bleeding site until bleeding stops
Phytonadione (Vitamin K)	EHL 26–193h, PRC C, Lact +
Generics *Inj 2mg, 10mg/ml*	**Hypoprothrombinemia:** 2.5–25mg PO/IM/SC; **Anticoagulant-induced hypoprothrombinemia:** 2.5–10mg PO/SC/IM; haemorrh. disease of the newborn: PRO: 0.5–1mg IM 1h after birth; Tx: 1mg SC/ IM
Sorafenib	EHL 25-48h, PRC C, Lact. ?
Nexavar *Tab 200mg*	**Advanced/metastatic Renal Cell (clear cell) Carcinoma:** 400mg PO bid
Sunitinib malate	EHL 80-110h, PRC C, Lact. ?
Sutent *Cap 12.5mg, 25mg, 50mg*	**Gastrointestinal stromal tumour, Metastatic Renal Cell (clear cell) Carcinoma:** 25-50mg PO qd

4 Respiratory

4.1 Bronchodilators

4.1.1 Systemic Beta Adrenergic Agonists

MA/EF: (orciprenaline) nonselective beta-adrenergic agonists
MA/EF: stimulation of beta-2 receptors ⇒ relaxation of bronchial smooth muscles, mucociliar clearance ↑
AE: N/V, nervousness, tremors, dizziness, drowsiness, anxiety, headache, tachyarrhythmias, extrasystoles, hypertension, angina pectoris, N/V
CI: hypertrophic obstructive cardiomyopathy, cardiac arrhythmias; hypersensitivity to the drug

Orciprenaline	EHL 3–6 h, PRC C, Lact ?
Orcipren *Syrup 10mg/5ml* **Generics** *Syrup 10mg/5ml*	**Asthma/COPD:** Syrup 20mg PO tid or qid; **CH** 4–12yrs: 10mg PO tid, >12yrs. 20g PO tid

Salbutamol	EHL 4h, PRC C, Lact ?
Apo-Salvent *Tab 2mg, 4mg* **Ventolin** *Inj 500mcg/ml, 1,000mcg/ml* *Oral soln 0.4mg/ml* **Ventolin Rotacaps** *Cap 200mcg, 400mcg* **Generics** *Tab 2mg, 4mg*	**Asthma/COPD:** 2–4mg PO tid–qid, max 16mg PO/d, IV: 5mcg/min, incr to 10mcg/min, max 20mcg/min, IM: 500mcg (8mcg/kg) q4h, max 20mg/d; **CH asthma** 2–6 y: 0.1mg/kg PO tid–qid, 6–12 y: 2mg PO tid–qid, max 8mg/d

4.1.2 Inhaled Alpha-Beta Adrenergic Agonists

MA/EF: stimulation of alpha- and beta-adrenergic receptors ⇒ relaxation of bronchial smooth muscles, mucosal vasoconstriction

Epinephrine racemic	EHL 4h, PRC C, Lact ?
Vaponefrin *Sol (inhal) 2.25%*	**Bronchospasm**: 0.5ml nebulized q3–4h; **Croup, CH** <4 y: 0.05ml/kg nebulized q2–4h, max 0.5ml/dose q1–2h

4.1.3 Inhaled Beta Adrenergic Agonists

MA/EF: selective stimulation of β_2-receptors ⇒ bronchial muscles relax, mucociliar clearance ↑; **MA/EF:** (orciprenaline) nonselective beta-agonist;
MA/EF: see Systemic Beta Adrenergic Agonists →83;
AE: nervousness, dizziness, dry mouth/throat, tachycardia, tremors, headache, N/V;
AE: nervousness/tremors, tachycardia, coughing, nausea, headache;
CI: hypersensitivity to the drugs, hypertrophic obsructive cardiomyopathy, cardiac arrhythmias; **CI** (formoterol): lactose allergy, **CI** (salmeterol): hypersensitivity to lecithin, soya, lactose; **CI:** hypersensitivity to the drug
Note: salmeterol: long-acting β_2-sympathomimetic, not for Tx of acute asthmatic reaction

Fenoterol	EHL 2–3h, PRC C, Lact ?
Berotec Inhalation Aerosol *MDI 100mcg/dose* **Berotec Inhalation Solution** *Sol (inhal) 1mg/ml, 0.625mg/ml, 0.25mg/ml*	**Asthma/COPD:** 1–2 puffs tid or qid, max 8 puffs/d; 0.5–1mg neb q6h
Formoterol	EHL 12h, PRC C, Lact -
Foradil *Cap 12mcg* **Oxeze Turbuhaler** *MDI 6mcg/dose, 12mcg/dose*	**Asthma/COPD:** 6–12mcg bid, max 48mcg/d
Terbutaline	EHL 11–26h, PRC B, Lact +
Bricanyl Turbuhaler *MDI 0.5mg/dose*	**Asthma/COPD:** 1 puff prn, max 6 puffs/d
Salbutamol	EHL 4h, PRC C, Lact ?
Airomir *MDI 120mcg/dose* **Apo-Salvent** *Resp. soln 5mg/ml, MDI 100mcg/dose, Sterules 1mg/ml, 2mg/ml, Tab 2mg, 4mg* **Ventolin** *Sol (inhal) 1.25mg/2.5 ml, 2.5mg/2.5ml, 5mg/2.5ml, 5mg/ml* **Ventolin Diskus** *Inhal 200mcg/blister* **Ventolin HFA** *MDI 100mcg/dose* **Generics** *MDI 100mcg/dose* *Sol (inhal) 5mg/ml, 0.5mg/ml, 1mg/ml, 2mg/ml*	**Asthma:** MDI: 1–2 puffs q4–6h, max 12 puffs/d; Sol (inhal): 2.5mg diluted in 3ml NS tid–qid; Cap inhal.: 200–400mcg q4–6h via Rotahaler; **PRO of exercise-induced asthma:** 180mcg (2 inhal) by MDI 15min prior to exercise; **CH asthma** MDI >4 y: 1–2 puffs q4–6h; Sol (inhal): 0.1mg/kg diluted in 3ml NS, max 2.5mg tid–qid; Cap inhal.: > 4 y: 200–400mcg q4–6h via Rotahaler
Salmeterol	EHL 5.5h, PRC C, Lact ?
Serevent *Diskhaler disks 50mcg/dose, MDI 25mcg/dose, Diskus 50mcg/dose*	**Asthma/COPD:** 50mcg inhal bid

4.1.4 Alpha-Beta-Adrenergic Agonists

MA/EF: stimulation of alpha- and beta-adrenergic receptors ⇒ bronchodilation; vasoconstriction, cardiac output ↑ ⇒ BP ↑
AE (ephedrine): CNS stimulation, HTN, palpitations, tremor, N/V
AE (epinephrine): HTN, N/V, headache, arrhythmias
CI: (ephedrine): hypersensitivity to ephedrine, angle closure glaucoma, anesthesia with cyclopropane or halothane, thyrotoxicosis, DM, HTN (in pregnancy), other CVS DO
CI (epinephrine): cardiac dilatation/coronary insufficiency, narrow angle glaucoma, hypersensitivity to epinephrine, shock, intra-arterial injection, labor

Ephedrine	EHL 3–6h, PRC C, Lact ?
Generics *Tab 8mg, 15mg, 30mg, Inj 50mg/ml*	**Asthma:** 25–50mg q3–4h or 25–50mg SC or 5–25mg/dose slow IV, max 150mg/d
Epinephrine	PRC C, Lact ?
Adrenalin *Inj 1mg/ml, Topical 1mg/ml* **Epipen** *Inj (IM) 0.3mg/delivery* **Epipen Jr.** *Inj (IM) 0.15mg/delivery* **Generics** *Inj 0.1mg/ml, 1mg/ml*	**Asthma:** 0.2–0.5ml of 1:1,000 Sol (0.2–0.5mg) SC q2h prn, rep q20min for a max of 3 doses. MDI: inhalation of 0.1% to 1% Sol prn

4.1.5 Inhaled Anticholinergics

MA/EF: anticholinergic ⇒ bronchodilating
AE: dry mouth, bitter taste, epistaxis, nasal dryness/congestion
CI: hypersensitivity to the drug, soya lecithin, soybean, peanut

Ipratropium	EHL no data, PRC B, Lact ?
Apo-Ipravent *Sol (inhal) 250mcg/ml, Spray (Nasal) 0.03%, 0.06%* **Atrovent** *MDI 20mcg/puff, Sol (inhal) 250mcg/ml, 125mcg/ml* **Novo-Ipramide** *Sol (inhal) 250mcg/ml* **Generics** *Sol (inhal) 125mcg/ml, 250mcg/ml*	**COPD, bronchospasms:** MDI: 40mcg inhal tid-qid, max 240mcg/d; Sol (inhal): 250–500mcg nebulized q4–6h prn, **CH** 5–12y: 125–250mcg inh q4–6h prn
Tiotropium	EHL 5–7d, PRC B, Lact ?
Spiriva *Cap 18mcg*	**COPD:** 18mcg inhal qd

4.1.6 Xanthines/Theophyllines

MMA: inhibition of intracellular phosphodiesterase ⇒ cAMP ↑
EF: bronchial spasmolysis, central stimulation of respiration, positive inotropic and chronotropic, vasodilation (except for brain vessels), diuresis ↑
AE: N/V, tremors, convulsions, nervousness, gastroesophageal reflux, chest pain, tachycardia, palpitations, hypotension, rapid breathing, headache
CI: symptomatic coronary artery disease, PUD,
CI: (oxtriphylline): untreated seizure disorder

Aminophylline (85% theophylline)	EHL no data, PRC C, Lact ?
Phyllocontin *Tab sust. rel. 225mg, 350mg* **Generics** *Sol (oral) 25mg/ml, 50mg/ml*	**Bronchospasm, asthma:** ini 6mg/kg IV over 20–30min., maint 0.5–0.7mg/kg/h IV inf; 16mg/kg/d PO div q6–8h, max 400mg/d
Oxtriphylline (64% theophylline)	PRC C, Lact +, serum level: 10–20 mcg/ml
Choledyl *Sol (oral) 100mg/5ml* **Generics** *Tab 100mg, 200mg, 300mg*	**Bronchospasm, asthma, COPD:** ini 200–400mg/d div q6–8h, maint 800–1200mg/d; **CH** 10–14 yrs.: ini 22mg/kg/d div q6h x 24h, maint 15–22mg/kg/d div q6h
Theophylline	PRC C, Lact +, serum level: 10–20 mcg/ml
Apo-Theo LA *Tab 100mg, 200mg, 300mg* **Novo-Theophyl SR** *Tab 100mg, 200mg, 300mg* **Theolair** *Sol (oral) 80mg/ 15ml, Tab 125mg* **Uniphyl** *Tab ext. rel. 400mg, 600mg* **Generics** *Elixir (oral) 80mg/15ml, Inj 0.8mg/ml, 1.6mg/ml, 4mg/ml*	**Asthma:** acute: ini 5mg/kg IV over 20–30min then maint 0.6mg/kg/h IV; 16mg/kg/d PO in div tid–qid; adjust dose based on serum level, max 400mg/d; DARF not req

4.2 Inhaled Corticosteroids

EF: suppression of inflammatory reactions ⇒ β_2-receptor sensitivity ↑
AE: hoarseness, oral and pharyngeal candidosis
CI: lung tuberculosis, fungal or bacterial respiratory tract infections, treatment of status asthmaticus,
CI (fluticasone): lactose allergy

Beclomethasone	EHL 3h, PRC C, Lact ?
QVar *MDI 50mcg/puff, 100mcg/puff* **Generics** *MDI 50mcg/puff*	**Asthma:** 50–400mcg inhal bid

Budesonide	EHL 2–3h, PRC C, Lact ?
Pulmicort Turbuhaler *Powder (inhal) 100mcg/inhal., 200mcg/inhal. , 400mcg/inhal., Nebuamp 0.125mg/ml, 0.25mg/ml, 0.5mg/ml*	**Asthma:** 200–400mcg inhal bid, max 2400mcg/d; 1–2mg neb bid; **CH** 6–12 y: 100–200mcg inhal bid; 0.25–0.5mg neb bid
Ciclesonide	EHL 5–6h, PRC C, Lact ?
Alvesco *Sol. (inhal) 100mcg/inhal., 200mcg/ inhal.*	**Asthma:** ini 400mcg inhal qd, maint. 100–800mcg inhal div qd–bid; CH: not recommended
Fluticasone	EHL 7.8h, PRC C, Lact ?
Flovent *MDI 50, 125, 250mcg/puff, Diskus (inhal) 50, 100, 250, 500mcg/inhal.*	**Asthma maint:** MDI/Diskus: 100–500mcg bid, max 1,000mcg bid; **CH** 4–16 y: 50–100mcg bid, max 200mcg bid

4.3 Asthma/COPD Combinations

Budesonide + Formoterol	
Symbicort Turbuinhaler *MDI 100+6mcg/inhal, 200+6mcg/inhal*	**Asthma, COPD:** 100+6mcg–200+6mcg q12h
Fluticasone + Salmeterol	
Advair Diskus *Powder (inhal) 0.1+0.05mg/inhal., 0.25+0.05mg/inhal., 0.5+0.05mg/ inhal.*	**Asthma:** maint inhalation of 0.1–0.5 + 0.05mg q12h
Ipratropium Bromide + Fenoterol	
Duovent UDV *Sol (inhal) 0.125mcg + 0.3125mg / ml*	**Asthma, COPD:** 4ml q6h prn
Ipratropium Bromide + Salbutamol	
Apo-Salvent Ipravent Sterules *Sol (inhal) 0.5 + 3mg/2.5ml* **Combivent** *MDI 0.020 + 0.120mg/puff, Sol (inhal) 0.5 + 3mg/2.5ml* **Gen-Combo Sterinebs** *Sol (inhal) 0.5 + 2.5mg/2.5ml* **ratio-Ipra Sal UDV** *Sol (inhal) 0.5 + 3mg/ 2.5ml*	**COPD:** 2 puffs (MDI) or 1 neb qid; max 12 puffs/d

4.4 Leukotriene Inhibitors

MA: blockage of leukotriene receptors
EF: bronchial dilatation, decrease of bronchial hyperreactivity
AE: headache, fever, diarrhea, nausea, sinusitis

Montelukast	EHL 2.7–5h, PRC B, Lact -
Singulair *Tab 10mg, Tab (chew) 4mg, 5mg, Granules 4mg/packet*	**Asthma:** 10mg PO qhs; **CH** 2–5 y: 4mg PO qhs; 6–14 y: 5mg PO qhs **Seasonal allergies:** 10mg PO qhs
Zafirlukast	EHL 10h, PRC B, Lact -
Accolate *Tab 20mg*	**Asthma:** 20mg PO bid (1h ac or 2h pc)

4.5 Mucolytics, Expectorants

MA/EF (acetyl cysteine): splits disulfide bridges in protein part of mucus molecules ⇒ sputum viscosity ↓
AE (acetyl cysteine): allergic skin reactions, nausea, heartburn
AE (guaifenesin): dizziness, headache, N/V, rash, urticaria
CI (acetyl cysteine): restricted use in children < 1
CI (guaifenesin): hypersensitivity to guaifenesin products

Acetylcysteine	EHL 11min–2.27h, PRC B, Lact ?
Mucomyst *Sol (inhal) 20%* **Parvolex** *Sol (inhal) 200mg/ml* **Generics** *Inj 200mg/ml*	**Mucolytic:** nebulization of 1–10ml (20%) or 2–20ml (10%) q2–6h prn; intratracheal instillation: 1–2ml ET (10–20%) prn up to qh
Guaifenesin	EHL 1h, PRC C, Lact ?
Balminil Expectorant *Syrup 100mg/5ml* **Benylin E Extra Strength** *Syrup 200mg/5ml* **Robitussin** *Syrup 100mg/5ml*	**Expectorant:** 100–400mg PO q4h or 600–1200mg PO q12h (ext.rel), max 2.4g/d; **CH** >12y: adult dose, 6–11y: 100–200mg PO q4h or 600mg PO q12h (ext.rel), max 1.2g/d, 2–5y: 50–100mg PO q4h or 300mg PO q12h (ext.rel), max 600mg/d

4.6 Mast Cell Stabilizers

MA/EF: stabilization of mast cell membranes ⇒ mediator release ↓
AE: bad taste, nausea, ocular burning, nasal congestion, cough
CI: hypersensitivity to the drug

Cromolyn Sodium	EHL 80–90min, PRC B, Lact ?
Nalcrom *Cap 100mg* **Generics** *Sol (inhal) 1%*	**Asthma:** MDI: ini 2mg inhal. qid, maint 2mg q4–6h; Spinecaps: 20mg inhal qid
Ketotifen	EHL 3–5h, PRC C, Lact +
Zaditen *Syrup 1mg/5ml, Tab 1mg* **Generics** *Syrup 1mg/5ml, Tab 1mg*	**Asthma: CH** >3y: 1mg PO bid, 6m–3y 0.05mg/kg bid
Nedocromil	EHL 1.5–3.3h, PRC B, Lact ?
Tilade *MDI 2mg/puff*	**Asthma:** 2 puffs qid, reduce dose after improvement; **CH** > 6y: 2 puffs qid, reduce dose after improvement

4.7 Antitussives - Single Ingredient Drugs

MA/EF (dextromethorphan): acts on cough center in medulla oblongata ⇒ threshold for coughing ↑
AE (dextromethorphan): restlessness, hallucination, GI symptoms and skin reactions
AE (chlophedianol): excitation, hyperirritability, nightmares,
AE (hydrocodone): respiratory depression, HTN, sedation, nausea, vomiting
CI (dextromethorphan): advanced respiratory insufficiency, use of MAO inhibitors
CI (codeine): hypersensativity, acute asthma/COPD, resiratory depression, cor pulmonale, acute alcoholism, delerium tremens, severe CNS depression, use of MAO inhibitors, increased ICP, convuslion disorder, **CI** (hydrocodone): intracranial lesion, increased ICP

Codeine phosphate	EHL 2.5–3.5h, PRC C, Lact +
Linctus codeine *Liq (oral) 0.2%* **Generics** *Syrup 5mg/ml, Tab 15mg, 30mg*	**Cough**: 10–20mg PO/ SC q4–6h prn; **CH** > 2y: 0.5–1mg/kg/dose PO/SC/IM q4–6h, 2–6y: 1mg/kg/d PO div qid, max 30mg/ 24h; 6–12y: 5–10mg PO q4–6h prn; max 60mg/24h; DARF: GFR (ml/min) > 50: 100%, 10–50: 75%, <10: 50%

Hydrocodone	EHL 3.8h, PRC C, Lact ?
Hycodan *Syrup 5mg/5ml, Tab 5mg*	**Cough**: 5mg po q4h prn, max 30mg/d, **CH** 2–12y 2.5mg po q4h prnmax 15mg/d, <2y 1.25mg po q4h prn, max 7.5mg/d
Chlophedianol	PRC C, Lact ?
Ulone *Syrup 25mg/5ml*	**Cough**: 25mg po 3–4x/d, **CH** 6–12y 12.5–25mg 3–4x/d, 2–6y 12.5mg po 3–4x/d
Dextromethorphan	EHL 1.5–4h, PRC C, Lact +
Balminil DM *Syrup 15mg/ml* **Benylin DM** *Syrup 15mg/5ml* **Koffex DM** *Syrup 15mg/5ml* **Triaminic Softchew Cough** *Tab (chew) 7.5mg*	**Cough**: 10–20mg po q4h or 30mg po q6–8h prn, max 120mg/d

4.8 Antitussives - Combinations

Ammonium chloride + Codeine + Diphenhydramine	
Balminil Codeine Night-Time + Expectorant *Syrup 125 + 3.3 + 12.5mg/5ml*	**Cough**: 5–10ml PO q6–8h PRN; **CH** 6–12y: 2.5–5ml PO q6–8h PRN; max 4 doses/d
Acetaminophen + Diphenhydramine + Pseudoephedrine	
Benadryl Allergy/Sinus/Headache *Cap 500 + 12.5 + 30mg* **Benadryl Total Allergy Regular Strength** *Cap 500 + 12.5 + 30mg* **Benadryl Total Allergy Extra Strength** *Cap 500 + 25 + 30mg*	**Cough**: 2 cap PO q6h, max 8/d, **CH** <12y: not rec
Acetaminophen + Dextromethorphan + Pseudoephedrine	
Triaminic Cough & Sore Throat *Syrup 160 + 7.5 + 15mg/5ml* **Triaminic Softchew Throat Pain & Cough** *Tab (chew) 160 + 5 + 15mg*	**Cough**: (Robitussin) 15ml PO q6–8h PRN; **CH** (Triaminic) 6–12y: 2 tabs or 10ml PO q6h PRN, 2–6y: 1 tab or 5ml PO q6h PRN; max 4 doses/d
Acetaminophen + Chlorpheniramine + Dextromethorphan + Pseudoephedrine	
Triaminic Cold, Cough & Fever *Syrup 160 + 1 + 7.5 + 15mg/5ml*	**Cough**: **CH** 6–12y: 10ml PO q6h PRN, max 4 doses/d

Chlorpheniramine + Dextromethorphan + Pseudoephedrine	
Triaminic Cold & Cough *Syrup 1 + 5 + 15mg/5ml* **Triaminic Cold & Night Time Cough** *Syrup 1 + 7.5 + 15mg/5ml* **Triaminic Softchews Cold & Cough** *Tab (chew) 1 + 5 + 15mg*	**Cough**: **CH** 6–12y: 2 tabs or 10ml PO q6h PRN, max 4 doses/d
Dextromethorphan + Pseudoephedrine	
Triaminic Cough *Syrup 7.5 + 15mg/5ml* **Triaminic Cough & Congestion** *Syrup 7.5 + 15mg/5ml*	**Cough**: (Robitussin) 15ml PO q6–8h PRN, **CH** 6–12y: 7.5ml PO q6–8h PRN, 2–6y: 3.75ml PO q6–8h PRN; (Triaminic) **CH** 6–12y: 10ml PO q6h PRN, 2–6y: 5ml PO q6h PRN; max 4 doses/d
Guaifenesin + Acetaminophen + Dextromethorphan + Pseudoephedrine	
Balminil Cough & Flu *Syr 100 + 325 + 15 + 30mg/15ml* **Benylin 1 Cold and Flu** *Cap 100 + 500 + 15 + 30* **Sudafed cold & flu** *Cap 100 + 250 + 10 + 30mg*	**Cough/nasal congestion:** 2 caps PO q4h prn, max 8/d
Guaifenesin + Bismuth	
Bismutal *Rectal supp 250 + 150mg*	**Sore throat:** 1 supp prn
Guaifenesin + Brompheniramine + Codeine + Phenylephrine + Phenylpropanolamine	
Dimetane expectorant-C *Syrup 100 + 2 + 10 + 5 + 5mg /5ml* **Dimetane expectorant-DC** *Syrup 100 + 2 + hydrocodone 1.8mg + 5 +5mg /5ml*	**Cough:** 5–10ml PO q6h prn; **CH** 6–12y: 2.5–5ml PO q6–8h prn
Guaifenesin + Codeine + Pheniramine	
Robitussin AC *Syrup 100 + 10 + 7.5mg / 5ml*	**Cough:** 5–10ml PO q4–6h prn; **CH** 6–12y: 2.5–5ml PO q4–6h prn

Guaifenesin + Codeine + Pseudoephedrine	
Balminil Codeine + Decongestant + Expectorant *Syrup 100 + 3.3 + 30mg/5ml* **Benylin codeine Syrup** *100 + 3.3 + 30mg/5ml* **Calmylin with codeine** *Syrup 100 + 3.3 + 30mg /5ml*	**Cough:** 10ml PO q4h prn, max 40ml/d
Guaifenesin + Codeine + Pseudoephedrine + Triprolidine	
CoActifed expectorant *Syrup 100 + 10 + 30 + 2mg /5ml* **ratio-Cotridin expectorant** *Syrup 100 + 10 + 30 + 2mg /5ml*	**Cough:** 10ml PO q4-6h prn, max 40ml/d
Guaifenesin + Dextromethorphan	
Balminil DM + expectorant *Syrup 200 + 15mg /5ml* **Benylin DM-E** *Syrup 100 + 15mg /5ml* **Koffex DM + expectorant** *Syrup 200 + 15mg /5ml* **Robitussin DM** *Syrup 100 + 15mg /5ml*	**Cough:** 10ml PO q4h prn, max 60ml/d or 1-2 Tab PO q12h, max 4 Tab/d, 1-2 cap PO q6h PRN; **CH** >12y: adult dose, 6-11y: 5ml PO q4h, max 30ml/d or 1 Tab PO q12h, max 2 Tab/d, 2-5y: 2.5ml PO q4h, max 15ml/d or ½ Tab PO q12h, max 1 Tab/d
Guaifenesin + Dextromethorphan + Pseudoephedrine	
Balminil DM + decongestant + expectorant *Syrup 200 + 15 + 30mg /5ml* **Benylin DM-D-E** *Syrup 200 + 15 + 30mg /5ml* **Koffex DM + decongestant + expectorant** *Syrup 200 + 15 + 30mg /5ml* **Robitussin cough & cold** *Cap 200 + 10 + 30mg*	**Cough:** 10ml PO q6h prn, max 40ml/d
Guaifenesin + Mepryramine + Potassium iodide + Theophylline	
ratio-Theo-bronc *Syrup 50 + 6 + 80 + 35mg /5ml*	**Bronchospasm:** 10ml PO qid prn; **CH** >6y: 2.5-5ml PO tid prn

Guaifenesin + Oxtriphylline	
Choledyl expectorant *Syrup 50 + 100mg / 5ml*	**Bronchospasm:** 10ml PO qid prn
Guaifenesin + Phenylpropanolamine	
Entex LA *Tab 600 + 75mg*	**Nasal congestion:** 1 tab PO bid prn; **CH** 6–12y: half tab PO bid prn
Chlorpheniramine + Pseudoephedrine	
Triaminic Cold and Allergy *Syrup 1mg + 15mg/5ml* **Triaminic Softchews Cold and Allergy** *Tab (chew) 1mg + 15mg*	**Nasal congestion: CH** 6–12: 10ml or 2 tab PO q4–6h PRN, max 4 doses/d
Pseudoephedrine + Ibuprofen	
Sudafed Sinus Advance *Cap 30mg + 200mg*	**Sinus congestion:** 1–2 cap PO q4h PRN, max 6 doses/d
Codeine + Pseudoephedrine + Triprolidine	
CovanSyrup *10mg + 30mg + 2mg/5ml* **Ratio-Cotridin** *Syrup 10mg + 30mg + 2mg/5ml*	**Cough:** 10ml PO q6h prn, max 40ml/d

4.9 Other Respiratory Drugs

MA/EF: cholinergic (parasympathomimetic) analogue of acetylcholine ⇒ stimulation of muscarinic, parasympathetic receptors ⇒ smooth-muscle contraction of airways, tracheobronchial secretions ↑
AE: cough, dyspnea, throat irritation, headache, lightheadedness
CI: hypersensitivity to methacholine

Methacholine	EHL no data, PRC C, Lact -
Provocholine *Sol (inhal) 100mg/vial, 160mg/vial, 320mg/vial, 1280mg/vial*	**Diagnosis of bronchial airway hyperreactivity:** inhalation of incr serial conc (0.025mg/ml–25mg/ml)

5 Gastroenterology

5.1 Antiulcer Drugs

5.1.1 H_2 Antagonists

MA: competitive antagonism at H_2-receptor on parietal cells
EF: inhibition of basal and histamine-stimulated acid secretion
AE: exanthema, headache, dizziness, confusion, agranulocytosis, gynecomastia, cholestasis, transaminases ↑
CI: hypersensativity to drug

Cimetidine	EHL 2h, PRC B, Lact +
Novo-Cimetine *Tab 200mg, 300mg, 400mg, 600mg, 800mg* **Nu-Cimet** *Tab 200mg, 300mg, 400mg, 600mg* **Peptol** *Tab 200mg, 400mg, 800mg* **Generics** *Tab 200mg, 300mg, 400mg, 600mg, 800mg, Sol (oral) 300mg/ 5ml*	**Active ulcers:** 800–1200mg/d div qd–bid, x 4–6wk; **ulcer (maint):** 400mg qhs or 300mg PO bid; **GERD:** 1200mg/d PO x 8–12wk; **hypersecretory conditions:** 300mg PO qid, max 2400 mg/d; **NSAID lesion:** 800mg/d div qd–bid, **PRO NSAID:** 400mg PO qd, DARF: GFR (ml/min) >50: 100%, 10–50: 75%, <10: 50%
Famotidine	EHL 2.59–4h, PRC B, Lact ?
Pepcid *Tab 20mg, 40mg, Inj 10mg/ml* **Pepcid AC** *Tab 10mg, Tab (chew) 10mg* **Generics** *Tab 10mg, 20mg, 40mg, Inj 10mg/ml*	**Active ulcers:** 20mg bid PO/IV or 40mg PO qhs x 4–8wk; **ulcer (maint):** 20mg PO/IV qhs; **GERD:** 20 PO bid; **esophagitis (due to GERD):** 20–40mg PO bid x 12wk; **hypersecretory conditions:** 20mg PO q6h, max 800mg/d; **PRO GERD:** 10mg PO 10–15min before meals, max 20mg/d; DARF: CrCl (ml/min) <50: 50% dose or q36–48h
Nizatidine	EHL 1–2.8h, PRC B, Lact -
Axid *Cap 150mg, 300mg* **Generics** *Cap 150mg, 300mg*	**Active ulcers:** 300mg PO qhs or 150mg PO bid x 8wk; **ulcer (maint):** 150mg PO qhs; GERD: 150mg PO bid x 12wk; **heartburn PRO:** prn 75mg PO 1h ac, max 150mg/d; DARF: GFR (ml/min), 20–50: 150mg qd, <20: 150mg qod

Ranitidine	EHL 2–2.5h, PRC B, Lact +
Novo-Ranidine *Tab 150mg, 300mg, Oral (sol) 168mg/10ml* **Nu-Ranit** *Tab 150mg, 300mg* **Zantac** *Tab 75mg, 150mg, 300mg, Syr 75mg/5ml, Inj 25mg/ml* **Generics** *Tab 75mg, 150mg, 300mg*	**Active ulcers:** 150mg PO bid or 300mg qhs or 50mg IV/ IM q6–8h or 6.25mg/h as continuous IV inf, max 400mg/d; **ulcer (maint):** 150mg PO qhs; GERD: 150mg PO bid; **hypersecretory conditions:** 150mg PO bid, max 6g/d; **Zollinger-Ellison syndrome:** ini 100mg IV (bolus), then ini 0.5mg/kg/h continuous IV inf, prn incr by 0.5 mg/kg/h, max 4mg/kg/h or 9,000mg/24h; **esophagitis (erosive, active):** 150mg PO qid; **esophagitis (erosive, maint):** 150mg PO bid; DARF: GFR (ml/min) <50: 150mg PO qd or 50mg IV q18–24h

5.1.2 Proton Pump Inhibitors

MA/EF: blockage of H^+/K^+-ATPase ⇒ greatest suppression of acid production
AE: dizziness, headache, diarrhea, constipation, flatulence, exanthema, liver enz. ↑

Esomeprazole	EHL 1.5h, PRC B, Lact ?
Nexium *Tab del. rel. 20mg, 40mg*	**GERD:** 20mg PO qd x 2–4wk; **Reflux esophagitis:** 40mg PO qd x 4–8wk, maint 20mg PO qd

Lansoprazole	EHL 0.9–1.5h, PRC B, Lact ?
PrevAcid *Cap del.rel. 15mg, 30mg*	**Gastric, duodenal ulcers:** 15mg PO ac qam x 2–4wk; **Erosive esophagitis (active):** 30mg PO qam x 4–8wk; **erosive esophagitis (maint):** 15mg PO ac qam; **Zollinger-Ellison syndrome:** 60mg PO ac qam, >120mg/d div bid, max 90mg ac bid; DARF: not req, **Liver impairment:** max 30mg/d

Omeprazole	EHL 0.5–1.5h, PRC C, Lact ?
Losec *Tab del. rel. 10mg, 20mg, 40mg* **Losec MUPS** *Tab del. rel. 10mg, 20mg* **Generics** *Tab 20mg, 40mg*	**GERD:** 20mg PO qd x 4–8–12wk; **active duodenal ulcers:** 20mg PO qd x 4–8wk; maint 20mg PO qd; **gastric ulcers:** 20mg PO ac qam x 4–8wk; **ulcer PRO:** 20mg PO/NG qd; **erosive esophagitis:** 20mg PO qd, maint 10mg PO qd; **hypersecretory conditions, Zollinger-Ellison syndrome:** 60mg PO qd, >80mg div prn, max 120mg PO tid; ini prn 60mg IV q8h; DARF: not req

Pantoprazole	EHL 1h, PRC B, Lact ?
Pantoloc *Tab ent.coat. 20mg, 40mg* **Panto IV** *Inj 40mg/vial* **Generics** *Inj 40mg/vial*	**Duodenal/gastric ulcer:** 40mg PO/IV ac qam x 4–8wk, max 80mg/d; **GERD/reflux esophagitis:** 40mg PO/IV ac qam x 4–6wk, maint 20–40mg PO qd; **PRO NSAID:** 20mg PO qam; **Hypersecretion:** 80mg IV bid; **Acute upper GI bleed:** 80mg IV x1, then 8mg/h x 72h; DARF: max 40mg/d

Rabeprozole	EHL 0.85–2h, PRC B, Lact ?
Pariet *Tab 10mg, 20mg*	**GERD/reflux esophagitis**: 20mg PO qd x for 4–8 weeks; maint 10–20mg PO qd; **gastric/duodenal ulcer**: 20 mg PO qd x 4–6 weeks; **Hypersecretory conditions**: 60 mg PO qd

5.1.3 Helicobacter pylori Treatment

Amoxicillin + Clarithromycin + Lansoprazole	PRC C , Lact ?
Hp-PAC *contains* *Prevacid, Cap 30mg (lansoprazole),* *Amoxicillin, Cap 500mg,* *Biaxin, Tab 500mg (clarithromycin)*	**Duodenal ulcers associated with H.p.:** Prevacid 1 Cap, Amoxicillin 1,000mg, Clarithromycin 500mg PO bid x 7d

Amoxicillin + Clarithromycin + Omeprazole	PRC C , Lact ?
Losec 1-2-3 A *Cap 1,000mg + 500mg + 20mg*	**Duodenal ulcers associated with H.p.:** Amoxicillin 1,000mg, Clarithromycin 500mg, Omeprazole 20mg PO bid x 7d

Amoxicillin + Clarithromycin + Esomeprazole	PRC C , Lact ?
Nexium 1-2-3 A *Amoxicillin, Cap 1,000mg,* *Clarithromycin, Tab 500mg* *Nexium, Tab. ext. rel. 20mg (esomeprazole)*	**Duodenal ulcers associated with H.p.:** Amoxicillin 1,000mg, Clarithromycin 500mg, Nexium 1 tab PO bid x 7d

Metronidazole + Clarithromycin + Omeprazole	PRC C , Lact ?
Losec 1-2-3 M *Cap 500mg + 250mg + 20mg*	**Duodenal ulcers associated with H.p.:** Metronidazole 500mg, Clarithromycin 250mg, Omeprazole 20mg PO bid x 7d

5.1.4 Other Antiulcer Drugs

MA/EF (misoprostol): prostaglandin E_1 analog ⇒ prostaglandin-mediated inhibition of acid secretion, activation of bicarbonate and mucus secretion; **MA/EF** (sucralfate): forming of an adherent, protective protein complex at ulcer site; **AE** (misoprostol): diarrhea, dizziness, headache, metrorrhagia; **AE** (sucralfate): constipation, raise of aluminum level in renal insufficiency; **CI** (misoprostol): children, epilepsy, women of childbearing potential have to use adequate contraception, infectious intestinal illnesses
CI (sucralfate): hypersensitivity to sucralfate

Misoprostol	EHL rapid, metabol. 20–40min, PRC X, Lact -
Generics *Tab 0.1mg, 0.2mg*	**NSAID-ind. gastric ulcers (PRO), peptic ulcers (Tx):** 200 mcg PO qid; if not tolerated: 100 mcg PO qid; DARF: not req

Sucralfate	PRC B, Lact +
Novo-Sucralate *Tab 1g* **Sulcrate** *Tab 1g, Susp 1g/5ml* **Generics** *Tab 1g*	**Duodenal ulcers:** 1g PO qid (1h ac and hs) x 6-8wk; ulcer (maint): 1g PO bid; DARF: risk of aluminium accumulation in chronic RF
see Propantheline →108	

5.2 Antacids

MA/EF: neutralization of stomach acid
AE (aluminium): constipation, ileus, phosphate deficiency;
AE (magnesium): diarrhea; **AE** (calcium): kidney stones, hypercalcemia, constipation
CI: hypersensitivity to antacids

Aluminium Hydroxide	PRC B, Lact ?
Amphojel *Tab 600mg, Sol (oral) 320mg/5ml*	**GERD, mild heartburn:** 500–1800mg PO tid–6 times/d between meals and hs; DARF: req in severe RF
Aluminium Hydroxide + Alginic acid	
Gaviscon Heartburn Relief *Susp (oral) 100mg+250mg/5ml*	**GERD, mild heartburn:** 10–20ml or 2–4 Tab PO qid, max 80ml or 16 tablets/d
Aluminium + Magnesium Hydroxide	PRC B, Lact ?
Diovol *Tab 184mg+100mg, Cap 200mg + 200mg, Susp (oral) 165mg+200mg/5ml, 494mg+300mg/5ml* **Gelusil** *Tab 153mg+200mg, 306mg+ 400mg, Susp (oral) 153mg+200mg/5ml* **Maalox** *Tab (chew) 600mg+300mg* **Mylanta DS Plain** *Susp (oral) 306mg+400mg/5ml*	**GERD, mild heartburn:** 10–20ml or 1–4 Tab PO qid; DARF: req in severe RF
Aluminium + Magnesium Hydroxide + Oxethazine	
Mucaine *Susp (oral) 300mg+100mg+ 10mg/5ml*	**GERD, mild heartburn:** 5–10ml PO qid
Aluminium + Magnesium Hydroxide + Simethicone	
Diovol Plus *Tab 184mg+100mg+25mg* **Maalox with Anti-Gas** *Susp(oral) 200mg+200mg+20mg/5ml, 400mg+400mg+40mg/5ml* **Mylanta Regular Strength** *Tab 153mg+200mg+20mg, Susp(oral) 153mg+200mg+20mg/5ml* **Mylanta DS** *Tab 306mg+400mg+30mg* **Mylanta Extra Strength** *Susp (oral) 497mg+350mg+30mg/5ml*	**GERD, mild heartburn:** 5–20ml or 2–4 Tab PO qid

ASA + Sodium Bicarbonate + Citric Acid	
Alka Seltzer *Tab 325mg + 1916mg + 1,000mg*	**Heartburn**: adults and **CH**>12y: 2 tabs PO q4h PRN, max 8 tabs/d; age>60 max 4 tabs/d
Calcium Carbonate	PRC B, Lact ?
Maalox *Tab (chew) 600mg, 1,000mg* **Tums** *Tab (chew) 500mg, 750mg, 1g*	**GERD, mild heartburn:** 0.5–1.5g PO prn, max 8g/d
Calcium Carbonate + Magnesium Carbonate + Sodium Alginate	
Maalox HRF *Susp (oral) 300mg+125mg+275mg/5ml*	**GERD, mild heartburn:** 5–10ml PO qid
Calcium Carbonate + Simethicone	PRC B, Lact ?
Maalox Quick Dissolve with Antigas *Tab (quick dissolve) 1,000mg+60mg*	**GERD, mild heartburn:** 1–2 Tab PO qid
Magnesium Carbonate + Alginic acid	PRC B, Lact ?
Gaviscon Heartburn Relief (aluminium free) *Tab 40mg+200mg, 63mg+313mg*	**GERD, mild heartburn:** 2–4 Tab PO qid

5.3 Laxatives

MA/EF (bisacodyl,castor oil, glycerin, picosulfate, senna): stimulant laxatives, increase intestinal motility and secretion
MA/EF (docusate mineral oil): detergent and stool softener
MA/EF (lactulose, magnesium citrate/hydroxide/oxide, polyethylene glycol, sodium phosphates): poorly absorbed, osmotic effect
MA/EF (methylcellulose, psyllium: stool bulking agent
AE: electrolyte loss (especially K^+)
AE (senna): melanosis coli
CI: ileus, gastroenteritis, acute surgical abdomen, appendicitis, intestinal obstruction, severe dehydration
CI (oral or rectal phosphates): renalfailure

Bisacodyl	PRC B, Lact ?
Carters Little Pills *Tab 5mg* **Dulcolax** *Tab 5mg, Supp 5mg,10mg, Microenema 10mg/5ml* **Gentlax** *Tab 5mg* **Generics** *Tab 5mg, Supp 10mg*	**Constipation, colonic evacuation:** 10–15mg PO hs prn, 10mg PR prn, max 30mg/d; **CH** <2 y: 5mg PR prn, max 5mg/d; **CH** 2–12 y: 5–10mg PR prn, max 10mg/d

Bisacodyl + Magnesium Citrate	
Royvac *Kit: Tab 5mg, Supp 10mg (Bisacodyl) + Soln 17.46g/bottle (Mg Citrate)*	**Constipation, bowel evacuation:** Day before colonic procedure: 1 bottle oral Sol po at 12:30 pm, then 1 Supp PR at 10:00 PM
Castor Oil	PRC N, Lact ?
Generics *Liquid (oral) 100%*	**Constipation:** 15ml PO prn on empty stomach; colonic evacuation: 15–30ml PO prn on empty stomach; **CH** < 2 y: 1–2ml, max 5ml PO; **CH** 2–11 y: 5–15ml PO
Docusate Calcium	PRC C, Lact ?
Generics *Cap 240mg*	**Constipation:** 240mg PO prn
Docusate + Sennosides	
Senokot-S *Tab 50mg + 8.6mg*	**Constipation:** 2–4 Tab PO qhs, max 4 Tab bid
Docusate Sodium	PRC C, Lact ?
Colace *Liquid (oral) 10mg/ml, Cap 100mg, Syr 20mg/5ml* **Selax** *Cap 100mg, Syr 20mg/5ml* **Soflax** *Cap 100mg, 200mg* **Generics** *Cap 100mg, Liquid (oral)10mg/ml, Syr 4mg/ml, 50mg/ml*	**Constipation:** 50–400mg/d PO qd–qid; **CH** <3 y: 10–40mg/d PO prn, **CH** 3–6 y: 20–60mg/d PO prn, **CH** 6–12 y: 40–150mg/d PO prn, **CH** >12 y: 50–200mg/d PO prn
Glycerin	PRC C, Lact ?
Generics *Supp 1.8g, 2.65g (90% glycerin)*	**Constipation:** 1 supp (2.65g) pr; **CH** >2y 1 supp (1.8g) pr qd
Glycerin + Natrium Citrate + Natrium Lauryl Sulfoacetate + Sorbic Acid + Sorbitol	PRC C, Lact ?
Microlax *Enema 5ml/tube*	**Constipation:** 1 tube pr
Lactulose	PRC B, Lact ?
Duphalac *Sol (oral) 10g/packet* **Laxilose** *Sol (oral) 667mg/ml* **Generics** *Sol (oral) 667mg/ml*	**Constipation:** 30–45ml PO qd–qid prn; infants: 2.5–10ml/d PO div tid–qid, **CH** adolescents: 40–90ml/d PO div tid–qid; **hepatic encephalopathy** (PRO/Tx): 30–45ml/dose PO q1h until effect, then 30–45ml PO tid–qid or 300ml PR with 700ml water, rep q4–6h prn

Magnesium Citrate	PRC B, Lact +
Citrodan *Sol (oral) 15g/bottle* **Citro-Mag** *Sol (oral) 15g/bottle*	**Bowel evacuation:** 150–300ml PO qd; **CH** 6–12y: 0.5ml/kg PO q4–6h
Magnesium Hydroxide	PRC N, Lact +
Phillips' Milk of Magnesia *Tab (chew) 300mg, Liquid (oral) 80mg/ml* **Generics** *Tab (chew) 311mg, Liquid 375mg/5ml, 400mg/5ml, 800mg/5ml, 2400mg/10ml*	**Laxative:** 15–40 ml PO qd or 6–8 Tab PO/d prn; **CH** <2 y: 0.5 ml/kg PO qd, 2–5 y: 5–15 ml/d PO qd or 1–2 Tab PO/d prn, 6–11 y: 15–30 ml PO qd, 3–4 Tab PO/d prn; DARF: req in severe RF
Methylcellulose	PRC N, Lact ?
Entrocel *Sol (oral) 1.8%*	**Laxative:** 1 tablespoon in 8 oz cold water PO qd–tid; **CH** 6–12 y: 50% of adult dose
Mineral Oil	PRC C, Lact ?
Fleet Enema Mineral Oil *Sol (rectal) 130ml/dose* **LansoÿL** *Liq (oral) 75% mineral oil* **LansoÿL sugar free** *Liq (oral) 75% mineral oil*	**Laxative:** 15–45ml PO or 120ml PR; **CH** 5–11 y: 5–15ml PO, **CH** 2–11 y: 30–60ml PR
Picosulfate + Magnesium Oxide + Citric Acid	PRC C, Lact ?
Picodan *Powder for Sol (oral) 10 mg + 3.5 g + 12 g/sachet* **Pico-Salax** *Powder for Sol (oral) 10 mg + 3.5 g + 12 g/sachet*	**Bowel preparation:** 1 sachet PO before 8 am and 1 sachet PO between 2 - 4 pm on the day before the procedure, drink with 250ml water q hour; **CH** 1-6 y: 1/4 sachet morning, 1/4 sachet afternoon; **CH** 6-12 y: 1/2 sachet morning, 1/2 sachet afternoon
Polyethylene Glycol with Electrolytes	PRC C, Lact ?
Colyte *Powder for Sol (oral) polyethylene glycol 240g/4L* **Klean-Prep** *Powder for Sol (oral) polyethylene glycol 236g/4L* **Peglyte** *Powder for Sol (oral) polyethylene glycol 238.18g/4L*	**Bowel preparation:** 250ml PO q 10min
Psyllium Hydrophilic Mucilloid	
Metamucil *Powder 0.3g, 0.5g, 0.6g /g*	**Constipation:** 1 tsp (3.4g psyllium) PO qd to tid; **CH** 6–12 y: 1/2 tsp PO tid prn; **Elevated serum cholesterol:** 1 tsp (3.4g) PO tid

Senna	EHL 4.0–12.1h, PRC C, Lact +
Senokot *Tab 8.6mg, Syr 1.7mg/ml, Gran 15mg/tsp., Supp 30mg* **X-prep** *Liq. 119mg/70ml, Powder 157.5mg/pouch* **Generics** *Tab 8.6mg, 12mg*	**Laxative or bowel preparation:** 1 tsp gran (15mg) in water or 10–15ml or 2 Tab (8.5mg) PO or 1 supp PR hs; max 4 tsp of gran or 30ml syrup or 8 Tab (34–50mg PO bid) or 2 supp/d; **CH** 6–12 y: 1 Tab or 1/2 tsp PO bid, 2–6 y: 1/2 Tab or 1/4 tsp PO qd

Sodium Phosphate	EHL 20h, PRC N, Lact ?
Fleet Enema *Enema 130ml/dose* **Fleet Phospho-Soda** *Sol (oral) monobasicsodium phosphate 2.4 g + dibasicsodium phosphate 0.9 g/5ml* **Phoslax** *Sol(oral) 3.3g/5ml* **Phosphates Solution** *Sol(oral) 3.3g/5ml*	**Laxative:** 1 adult enema (118ml) PR prn or 20–45ml oral sol PO prn; **CH** 2–11 y: 1 pediatric enema (59ml) PR prn or 5–9 y: 5–10ml oral sol PO prn, 10–11 y: 10–20ml oral sol PO prn; DARF: contraind.

5.4 Antidiarrheals

MA/EF (attapulgite): swelling agent ⇒ inhibition of peristalsis; **MA/EF** (bismuth subsalicylate): direct binding of bacteria toxines ⇒ antimicrobial, antisecretory
MA/EF (loperamide, diphenoxylate): stimulation of peripheral opium rec. ⇒ peristalsis↓
AE (loperamide): headache, tiredness, dizziness, dry mouth, nausea
CI (bismuth): hypersensitivity to salicylates, varicella/influenza infection in children
CI (loperamide): ileus, children <2 y, acute dysentry, acute ulcerative colitis or pseudomembranous colitis

Atropine + Diphenoxylate	EHL 2.5h (D.), 4h (A.), PRC C, Lact ?
Lomotil *Tab 0.025mg + 2.5mg,*	**Diarrhea:** 15–20mg PO div tid–qid; **CH** >2 y: 0.3–0.4mg/kg/d div bid–qid

Attapulgite	PRC N, Lact ?
Kaopectate *Tab 600mg, 750mg, Liquid (oral) 600mg/15ml, 750mg/15ml*	**Diarrhea:** 1.200–1.300mg PO; max 9,000mg/d; **CH** 3–6 y: 300mg/dose PO, max 2.250 mg/d, 6–12 y: 600–750 mg/ dose PO; max 4.500mg/d

Bismuth Subsalicylate	EHL 21–72d, PRC D, Lact -
Pepto-Bismol *Tab (chew) 262mg, Liquid (oral) 262mg/15ml, 525mg/ 15ml, 525mg/oz, 1050mg/oz* **Generics** *Tab 262mg, Tab (chew) 262mg, Liquid (oral) 262mg/ 15ml, 130mg/15ml*	**Diarrhea:** 2 Tab or 30 ml PO q 30–60min max 8 doses/d; **CH** 3–6 y: 1/3 Tab or 5ml q30–60min prn, 6–9 y: 2/3 Tab or 10ml q30–60min prn, 9–12 y: 1 Tab or 15ml q30–60min prn

Loperamide	EHL 7–15h, PRC B, Lact +
Diarr-Eze *Cap 2mg, Sol (oral) 0.2mg/ml* **Imodium** *Tab (quick dissolve) 2mg,Cap 2mg* **Loperacap** *Tab 2mg* **Generics** *Tab 2mg, Cap 2mg,Sol (oral) 0.2mg/ml*	**Diarrhea:** 4mg PO ini, then 2mg after each loose stool, max 16mg/d; **CH** 2–5 y: 1mg tid, 6–8 y: 2mg bid, 8–12 y: 2mg tid
Loperamide + Simethicone	EHL 7–15h, PRC B, Lact +
Imodium Advanced *Tab (chew) 2mg+125mg*	**Diarrhea:** 2 Tab PO ini, then 1 Tab after each loose stool, max 4 Tab/d; **CH** 6–11 y: 1 Tab PO ini, then 1/2 Tab after each loose stool, max 3 Tab/d (9–11y), max 2 Tab/d (6–8y)

5.5 Antiemetics

5.5.1 Antiemetics - 5-HT3 Receptor Antagonists

MA/EF: selective blockage of central 5-HT_3-receptors ⇒ antiemetic
AE: headache, constipation, tiredness; **CI:** children

Dolasetron	EHL <10min, PRC B, Lact ?
Anzemet *Tab 50mg, 100mg, Inj 20mg/ml*	**N/V with chemo:** 1.8mg/kg or 100mg IV 30min before chemo or 100mg PO 60min before chemo; **CH** 2–16 y: 1.8mg/kg, max 100mg IV/PO; **postop N/V:** 12.5mg IV, 100mg PO 2h prior to surgery; **CH** 2–16 y: 0.35mg/kg IV, max 12.5mg or 1.2mg/kg PO, max 100mg 2h prior to surgery;DARF:notreq
Granisetron	EHL 10–11h, PRC B, Lact ?
Kytril *Tab 1mg, Inj 1mg/ml*	**N/V with chemo:** 10mcg/kg IV 30min before chemo or 1mg PO 1h before and 12h after chemo; **CH** 2–16 y: 10mcg/kg IV 30min before chemo; **postop N/V:** 1–3mg IV; DARF: not req
Ondansetron	EHL 3h, PRC B, Lact ?
Zofran *Tab 4mg, 8mg, Tab (orally disint) 4mg, 8mg, Sol (oral) 4mg/5ml, Inj 2mg/ml* **Generics** *Tab 4mg, 8mg, Inj 2mg/ml*	**N/V with chemo:** 8mg IV, rep in 8h or 8mg PO 30min before chemo, rep in 8h; **CH** >4 y: 0.15mg/kg IV, rep in 4h and 8h after first dose, 4–11 y: 4mg PO, rep in 4h and 8h after first dose; **N/V with radiation:** 8mg PO tid; **postop N/V:** 4mg IV;

5.5.2 Antiemetics - Anticholinergics

MA/EF: antimuscarinic ⇒ antiemetic;
AE: tachycardia, dizziness, hallucinations, dry mouth, constipation, blurred vision;
CI: angle closure glaucoma, hypersensitivity to scopolamine, tachycardia secondary cardiac insufficiency or thyrotoxicosis, prostatic hypertophy, pyloric obsruction, paralytic ileus

Scopolamine	PRC C, Lact +
Transderm-V *Film (ext.rel, TD) 1mg/72h* **Generics** *Inj 0.4mg/ml, 0.6mg/ml*	**Motion sickness, postop vomiting:** 0.6–1mg PO/SC, 1 patch behind ear q3d; **pre-med:** 1mg IM/IV/SC 1–4h prior to anesthesia or 0.4–0.6mg IM/IV/SC 45–60min prior to anesthesia

5.5.3 Antiemetics - Antihistamines

MA/EF: inhibition of histamine receptors ⇒ antiemetic (see antihistamines →251, →288, →289)
AE (dimenhydrinate): sedation, drowsiness, thickening of bronchial secretions, blurred vision, glaucoma, dry mouth/nose/throat, appetite loss, difficult urination;
AE (promethazine): drowsiness, dizziness, nervousness, blurred vision, difficult painful urination, dry mouth/nose/throat, hypotension, tachycardia;
CI (dimenhydrinate): prostate hypertrophy, glaucoma, chronic lung disease;
CI (promethazine): coma, urinary retention, glaucoma

Dimenhydrinate	PRC B, Lact +
Gravol *Tab 15mg, 25mg, 50mg, Tab (chew) 15mg, 50mg, Liquid (oral) 15mg/5ml, Supp 25mg, 50mg, 100mg, Cap 25mg, 50mg, Inj 50mg/ml* **Generics** *Tab 50mg, Supp 50mg, 100mg, Inj 10mg/ml, 50mg/ml*	**PRO of motion sickness:** 50–100mg PO 30min prior to travel, q4–6h; **nausea:** 50–100 mg/dose PO/IM/IV q4–6h; DARF: not req
Promethazine	EHL 7–15h, PRC C, Lact ?
Generics *Inj 25mg/ml*	**Nausea, motion sickness:** 12.5–25mg PO/IM/PR q4–6h prn; DARF: not req

5.5.4 Other Antiemetics

MA/EF (metoclopramide, prochlorperazine): inhibition of dopamine receptors ⇒ antiemetic; **MA/EF** (aprepitant): antagonist at human substance P neurokinin 1 (NK1) receptor; **AE** (dronabinol/nabilone): drowsiness, dizziness, impairment of sensory perception; **AE** (metoclopramide): dizziness, drowsiness, tiredness, headache, prolactin ↑, breast tenderness, gynecomastia, dry mouth, diarrhea, constipation; dyskinesias (children), Parkinsonism; **AE** (prochlorperazine): extrapyramidal effects, drowsiness, blurred vision, orthostatic hypotension, fainting, dry mouth/nose, constipation; **CI** (chlorpromazine/ perphenazine): severe CNS depression, blood dyscrasias, severe liver disease; **CI** (dronabinol/nabilone): hypersensativity to marijuana, sesame oil, psychotic disorder; **CI** (metoclopramide): pheochromocytoma, GI hemorrhage, obstruction or perforation, epilepsy, mental illness, Parkinson's disease; known hypersensitivity to the drug, combination with MAO inhibitors, caution with children <14, and RF; **CI** (prochlorperazine): coma, stupor, severe cardiovascular disease; after a large amount of depressants (including alcohol); hypersensitivity to the drug; **CI** (aprepitant): hypersensitive to this drug, use with pimozide, terfenadine, astemizole, or cisapride

Aprepitant	EHL 9-13h, PRC B, Lact ?
Emend *Cap 80mg, 125mg*	**Nausea prevention (chemo-induced):** 125 mg PO 1 h prior to chemother. treatment (Day 1) and 80 mg qam on Days 2 and 3; must be administered with other anti-emetic agents
Chlorpromazine	EHL 6h, PRC C, Lact ?
Generics *Inj 25mg/ml*	**Nausea:** 30–100mg PO qd, div dose; 25–50mg IV/IM 3–4x/d; 100–300mg PR qd
Doxylamine + Pyridoxine	
Diclectin *Tab del. rel. 10mg + 10mg*	**Nausea of pregnancy:** 2 Tab PO qhs and 1 Tab PO bid PRN
Dronabinol	EHL 19–36h, PRC C, Lact ?
Marinol *Cap 2.5mg, 5mg, 10mg*	**Postop nausea:** 5–15mg/m2 PO q3–6h; **chemo-induced nausea:** 5mg/m2 PO 1–3 h prior to chemo, then 5mg/m2/ dose q2–4h after chemo for 4–6 doses/d; DARF: not req
Droperidol	PRC C
Generic *Inj 2.5mg/ml*	**Nausea:** 2.5–5 mg IV
Metoclopramide	EHL 2.5–5h, PRC B, Lact ?
Apo-Metoclop *Tab 5mg, 10mg* **Generics** *Tab 5mg, 10mg, Inj 5mg/ml*	**GERD:** 10–15mg PO qid; **postop nausea:** 10mg IV/PO; **chemo-induced nausea:** 1–2mg/kg/dose IV q2–4h; DARF: GFR (ml/ min) >50: 100%, 10–50: 75%, <10: 50%

Nabilone	EHL 2h, PRC C, Lact -
Cesamet *Cap 1mg*	**Nausea:** 1–2mg PO bid
Perphenazine	PRC C, Lact ?
Trilafon *Inj 5mg/ml* **Generic** *Tab 2mg, 4mg, 8mg, 16mg*	**Nausea:** 5–10mg IV
Trifluoperazine	
Generic *Tab 1mg, 2mg, 5mg, 10mg, 20mg*	**Nausea:** 2–5 mg PO
Prochlorperazine	EHL 6.8–9h, PRC C, Lact -
Nu-Prochlor *Tab 5mg, 10mg* **Stemetil** *Inj 5mg/ml, Liq 5mg/5ml, Supp 10mg, Tab 5mg, 10mg* **Generics** *Tab 5mg, 10mg*	**Nausea:** 5–10mg PO/IM tid/qid, max 40 mg/d or 25mg PR bid or 5–10mg IM q3–4h prn

5.6 Anti-Inflammatory Drugs, Bowel

MA: influence on prostaglandin biosynthesis, inhibition of leukotriene synthesis
EF: locally anti-inflammatory; **AE:** headache, dizziness, nausea, agranulocytosis, pancytop., allerg. reactt., renal functi. impairment; **CI:** gastric/duodenal ulcer, intest. obstruct., hypersens. to salicylates, hemmorhagic diathesis, **CH** < 2y; **CI** (sulfasalazine): porphyria

Mesalamine/5-ASA	EHL 0.6–1.4h, PRC B, Lact ?
Asacol *Tab ent. coat. 400mg, 800mg* **Mesasal** *Tab 500mg* **Mezavant** *Tab (MMX) 1.2g* **Novo-5-ASA** *Tab 400mg* **Pentasa** *Tab del. rel. 500mg, Enema 1g, 4g, Supp 1g* **Salofalk** *Enema 2g, 4g, Supp 250mg, 500mg, Tab 500mg, 1,000mg*	**Ulcerative colitis:** ini 800–3200mg/d PO div, maint 1600mg/d PO div, max 4800mg/d or 1.5-3g/d div; Enema: 1–4g PR qhs; (Pentasa) Supp. 1g pr qhs, (Salofalk) 1g PO tid–qid, 500mg PR bid–tid or 1g PR qd; (Mezavant): induction of remission mild-mod UC: 2.4-4.8 g PO qd; **Crohn's disease**: Tab ext. rel. 1g PO qid, maint 750mg PO qid, (Salofalk) 3g/d PO div
Olsalazine	EHL 0.9h, PRC C , Lact ?
Dipentum *Cap 250mg*	**Ulcerative colitis:** 500 mg PO qid, max 3g/d, maint 500mg po bid
Sulfasalazine	EHL 7.6h , PRC B , Lact ?
Salazopyrin *Tab 500mg, Tab ent. coat. 500mg* **Generics** *Tab 500mg, Tab ent. coat. 500mg*	**IBD:** 1–2g PO tid–qid, **CH** (25–35kg): 500mg PO tid, (35–50kg): 1g PO bid–tid; **PRO UC:** 1g PO bid–tid, **CH** (25–35kg): 500mg PO bid, (35–50kg): 500mg PO bid–tid

5.7 GI Enzymes

MA/EF (pancrelipase): mixture of amylase, trypsin, and lipase
AE (pancrelipase): skin rash, hypersensitivity, nausea/diarrhea with large doses, hyperuricemia, hyperuricosuria
CI (pancreatic enzymes): hypersensitivity to pork protein

Lactase Enzyme	PRC N, Lact ?
Dairyaid *Tab 3,000 FCC, Cap 4,500 FCC* **Dairy Free** *Tab 3,000 FCC, Tab 4,500 FCC* **Lactaid** *Tab (original strength) 3,000 FCC U of enzyme, Tab (extra strength) 4,500 FCC U of enzyme, Cap (ultra) 9,000 FCC U of enzyme, Cap (ultra, chew) 9,000 FCC U of enzyme, Gtt lactase* **Lactrase** *Cap 250mg*	**Lactose intolerance:** 3 Cap PO (original strength), 2 Cap PO (extra strength), 1 Cap PO (ultra), swallow Cap with first bite of dairy foods or 5–7 Gtt, max 15gtt PO/liter of milk
Pancrealipase (lipase+protease+amylase)	PRC C, Lact ?
Cotazym *Cap 8,000U+3,0000U+30,000U* **Cotazym 65B** *Cap 8,000U+30,000U + 30,000U + 65mg conj. bile salts* **Creon 5, Creon 10, Creon 20, Crean 25** *Cap 5,000U+18,750U+16,600U, 10,000U+37,500U+33,200U, 20,000U+75,000U+66,400U, 25,000U+62,500U+74,000U* **ECS 4, ECS 8, ECS 20** *Cap 4000U +11,000U +11,000U, 8,000U +30,000U +30,000U, 20,000U+55,000U+55,000U* **Pancrease** *Cap 4,500U+25,000U+20,000U* **Pancrease MT** *Cap 4,000U +12,000U +12,000U, 10,000U+30,000U+30,000U, 16,000U+48,000U+48,000U* **Ultrase** *Cap 4,500U+25,000U+20,000U* **Ultrase MT12, MT20** *Cap 12,000U +39,000U+39,000U, 20,000U +65,000U +65,000U* **Viokase** *Powder 16,800U+70,000U +70,000U/ 1/4 tsp* **Viokase-8,-16** *Tab 8,000U+30,000U +30,000U, 16,000U+60,000U+60,000U*	**Pancreatic enzyme deficiency:** 1–4 Tab/Cap PO with each meal, 1 Tab/Cap with snacks; (Creon): **CH** 6–12mo: 2,000 U lipase, 1–6y: 4,000–8,000 U lipase, 7–12y: 4,000–12,000 U lipase (always with meals, feedings)

5.8 Gallstone Dissolving Drugs

MA/EF: inhibition of biliary cholesterol secretion and intestinal cholesterol resorption; inhibition of HMG-CoA-reductase ⇒ cholesterol synthesis ↓⇒ dissolving of cholesterol stones
AE: diarrhea, transaminases↑
CI: infx of the gall bladder and ducts, common bile duct or cystic duct occlusion, disturbed contractility of the gall bladder, calcified gall stones

Ursodiol	PRC B, Lact ?
Urso *Tab 250mg, 500mg* **Generics** *Tab 250mg, 500mg*	**Cholestatic liver disease, PBC:** 13–15mg/kg/d PO div bid-qid

5.9 Antispasmodics (Parasympatholytics)

MA/EF (dicyclomine): antimuscarinic ⇒ antispasmodic, smooth muscle relaxation
MA/EF (hyoscyamine): competitive inhibition of muscarinic acetylcholine receptors ⇒ antisecretory (exocrine glands, intestinal mucosa), smooth muscle relax, vagolytic effects
MA/EF (propantheline): anticholinergic, antispasmodic, bladder capacity↑, urinary frequency↓, gastric acid secretion↓
AE (dicyclomine, hyoscyamine): urinary retention, constipation, blurred vision, dry mouth, tachycardia, dizziness, headache, nausea
AE (propantheline). urinary retention, constipation, blurred vision, dry mouth, tachycardia, dizziness, headache, sexual dysfunction
CI (dicyclomine, hyoscyamine): obstructive uropathy, GI obstruction, ulcerative colitis, glaucoma, children (<6m dicyclomine, <2 y hyoscyamine), reflux esophagitis, myasthenia gravis, megacolon
CI (hyoscine): myasthenia gravis, megacolon, glaucoma, obsructive prostatic hypertrophy
CI (hyoscyamine): hepatic, renal, or pulmonary insufficiency, intestinal atony in elderly or debilitated patients, myasthenia gravis, cardiospasm, unstable CVS status
CI (propantheline): hypersensitivity to anticholinergic drugs, myasthenia gravis, narrow-angle glaucoma, obstructive GI disease, paralytic ileus, reflux esophagitis, ulcerative colitis, obstructive uropathy, unstable CVS status in acute hemorrhage

Dicyclomine	EHL 1.8h, PRC B, Lact ?
Bentylol *Tab 20mg, Tap 10mg, Syr 10mg/5ml, Inj 10mg/ml* **Formulex** *Cap 10mg* **Lomine** *Cap 10mg*	**Functional bowel syndrome:** ini 10–20mg PO tid-qid, max 160mg/d, 20mg IM qid (max 2d); **CH** 6 mo–2 y: 5–10mg PO 15min ac tid-qid, max 40mg/d, 2–12 y: 10mg/d PO tid-qid

Hyoscine	EHL 2-3min, PRC C, Lact ?
Buscopan *Tab 10mg, Inj 20mg/ml* **Generics** *Inj 20mg/ml*	**GI hypermotility, functional bowel syndr.:** 10-20mg/d, max 60mg/d, 10-20 IV/SC/IM, max 100mg/d
Hyoscyamine	EHL 3.5h, PRC C, Lact -
Levsin *Tab 0.125mg*	**GI hypermotility, functional bowel syndr.:** 0.125-0.25mg PO/SL q4h or prn, max 1.5mg/d or 0.375-0.75mg PO q12h, max 1.5mg/d (ext. rel); **CH** 2-12 y: 0.0625-0.125mg q4h prn or 0.375mg (ext. rel) PO q12h, max 0.75mg/24h, >12 y: adult dose
Propantheline	EHL (biphasic) 57.9min, 2.93h, PRC C, Lact ?
Pro-Banthine *Tab 7.5mg, 15mg*	**GI antispasmodic, peptic ulcer:** 15mg tid 30min ac, 30mg qhs; UT

5.10 Antiflatulents

MA/EF: altering surface tension of gas bubbles, antifoaming
AE: mild diarrhea, regurgitation

Simethicone	PRC B, Lact ?
Ovol *Drops 40mg/ml, Cap 180mg, Tab 80mg, 160mg* **Phazyme** *Softgel 95mg, 125mg, 180mg*	**GI discomfort due to gas:** 180mg PO pc or qhs, 80-160mg PO qid or 180mg PO bid, max 540mg/d; **CH** <12 y: 10-20mg PO tid

5.11 Other GI Drugs

MA/EF (clinidium): anticholinergic, bladder capacity↑, urinary frequency↓, gastric acid secretion↓, antispasmodic
MA/EF (chlordiazepoxide): see Benzodiazepines →249
MA/EF (domperidone): peripheral dopamine antagonist, increases gastric motility
MA/AF (infliximab): IgG monoclonal Ab against TNF-alpha
MA/EF (pinaverium): calcium channel antagonist
MA/EF (octreotide): similar to somatostatin ⇒ secretory inhibition of some anterior pituitary hormones (growth hormone), suppression of pancreatic endocrine and exocrine function, inhibition of gastric acid and GI hormone secretion, suppression of serotonin secretion, inhibition of GI motility and splanchnic blood flow
MA (adalimumab): human antibody, binds TNF-alpha
MA (tegaserod): serotonin type 4 (5-HT4) receptor partial agonist
MA (vasopressin): stimulation of smooth muscle receptors ⇒ vasoconstriction
AE (adalimumab): serious infections, neurologic events, malignancies, injection site reactions, dyspnea, urticaria, headache, infusion reaction;
AE (domperidone): dry mouth, headache, abdominal cramps, diarrhea
AE (infliximab): dyspnea, urticaria, headache, infusion reaction
AE (octreotide): N/V, diarrhea, stomachache, hepatitis
AE (tegaserod): diarrhea, headache
AE (vasopressin): tremor, sweating, vertigo, N/V, metabolic acidosis, cardiac arrhythmias
CI (adalimumab): hypersensitivity to adalimumab, severe infections
CI (budesonide): systemic infection, actuve TB
CI (domperidone): mechanical obstruction
CI (clinidium): hypersensitivity to anticholinergic drugs, Myasthenia gravis, narrow-angle glaucoma, obstructive GI disease, paralytic ileus, reflux esophagitis, ulcerative colitis, obstructive uropathy, unstable CVS status in acute hemorrhage
CI (infliximab): severe infections, Class III/IV CHF, hypersensativity to murine proteins
CI (vasopressin): chronic nephritis with nitrogen retention, use with caution in epilepsy, migraine, asthma, heart failure, vascular diseases

Adalimumab — EHL 14d, PRC B, Lact ?

Humira *Inj 40mg/0.8ml*	**Moderately to severely active Crohn's disease:** ini 160 mg SC at week 0 (4 inj x 1day or 2 inj/d x 2days), then 80 mg SC at week 2, maint 40 mg SC every other week beginning at week 4

Azathioprine	EHL 3h, PRC D, Lact -
Imuran *Tab 50mg, Inj 100mg/20ml* **Generics** *Tab 50mg*	**Crohn's disease, Ulcerative colitis:** ini 50mg PO qd, maint 100-250mg PO qd, max 2.5mg/kg/d; DARF: GFR (ml/min) >50: 100%, 10–50: 75%, <10: 50%
Budesonide	
Entocort *Cap 3mg, Enema 2mg*	**Crohn's disease:** 9mg PO qd for upto 8wk, maint 6mg PO qam; **Distal UC**: 2mg enema qhs for upto 8wk; DARF: not req
Clinidium + Chlordiazepoxide	PRC D, Lact -
Apo-Chlorax *Cap 2.5mg + 5mg* **Librax** *Cap 2.5mg+5mg*	**Irritable bowel syndrome:** 1 Cap PO tid–qid, DARF: 50% in severe RF
Diltiazem	EHL 3–6.6h, PRC C, Lact -
Generics *Crm 2%*	**Chronic anal fissure:** 2% cream PR bid
Domperidone	PRC B, Lact +
Generics *Tab 10mg*	**Diabetic gastroparesis:** 10mg PO tid–qid, max 20mg PO qid
Erythromycin Base	PRC B, Lact ?
Apo-Erythro Base *Tab 250mg* **Apo-Erythro E-C** *Cap 250mg, 333mg* **Erybid** *Tab ext. rel. 500mg* **Eryc** *Cap ext.rel. 250mg, 333mg* **PCE** *Tab 333mg*	**GI prokinetic:** ini 3mg/kg IV over 60min, maint. 20mg/kg/d PO div tid–qid
Erythromycin Lactobionate	EHL no data, PRC B, Lact +
Generics *Inj 500mg/vial, 1g/vial*	**GI prokinetic:** ini 3mg/kg IV over 60min, maint. 20mg/kg/d PO div tid–qid
Hydrocortisone	EHL 9.5d, PRC B, Lact ?
Cortenema *Enema 100mg*	**IBD:** 100mg pr qd
Infliximab	EHL 9.5d, PRC B, Lact ?
Remicade *Inj 100mg/vial*	**Crohn's disease:** 5mg/kg IV at 0, 2, and 6weeks, then q8wks; **fistulizing Crohn's disease:** 5mg/kg IV at 0, 2, and 6wk; **Ulcerative colitis:** 5mg/kg IV at 0, 2, and 6wk , then q8wks

Mercaptopurine (6-MP)	PRC D, Lact ?
Purinethol *Tab 50mg*	**Crohn's disease, Ulcerative colitis:** ini 50mg PO qd, maint 75-125mg PO qd, max 1.5mg/kg/d
Methotrexate	EHL no data, PRC X, Lact -
Generics *Tab 2.5mg, 10mg* *Inj 10mg/ml, 25mg/ml*	**Crohn's disease:** ini 25mg IM qweek x 16 weeks, maint 15mg IM qweek
Nitroglycerin	PRC C, Lact ?
Nitrol *Oint. 2%*	**Chronic anal fissure:** 0.2%-0.4% PR bid
Octreotide	EHL 1.5h, PRC B, Lact ?
Sandostatin *Inj 50mcg/ml, 100mcg/ml, 200mcg/ml, 500mcg/ml* **Sandostatin LAR Depot** *Inj 10mg, 20mg, 30mg/vial*	**Acromegaly:** 100-300mcg SC bid, depot 20mg IM q4wk x 3mo, then q4wk according to GH level; **carcinoid tumors**: 100-600 mcg/d SC bid-qid or depot 20mg IM q4wk x 2 mo, then q4wk prn; **Vipomas:** 200-300 mcg/d SC bid-qid or depot 20mg IM q4wk x 2 mo, then q4wk prn; **Bleeding varices:** 50mcg/h IV x 1 then 50mcg/h IV for 48h, max 5d; DARF: req in severe RF
Pinaverium	PRC B, Lact+
Dicetel *Tab 50mg, 100mg*	**IBS:** 50mg PO tid, max 100mg PO tid
Pentoxifylline	EHL 0.4-1h, PRC C, Lact ?
Generics *Tab sust. rel. 400mg*	**Alcohol hepatitis:** 400mg PO tid
Tegaserod	EHL 11h, PRC B, Lact?
Zelnorm *Tab 6mg*	**IBS with constipation in women and men:** 6mg PO bid
Vasopressin	EHL 10-20min, PRC C, Lact ?
Pressyn *Inj 20 U/ml* **Generic** *Inj 20 U/ml*	**GI hemorrhage/esophageal varices:** ini 0.2-0.4 U/min IV, incr by 0.2 U/min q1h, max 0.9 U/min; diabetes insipidus: 5-10U SC/IM bid-tid prn (ǂ125)

6 Metabolic, Endocrine

6.1 Antigout Drugs

6.1.1 Uricosurics

MA/EF: inhibition of tubular uric acid reabsorption ⇒ uricosuric agent
AE: initial gout attack, N/V, headache, urate calculus, GI distress, rash, blood dyscrasias, nephrotic syndrome
CI: kidney stones, renal insufficiency, hypersensitivity to bromide + probenecid, < 2y, salicylate use, initiation-gouty attack, blood dyscrasias

Probenecid	EHL 3–17h, PRC B, Lact ?
Benuryl *Tab 500mg*	**Gout:** 250mg PO bid for 7d, then 500mg PO bid; **Penicillintherapy:** 2g/d PO in div doses; **CH** 2–14 y: ini 25mg/kg PO, then 40mg/kg div qid; DARF: GFR (ml/min) >50: 100%, <50: not rec
Rasburicase	EHL 18h, PRC C, Lact ?
Fasturtec *Tab 1.5mg/vial*	**PRO hyperuricemia secondary chemotherapy:** 0.2mg/kg IV qd for upto 7days
Sulfinpyrazone	EHL 2.7–6h, PRC C(D near term), Lact ?
Generics *Tab 100mg, 200mg*	**Gout:** ini 100–200mg/d PO in div doses, incr dose by 100–200mg every few days; max 800mg/d

6.1.2 Xanthine Oxidase Inhibitors

MA/EF: inhibition of xanthine oxidase ⇒ uric acid formation↓ (uricostatic agent)
AE: N/V, allergic reactions, leukopenia, xanthic calculus, pruritus, rash, myelosuppression, hepatotoxicity, **CI:** hypersesativity to drug, lactation

Allopurinol	EHL 1-2h, PRC C, Lact ?
Zyloprim *Tab 100mg, 200mg, 300mg* **Generics** *Tab 100mg, 200mg, 300mg*	**Gout:** ini 100-200mg PO/d div qd-tid, incr. 100mg/d at weekly interval, aim [uric acid]<360umol/L, max 300mg/dose, max 800mg/d; **PRO renal calcium stones:** 200-300mg PO/d; **chemother. with expected cell lysis:** 600-800mg PO/d dix qd-tid for 2-3d, start 1-2d before treatment; **CH** <10y: 10mg/kg/d PO div bid-tid; **CH** <6y: 150mg PO /d div tid; DARF: GFR (ml/min):10-20: 200mg/d, <10:100mg/d

6.1.3 Other Antigout Drugs

MA/EF (colchicine): prevention of phagocytosis of deposited urate crystals by leukocytes which release of inflammatory agents ⇒ antimitotic agent
AE (colchicine): diarrhea, N/V, epigastric pain, leukopenia, myelosuppression, myoneuropathy, alopecia
CI (colchicine): hypersensitivity to colchicine, blood dyscrasias, children < 2y, active PUD, serious GI, renal, hepatic, or cardiac disease

Colchicine	EHL 4.4h, PRC D, Lact +
Colchicine-Odan *Tab 0.6mg, 1mg*	**Acute gout:** ini 1-1.2mg PO, then 0.5-0.6mg PO q1-2h until symptoms abate or **AE** occur, max 8mg/d PO; **PRO gouty arthritis:** 0.5mg 1-4x/wk to 1.8mg PO qd; **Acute Familial Mediterranean Fever:** ini 0.6mg PO, then 0.6mg q1h x 3, then 0.6mg q2h x 2, then 0.6-1.2mg q12h until relief; **PRO FMF:** 1-2mg PO/d div, **CH** <5y: 0.5mg PO qd, >5y 1-1.5mg/d PO div bid-tid; DARF: CrCl 10-50: 50%, <10 avoid, Hepatic impairment: reduce

6.2 Ions, Minerals

6.2.1 Potassium

AE: N/V, belching, heartburn, flatulence, abdominal pain, diarrhea, mucosal ulcers, GI hemorrhage, ECG changes
CI: hyperkalemia, hyperchloremia, renal insufficiency, Addison's disease, acute dehydration, heat cramps

Potassium Chloride	PRC C, Lact ?
Apo-K *Tab (ext. rel) 8mEq* **K-10** *Liquid 20mEq/15ml* **K-Dur** *Tab (ext. rel) 20mEq* **K-Lor** *Powder 20mEq/pkt* **K-Lyte/Cl** *Powder 25mEq/7.8g* **Micro-K Extencaps, Micro-K-10 Extencaps** *Cap (ext.rel) 8mEq, 10mEq* **Roychol** *Liquid 20mEq/15ml* **Slow-K** *Tab (ext.rel), 8mEq*	**Hypokalemia Tx:** 40–100mEq/d PO; 40–300mEq/d IV, max 40mEq/liter, max 15mEq/h; **Hypokalemia PRO:** 20–40mEq/d PO qd–bid

Potassium Citrate	Lact +
K-Lyte *Tab (efferv) 25mEq* **Polycitra-K** *Crystals 30mEq/pkt, Sol (oral) 10mEq/5ml*	**Hypokalemia Tx:** 40–100mEq/d PO; 40–300mEq/d IV, max 40mEq/liter, max 15mEq/h; **Hypokalemia** PRO: 20–40mEq/d PO qd–bid

Potassium Gluconate	PRC A
Generics *Tab 550mg, 1,000mg, Liquid 20mEq/15ml*	**Hypokalemia Tx:** 40–100mEq/d PO; 40–300mEq/d IV, max 40mEq/liter, max 15mEq/h; **Hypokalemia** PRO: 20–40mEq/d PO qd–bid

6.2.2 Calcium

AE (calcium IV): sensation of heat, fits of perspiration, BP ↓, N/V, arrhythmias
CI (calcium IV): hypercalcemia, nephrocalcinosis, digitalis intoxication, severe renal insuff.

Calcium Carbonate	PRC C, Lact +
Apo-Cal *Tab 250mg, 500mg* **Calcite 500** *Tab 1250mg (500mg Ca)* **Calcium 500** *Tab 1250mg (500mg Ca)* **Calcium Oyster Shell** *Tab 650mg (250mg Ca), 1250mg (500mg Ca)* **Caltrate 600** *Tab 1500mg (600mg ca)* **Os-Cal** *Tab 1250mg (500mg Ca)* **Tums** *Tab (chew) 500mg, 750mg, 1,000mg* **Generics** *Cap 500mg*	**Hypocalcemia:** 1–2g PO qd; **osteoporosis PRO:** 1–1.5g PO qd; **RDA:** 1200mg PO qd
Calcium Chloride	PRC C, Lact ?
Generics *Inj 10% (1.36 mEq/ml)*	**Hypocalcemia:** 500–1,000mg IV q1–3d; **magnesium intoxication:** 500mg IV; **Hyperkalemia:** dose must be titrated by ECG-changes
Calcium Citrate	PRC C, Lact ?
Generics *Tab 150mg, 300mg, 350mg*	**Dietary supplement**: 500–2,000mg PO 2–4 times/day
Calcium Glucoheptonate	EHL n/a
Generics *Syr 100mg/5ml, 110mg/5ml, 125mg/ml*	**Dietary supplement**: 10 mL PO 1–3 times daily **CH**: 2.5–5 mL PO tid.
Calcium Gluconate	PRC C, Lact ?
Generics *Inj 10% Sol (0.465mEq/ml)*	**Hypocalcemia:** 0.5–2g slowly IV; 500–1,000mg PO bid–qid

6.2.3 Calcium Combinations

Calcium Carbonate + Cholecalciferol	
Os-Cal D *Tab 1250mg (500mg Ca) + 125 IU* **Viactiv** *Softchew1250mg(500mgCa)+100IU*	**Dietary supplement**: 1–2 tab PO qd

Calcium Carbonate + Cholecalciferol + Magnesium	
Calcium + *Liq 1250mg (500mg Ca) + 200 IU + 200mg/2 tsp*	**Dietary supplement**: 1–2 tsp PO qd
Calcium Carbonate + Copper + Manganese + Magnesium + Vitamin D + Zinc	
Caltrate Plus *Tab 1500mg (600mg Ca) + 1mg + 1.8mg + 50mg + 200 IU + 7.5mg*	**Dietary supplement**: 1–2 tab PO qd
Calcium Carbonate + Etidronate	
Didrocal *Calcium Carbonate: Tab 1250mg (500mg Ca)* **Etidronate:** *Tab 400mg*	**Osteoporosis:** 90-d cycle, 400mg etidronate PO qd x 14d then 500mg calcium PO qd x 76d
Calcium Carbonate + Risedronate	
Actonel Plus Calcium *Calcium Carbonate: Tab 1250mg (500mg Ca), Risedronate: Tab 35mg*	**Osteoporosis:** 28-d cycle, 35mg risendronate PO day 1, then 500mg calcium PO qd days 2-7, repeat x 4weeks
Calcium Carbonate + Vitamin D	
Calcite D-500 *Tab 1250mg (500mg Ca) + 125 IU* **Calcium 500 with Vitamin D** *Tab 1250mg (500mg Ca) + 125 IU* **Calcium D 500** *Tab 1250mg (500mg Ca) + 125 IU* **Caltrate Select** *Tab 1500mg + 400U* **Caltrate 600 + D** *Tab 1500mg (600mg Ca) 200IU, 1500mg (600mg Ca) + 400 IU* **Generics.** *Cap 500mg + 200 IU*	**Dietary supplement**: 1–2 tab PO qd
Calcium Citrate + Cholecalciferol + Magnesium + Silicon	
Active Calcium Plus *Tab 200mg + 100IU + 100mg + 2.25mg*	**Dietary supplement**: 2 tab PO bid
Calcium Glucoheptonate + Calcium Gluconate	
Calcium Stanley *Liq 132 + 112 mg/ml* **ratio-Calcium** *Syr 172.1 + 58.7mg/ml*	**Dietary supplement**: 10 mL PO 1–3 times daily **CH**: 2.5–5 mL PO tid
Vitamin D3 (cholecalciferol) + Alendronate	
Fosavance *Tab 2800IU + 70mg*	**Osteoporosis:** 1 tab PO qwk

6.2.4 Magnesium

AE: sleepiness, diarrhea, CNS disturbances, arrhythmias, muscle weakness, respiratory depression, flushing, hypotension;
CI: restricted use in case of depressed renal function, 2 hrs preceding delivery, heart block; IV: AV block, myasthenia gravis

Magnesium Chloride	EHL n/a
Formule 454 *Liq 180mg/5mlFormule 575Liq 400mg/ml* **Magnonat** *Liq 200mg/ml* **Generics** *Tab 606.5mg*	**Hypomagnesemia:** 100–600mg/d elemental magnesium PO div
Magnesium Glucoheptonate	EHL n/a
ratio-Magnesium *Sol (oral) 100mg (5mg Mg)/ml*	**Hypomagnesemia:** 15–30ml PO 1–3x/d
Magnesium Gluconate	PRC A, Lact +
Maglucate *Tab 500mg (29.3mg Mg), Liquid 54mg Mg/5ml*	**Hypomagnesemia:** 100–600mg/d elemental magnesium PO div tid
Magnesium Oxide	PRC B, Lact ?
Generics *Tab 252mg, 420mg, 835mg, Powder 240mg/ml, 750mg/1.25ml*	**Hypomagnesemia:** 100–600mg/d elemental magnesium PO div tid
Magnesium Sulfate	PRC A, Lact +
Generics *Inj 500mg/ml*	**Ventricular arrhythmias:** 1–6g IV over several min, then 3–20mg/min IV for 5–48h; **preeclampsia, eclampsia:** 4g IV, simultaneously 4–5g IM each buttock; preterm labor: 4–6g IV over 20min, then 1–3g/h IV

6.2.5 Fluoride

AE: N/V, diarrhea
CI: areas where water fluoride content is greater than 0.7ppm

Fluoride	PRC no data currently available , Lact ?
Fluor-A-Day *Drops 1mg/ml, Lozen 1mg, Tab (chew) 0.25mg, 0.5mg, 1mg* **Fluotic** *Tab 20mg*	**Osteoporosis:** 25mg PO bid (in combination with calcium citrate 400mg bid)

6.2.6 Phosphorous

Potassium Phosphate	PRC no data, Lact no data
Generics *Inj 3mmol/ml*	**Severe hypophosphatemia (< 1mg/dl):** 1–3g PO/PR; **CH:** 2–4mmol/kg/d PO; 25mmol IV over 24 hours

6.2.7 Iron

AE: N/V, diarrhea, constipation, dark-colored stools, when used intravenously: headaches, thrombophlebitis, allergic reactions, collapse; **CI:** hemochromatosis, hemolytic anemia, hemosiderosis, premature infants with vit. E deficiency

Ferrous Fumarate (33% elem. iron)	PRC C, Lact +
Palafer *Cap 300mg (100mg), Susp 300mg/5ml (100mg)* **Palafer CF** *Cap 300mg (100mg)*	**Iron deficiency:** 2–3mg/kg/d elemental iron PO div bid–tid
Ferrous Gluconate (11.6% elem. iron)	PRC C, Lact +
Generics *Tab 300mg (35mg)*	**Iron deficiency:** 2–3mg/kg/d elemental iron PO div bid–tid
Ferrous Polysaccharide (100% elem. iron)	PRC C, Lact +
Triferexx *Cap 150mg*	**Iron deficiency:** 2–3mg/kg/d elemental iron PO div bid–tid
Ferrous Sulfate (20% elem. iron)	PRC C, Lact +
Fer-In-Sol *Drops 75mg/ml (15mg), Syr 150mg/5ml (30mg)* **Ferodan Infant Drops** *Drops 75mg/ml (15mg)* **Ferodan** *Tab 300mg, Syr 150mg/5ml (30mg)* **Generics** *Tab 300mg (60mg)*	**Iron deficiency:** 2–3mg/kg/d elemental iron PO div bid–tid
Iron Dextran (100% elem. iron)	PRC C, Lact +
Dexiron *Inj 50mg/ml* **Infufer** *Inj 50mg/ml*	**Iron deficiency anemia:** total dose (ml) = 0.0442 x (desired Hb – observed Hb) x kg + [0.26 x kg] IV
Iron Sucrose (100% elem. iron)	EHL 6h, PRC C, Lact ?
Venofer *Inj 20mg/ml*	**Iron deficiency anemia in chronic hemodialysis:** 100mg IV 1–3x/wk up to 1g. rep prn

6.3 Drugs Affecting Electrolyte Imbalances

6.3.1 Biphosphonates

MA/EF: osteoclastic activity ↓⇒ osteal release of calcium ↓, bone degradation ↓
AE: allergic skin reactions, hypocalcemia, GI DO
AE (alendronate): abdominal pain, musculoskeletal pain, headache, diarrhea, constipation
AE (etidronate): loss of taste, osteomalacia, GI complaints, bone pain
AE (pamidronate): myelosuppression, HTN, thrombophlebitis, malaise, N/V
AE (risedronate): flu like syndrome, diarrhea, arthralgia, headache, abdominal pain, rash
CI: renal insufficiency, acute GI inflammation, children
CI (alendronate): hypersensitivity to alendronate products, esophageal abnormalities, inability to stand or sit upright for 30min, CrCl <35ml/min
CI (clodranate): Cr>440umol/L, severe inflammation of GI tract
CI (etidronate): hypersensitivity to etidronate products, osteomalacia
CI (pamidronate): hypersensitivity to biphosphonates
CI (risedronate): hypocalcemia, hypersensitivity to risedronate products

Alendronate	EHL up to 10y, PRC C, Lact ?
Fosamax *Tab 5mg, 10mg, 40mg, 70mg, Oral (sol) 70mg/75ml* **Generic** *Tab 5mg, 10mg, 70mg*	**Postmenopausal osteoporosis PRO:** 5mg PO qd or 35mg qwk; **postmenopausal osteoporosis Tx:** 10mg PO qd or 70mg qwk; **osteoporosis Tx men:** 10mg PO qd; **steroid-induced osteoporosis PRO + Tx:** 5mg PO qd (men and pre-menopausal women) or 10mg PO qd (postmenopausal women not taking estrogen); **Paget's disease:** 40mg PO qd for 6mo; DARF: GFR (ml/ min) 35–60: 100%, <35: not rec

Clodronate	EHL 13h, PRC C, Lact ?
Clasteon *Cap 400mg, Inj 30mg/ml*	**Hypercalcemia of malignancy, osteolytic bone lesions:** ini 300mg/d IV, maint 1600–2400mg PO qd or div bid, max 3200mg PO qd; DARF: dose should be reduced in severe renal failure

Etidronate	EHL 1-6h (or); 5.3-6.7h (IV), PRC C, Lact -
Didronel *Tab 200mg, 400mg* **Generics** *Tab 200mg*	**Paget's disease:** 5mg/kg/d PO upto 6mo, max 20mg/kg/d; **Tx/PRO steroid inducted osteoporosis, PRO post-menopausal osteoporosis:** 90d cycle: 400mg PO qd x 14d, then CaCO3 1250mg/d x 76d; **heterotopic ossification with hip replacement:** 20mg/kg/d PO 1mo before and 3mo after surgery; **heterotopic ossification with spinal cord injury:** 20mg/kg/d PO for 2wk, then 10mg/kg/d PO for 10wk; **hypercalcemia of malignancy:** 7.5mg/kg IV for 3d, then 20mg/ kg/d for 20-90d; DARF: creatinine >5 mg/dl: not rec
Pamidronate	EHL no data, PRC C, Lact ?
Aredia *Inj 30mg/vial, 90mg/vial* **Generics** *Inj 3mg/ml, 6mg/ml, 9mg/ml*	**Hypercalcemia:** (Ca >3mmol/l): 30mg IV; (3-3.5mmol/l): 30-60mg IV; (3.5-4mmol/l): 60-90mg IV; (>4mmol/l): 90mg IV, max inf. 22.5mg/h IV; **Paget's disease:** 30mg IV qwk x 6wks or 30mg IV, then 60mg wk 3,5,7 or 60mg q2wk x 3; **osteolytic bone lesions, multiple myeloma:** 90mg IV over 4h q4wk; DARF: not req in patients who receive 90mg monthly
Risedronate	EHL 1.5h, PRC C, Lact ?
Actonel *Tab 5mg, 30mg, 35mg*	**Paget's disease:** 30mg PO qd for 2 mo; **Tx/ PRO postmenopausal and steroid-induced osteoporosis:** 5mg PO qd or 35mg PO qwk; DARF: GFR (ml/min): >30: 100%, <30: not rec
Teriparatide	EHL 5min (IV), 1h (SC), PRC C, Lact ?
Forteo *TInj 250mcg/ml*	**Osteoporosis:** 20mcg SC qd

Zoledronic Acid	EHL 1.87h, PRC C, Lact ?
Zometa *Inj 4mg/vial*	**Hypercalcemia of malignancy, multiple myeloma, osteolytic bone lesions:** 4mg IV over 15min., rep. q3–4wks

6.3.2 Calcitonin

MA/EF: calcium and phosphate uptake in bone ↑, renal calcium and phosphate excretion ↑
AE: sensation of heat, flush, N/V, diarrhea, rash, depression, flu-like symptoms
CI: hypersensitivity to salmon calcitonin products

Calcitonin-Salmon	EHL 1h, PRC C, Lact ?
Calcimar *Inj 200 U/ml* **Caltine** *Inj 100 U/ml* **Miacalcin NS** *Spray (nasal) 200 U/spray* **Sandoz Calcitonin NS** *Spray (nasal) 200 U/spray*	**Postmenopausal osteoporosis:** 100 U SC/IM qd or qod; 200 U intranasal qd; **Paget's disease:** 50–100 U SC/IM qd or qod; **hypercalcemia:** 4 U/kg SC/IM q12h, incr prn to max 8 U/ kg q6–12h

6.3.3 Phosphate Binding Substances

MA/EF (sevelamer): polymer, free of calcium and aluminum, inhibition of enteral phosphate resorption; **MA/EF** (calcium acetate, lanthanum: binds to phosphate to form insoluble calcium phosphate which is excreted in the feces
AE (lanthanum, sevelamer): pain, N/V, diarrhea, constipation, flatulence, dyspepsia, dyspnea
AE (calcium acetate): hypercalcemia
CI (sevelamer): hypophosphatemia, ileus, bowel obstruction, hypersensitivity to sevelamer products
CI (calcium acetate): hypercalcemia

Calcium Acetate	PRC C, Lact ?
PhosLo *Tab 667mg (169mg calcium)*	**Hyperphosphatemia:** 2 tab PO with meals, maint 3–4 tab with meals

Sevelamer	PRC C, Lact ?
Renagel *Tab 400mg, 800mg*	**Hyperphosphatemia:** (Phosphate: 1.9–2.4mmol/l): 2.4g/d div tid with meals; (2.4–2.9mmol/l): 2.4–3.6g/d; (>2.9mmol/l): 4.8g/d

Lanthanum	EHL 53h, PRC C, Lact ?
Fosrenol *Tab 250mg, 500mg, 750mg, 1000mg*	**Hyperphosphatemia:** ini 750-1500 mg PO daily, div doses

6.3.4 Potassium Binding Resins

MA: enteral application of an insoluble synthetic material with sulphonic acid as basic structure; exchange of cations for neutralization of acid according to the cation concentrations in the intestinal lumen ⇒ binding and removal of potassium
AE: colonic necrosis, electrolyte abnormalities, constipation, hypocalcemia, N/V
CI: hypersensitivity to sodium polystyrene sulphonate, hypokalemia, conditions associated with hypercalcemia, bowel obsruction

Calcium Polystyrene Sulfonate	PRC C, Lact ?
Resonium Calcium *Powder (oral, rect) 300g/pack*	**Hyperkalemia:** 15g PO tid–qid; 30g retention enema qd, retain for > 9h; **CH:** ini 1g/kg PO qd in div doses, maint 0.5g/kg PO qd in div doses
Sodium Polystyrene Sulfonate	PRC C, Lact +
Kayexalate *Powder (oral, rect) 454g/bot* **Generics** *Susp (oral) 15g/60ml, Powder (oral, rect) 454g/bot, Enema 30g/120ml*	**Hyperkalemia:** 15g PO qd–qid; 30–50g retention enema q6h, retain for at least 30–60min

6.4 Vitamins

6.4.1 Vitamin B Group

AE (thiamine/vitamin B1): IV injection site reaction; **AE** (riboflavin/vitamin B2): urine discoloration; **AE** (pyridoxine/vitamin B6): neuropathy, N/V; **CI:** hypersensitivity product ingredients; **CI** (cyanocobalamin/vitamin B12): diarrhea, urticaria, pruritus, rash

Vitamin B1 (Thiamine)	EHL , PRC A, Lact +
Generics (thiamine) *Tab 50mg, 100mg, 500mg, Inj 100mg/ml*	**RDA:** 1–1.6mg PO qd; **Wernicke's encephalopathy:** ini 100mg IV, then 50–100mg IV/IM qd; **beriberi:** 10–20mg IM tid for 2wk, then 5–30mg PO qd; **wet beriberi with heart failure:** 10–30mg IV tid
Vitamin B2 (Riboflavin)	EHL 1.4h, PRC A, Lact +
Generics *Tab 50mg, 100mg*	**RDA:** 1.2–1.8mg PO qd; **Riboflavin deficiency:** 5–25mg/d PO qd

Vitamin B6 (Pyridoxine)	EHL 15–20d, PRC A, Lact +
Generics *Tab 10mg, 25mg, 50mg, 100mg, 250mg, Inj 100mg/ml*	**RDA:** 1.6–2.5mg PO qd; **pyridoxine def.:** 10–20mg PO qd for 3wk, then 2–5mg PO qd; **PRO of isoniazid neurop.:** 25–50mg PO qd; **Tx of isoniazid neurop.:** 50–200mg PO qd

Vitamin B12 (Cyanocobalamin)	PRC A, Lact +
Generics *Tab 0.1mg, 0.25mg, 0.5mg, 1mg, Inj 0.1mg/ml, 1mg/ml, 5mg/ml*	**RDA:** 2mcg PO qd; **vitamin B12 deficiency:** 25–250 mcg qd PO/intranasal; **pernicious anemia:** 100mcg/d IM/SC for 6–7d, then 100 mcg/d IM/SC qod for 7d, then 100mcg/d M/SC q3–4d for 2–3wk, then 100mcg q mo IM/ SC

6.4.2 Vitamin C

AE: occasional osmotic diarrhea, kidney stones, renal insufficiency
CI: restricted use in oxaluric urolithiasis, thalassemia and hemochromatosis, hypersensitivity to vitamin C products

Ascorbic Acid (Vitamin C)	EHL , PRC C, Lact ?
Proflavanol C *Tab 100mg* **Vitamin C Timed Release** *Cap (ext rel) 500mg, 1,000mg, 1500mg* **Generics** *Tab 500mg, Inj 500mg/ml*	**RDA:** 60–95mg/d PO; **scurvy:** 300mg/d IV/PO for 7d, then 100mg PO qd

6.4.3 Vitamin D

AE (calcitriol): hypercalcemia, N/V, polydipsia, polyuria; **AE** (dihydrotachysterol): hypercalcemia, renal impairment, N/V; **AE** (doxercalciferol): headache/malaise, edema, dyspnea, hypercalcemia; **CI** (calcitriol): hypercalcemia, vitamin D toxicity, hypersensitivity to calcitriol products; **CI** (dihydrotachysterol): hypercalcemia, hypersensitivity to dihydrotachysterol products ; **CI** (doxercalciferol): hypercalcemia or vitamin D toxicity

Alfacalcidol (Vitamin D3)	EHL 3h, PRC C, Lact +
One-Alpha *Cap 0.25mcg, 0.5mcg, 1mcg, Drops 2mcg/ml, Sol (oral) 0.2mcg/ml*	**Hypocalcemia in dialysis patients:** ini 0.25mcg PO qd, incr by 0.25mcg q4–8 wk until normocalc., most dialysis pat. respond to 0.5–1mcg/d PO or 1–2mcg IV 3x/wk

Calcitriol (Vitamin D3)	EHL 5-8h, PRC C, Lact ?
Calcijex *Inj 1mcg/ml, 2mcg/ml* **Rocaltrol** *Cap 0.25mcg, Cap 0.5mcg, Sol (oral) 1mcg/ml*	**Hypocalcemia in dialysis patients:** ini 0.25mcg PO qd, incr by 0.25mcg q4-8 wk until normocalcemic, most dialysis patients respond to 0.5-1mcg/d PO or 1-2mcg IV 3x/wk; **hypoparathyroidism:** 0.25mcg PO qd; incr prn q2-4wk up to 2mcg/d
Cholecalciferol (Vitamin D3)	PRC C
D-Vi-Sol *Liq (oral) 400 U/ml* **Generics** *Tab 400 U, 1,000 U*	**Supplement for breast-fed infants:** 400 U PO qd; supplement: 400-800 U PO qd
Dihydrotachysterol (Vitamin D2)	EHL no data, PRC C, Lact ?
Hytakerol *Cap 0.125mcg*	**Hypoparathyroidism:** ini 0.8-2.4mg PO qd for several d, maint 0.2-1mg PO qd
Doxercalciferol	EHL alpha,25-(OH)2D2 32-37h, PRC B, Lact ?
Hectorol *Cap 2.5mcg*	**Secondary hyperparathyroidism:** 10mcg PO 3x/wk
Ergocalciferol (Vitamin D2)	PRC A
Drisdol *Liq (oral) 8,288 U/ml* **Ostoforte** *Cap 50,000 U*	**Vitamin D resistant rickets:** 12,000-500,000 U PO daily, **Hypoparathyroidism**: 50,000-200,000 U plus 4g calcium lactate PO 6x/d
Paricalcitol	PRC C, Lact ?
Zemplar *Inj 5mcg/ml*	**Secondary hyperparathyroidism associated with chronic renal failure:** ini 0.04 µg/kg to 0.1 µg/kg IV, target PTH levels

6.4.4 Vitamin E

AE: bleeding DO
CI: hypersensitivity to vitamin E products, IV use in low birthweight infants, caution in coagulation DO or anticoagulant Tx, topical use in recent chemical peel or dermabrasion

Tocopherol (Vitamin E)	EHL , PRC A, Lact +
Generics *Cap 100mg (100 U vit E), 200mg (200 U vit E), 400mg (400 U vit E), 800mg (800 U vit E)*	**RDA:** 8-10mg PO qd; **vitamin E deficiency:** qid-5 times the RDA

6.4.5 Vitamin K

AE: when given intravenously anaphylactic reactions with apnea, dermatitis at injection site, hemolytic anemia with excessive doses; **CI:** hypersensitivity to Vitamin K, menadione (K3) administration in individuals with glucose-6-phosphate dehydrogenase deficiency

Phytonadione (Vitamin K)	EHL 26–193h, PRC C, Lact +
Generics *Inj 2mg, 10mg/ml*	**Hypoprothrombinemia:** 2.5–25mg PO/IM/SC; **anticoagulant-induced hypoprothrombinemia:** 2.5–10mg PO/SC/IM; **haemorrhagic disease of the newborn:** PRO: 0.5–1mg IM 1h after birth; Tx: 1mg SC/ IM

6.4.6 Folic Acid

AE: occasional CNS impairment, GI impairment, irritability, urticaria, pruritus
CI: megaloblastic anemia due to vit. B12 deficiency, hypersensitivity to folic acid products

Folic Acid	EHL , PRC A, Lact +
Generics *Tab 0.4mg, 1mg, 5mg, Inj 5mg/ml*	**RDA:** 0.18–0.4mg PO qd; **megaloblastic anemia:** 1mg PO/IM/SC/IV qd

6.5 Sex Hormones

6.5.1 Androgens, Anabolic Steroids

MA/EF: development and upkeep of secondary male sexual characteristics, regulation of spermatozoon production, libido, potentia coeundi, protein anabolism, sebum production
AE (androgens): cholestasis, inhibited spermatogenesis, accelerated bone maturation, virilization in women; **AE** (nandrolone decanoate): edema, HTN, virilization, hypoglycemia, lipid abnormalities; **AE** (testosterone): scrotal itching (Testoderm), clotting factor suppression, cholestatic jaundice; **CI** (androgens): prostate CA; **CI** (nandrolone decanoate): hypersensitivity to nandrolone products, male breast/prostate CA, nephrosis/nephrotic phase of nephritis, severe liver disease, pregnancy, cardiac or renal failure
CI (testosterone): prostate/breast CA, hypersensitivity to testosterone products, women of child-bearing potential

Nandrolone Decanoate	EHL 6–8d, PRC X, Lact ?
Deca-Durabolin *Inj 100mg/ml*	**Adj. tx for osteoporosis, Catabolic conditions:** 50–100mg IM q3–4wks, **CH** 2–13y: 25–50mg IM q3–4wks

Testosterone	EHL 10–100min (IM: approx. 8d), PRC X, Lact ?
Andriol *Cap 40mg* **Androderm** *Film (ext.rel, TD) 2.5mg/24h* **Androgel** *Gel 1%, Meter dose pump 1.25g/actuation* **Delatestryl** *Inj 200mg/ml* **Depo-Testosterone** *Inj 100mg/ml* **Testim** *Gel 1%*	**Hypogonadism:** (Film): 5mg/24h; (Gel): 5g topical qd; (Depo): 200–400mg IM q3–4wk; ini 120–160mg PO/d div bid, maint 40–120mg PO/d

6.5.2 Female Sex Hormones

see Gynecology, Obstetrics →287

6.6 Systemic Corticosteroids

EF: activation of gluconeogenesis, protein catabolism and lipolysis, inhibition of mesenchymal reactions (inflammation, exudation, proliferation), immunosuppression and anti-allergic effects (lymphopenia, eosinopenia, atrophy of lymphoid tissue, suppression of B and T cell activity); see also side effects
AE (corticosteroids):
Diabetogenic EF: hyperglycemia, glucosuria, steroid diabetes;
Catabolic EF: negative nitrogen balance, growth inhibition, osteoporosis;
DO in fat metabolism: truncal obesity, moon face, serum fatty acids ↑;
Complete blood count: thrombocytes ↑, erythrocytes ↑, neutrophils ↑, eosinophils ↓, basophils ↓, lymphocytes ↓;
Ulcerative EF: gastric acid ↑, gastric mucus protection ↓;
Eyes: corneal ulcer, glaucoma, cataract;
Skin: atrophy, striae rubrae, acne;
Capillary fragility ↑: petechiae, ecchymosis, purpura;
Mineralocorticoid EF: H_2O + Na+ retention, hypokalemia, BP ↑, alkalosis;
Immunodeficiency: susceptibility to infections ↑, reactivation of tuberculosis;
Endocrine neuropsychologic DO: euphoria, depression, confusion, hallucinations;
Muscles: weakness, atrophy;
Suprarenal gland atrophy: withdrawal syndrome (weakness, dizziness, shock)
AE (fludrocortisone): HTN, CHF, edema, hypokalemia
CI (corticosteroids, when used for longer periods): GI ulcerations, severe osteoporosis, acute viral and bacterial infx, systemic fungal infection, glaucoma, history of psychiatric diseases
CI (fludrocortisone): hypersensitivity to fludrocortisone, systemic fungal infections

Betamethasone	EHL 36–54h, PRC C, Lact -	Glu	Min
Betaject *Inj 3mg/ml* **Celestone Soluspan** *Inj 3mg/ml*	**Inflamm. disease:** 3–6mg IM qwk prn, **Intraarticular RA/OA:** (Hip): 3–6mg IA; (Knee/shoulder): 3mg IA; (Elbow/wrist): 1.5–3mg IA; (Hand): 0.75–1.5mg IA; **Periarticular:** 1.5–3mg prn; **fetal lung maturation, maternal antepartum:** 12mg IM q24h x 2 doses	30	0
Cortisone	EHL 8–12h, PRC C, Lact ?	0.8	2
Generics *Tab 25mg*	**Adrenal insufficiency, inflamm. disease:** 25–300mg PO qd **CH adrenal insufficiency:** 0.5–0.75mg/kg/d PO; **CH inflamm. disease:** 2.5–10mg/ kg/d PO; DARF not req		
Dexamethasone	EHL 36–54h, PRC C, Lact -	30	0
Dexasone *Tab 0.5mg, 0.75mg, 4mg* **Generics** *Tab 0.5mg, 0.75mg, 4mg, Elixir 0.5mg/5ml, Inj 4mg/ml, Inj 10mg/ml*	**Inflamm. disease:** 0.75–9mg/d PO/IM/IV div bid–qid; **cerebral edema:** ini 10mg IV, then 4mg IM q6h or 2mg PO bid–tid; **CH inflamm. disease:** 0.08–0.3mg/kg/d PO/ IM/IV div bid–qid; **CH cerebral edema:** ini 1.5mg/kg IV, then 1.5mg/kg/d IV div q4–6h; **fetal lung maturation, maternal antepartum:** 6mg IM q12h x 4 doses; DARF: not req		
Fludrocortisone	EHL 12–24h, PRC C, Lact ?	2	125
Florinef *Tab 0.1mg*	**Addison's disease, salt-losing adrenogenital syndrome:** 0.1–0.2mg PO qd		

Hydrocortisone	EHL 8–12h, PRC C, Lact -	Glu	Min
Cortef *Tab 10mg, 20mg* **Cortenema** *Enema 100mg* **Cortifoam** *Foam 80mg/application* **Hycort** *Enema 100mg* **Solu-Cortef** *Inj 100mg/vial, 250mg/vial, 500mg/vial, 1g/vial* **Generics** *Inj 100mg/vial, 250mg/vial, 500mg/vial, 1g/vial*	**Adrenal insufficiency:** 5–30mg PO bid–qid; **inflamm. disease:** 10–320mg/d PO div tid–qid or 100–500mg IV/IM q12h; **IBD:** 80–100mg PR qd–bid x 2–3wk, then qod; **CH adrenal insufficiency:** 0.5–0.75mg/kg/d PO div tid; **CH inflamm. disease:** 2.5–10mg/kg/d PO div tid–qid; DARF: not req	1	2
Methylprednisolone	EHL 18–36h, PRC C, Lact ?	5	0
Depo-Medrol *Inj (M.-acetate) 20mg/ml, 40mg/ml, 80mg/ml* **Depo-Medrol with Lidocaine** *Inj 40mg (plus 10mg lidocaine)/ml* **Medrol** *Tab 4mg, 16mg* **Solu-Medrol** *Inj (M.-succinate) 40mg/vial, 125mg/vial, 500mg/vial, 1g/ vial* **Generics** *Inj 500mg/vial, 1g/vial*	**Inflamm. disease:** 10–250mg IV/IM q4h; 4–48mg PO/d; 4–80mg intraarticular (methylprednisolone acetate), may be repeated after 1–5wk; **lupus nephritis:** 1g IV qd for 3d; **Acute IBD:** 20mg IV q8h; **CH inflamm. disease:** 0.5–1.7mg/kg/d PO/IV/IM div q6–12h;		
Prednisolone	EHL 18–36h, PRC C, Lact ?	4	1
Pediapred *Sol (oral) 5mg/5ml* **Generics** *Sol (oral) 5mg/5ml, Tab 5mg*	**Inflamm. disease:** 5–60mg PO/d; **CH:** 0.1–2mg/kg/ d PO div qd–qid; DARF: not req		
Prednisone	EHL 18–36h, PRC C, Lact +	4	1
Winpred *Tab 1mg* **Generics** *Tab 1mg, 5mg, 50mg*	**Inflamm. disease:** 5–60mg/d PO qd or div bid–qid; **CH:** 0.05–2mg/kg/d div qd–qid; DARF: not req		
Triamcinolone	EHL 18–36h, PRC C, Lact +	**Glu**	**Min**
Aristospan *Inj 20mg/ml* **Kenalog** *Inj (T.acetonide) 10mg/ml, 40mg/ml* **Generics** *Inj 10mg/ml, 40mg/ml*	**Inflamm. disease:** 4–48mg/d PO div qd–qid; 2.5–15mg, max 40mg **Intraarticular RA/OA:** 2–20mg IA q3–4wk prn; DARF: not req	5	0

Glu: relative glucocorticoid potency, **Min:** relative mineralocorticoid potency

6.7 Oral Antidiabetics

6.7.1 Sulfonylureas - 1st Generation

MA/EF: blockage of ATP-dependent K^+ channels ⇒ release of insulin from pancreatic β-cells ↑, sensitivity of peripheral tissues to insulin ↑
AE (sulfonylureas): N/V, hypoglycemia, cholestatic jaundice, pancytopenia
AE (chlorpropamide): hypoglycemia, N, allergic skin reactions
AE (tolbutamide): hypoglycemia, nausea, heartburn, allergic skin reactions
CI (sulfonylureas): type 1 DM, ketoacidosis, renal insufficiency, coma, severe infection, severe thyroid or liver disease, trauma or surgery

Chlorpropamide	EHL 36h, PRC C, Lact -
Novo-Propamide *Tab 250mg* **Generics** *Tab 100mg, 250mg*	**DM:** ini 250mg PO qd, maint 100–500mg, max 750mg PO qd; DARF: GFR (ml/min) >50: 50%, <50: not rec
Tolbutamide	EHL 4.5–6.5h, PRC C, Lact ?
Generics *Tab 500mg*	**DM:** ini 1g PO qd, maint 500mg–3g PO qd, max 3g/d

6.7.2 Sulfonylureas - 2nd Generation

MA/EF: see Sulfonylureas - 1st Generation →130 ; **AE** (glimepiride): hypoglycemia, N; **AE** (glyburide): hypoglycemia, N, heartburn, allergic skin reactions; **CI**: as above

Gliclazide	EHL 10.4h, PRC ?, Lact ?
Diamicron *Tab 80mg* **Diamicron MR** *Tab (modified release) 30mg* **Generics** *Tab 80mg*	**DM:** ini 80mg PO bid, maint 80–320mg PO/d (div doses of > 160mg bid), max 320mg/d; (Modified release): ini 30mg PO qd, maint 30–120mg PO qd
Glimepiride	EHL 5h, PRC C, Lact -
Amaryl *Tab 1mg, 2mg, 4mg* **Generics** *Tab 1mg, 2mg, 4mg*	**DM:** ini 1–2mg PO qd, main. 1–4mg PO qd, max 8mg/d
Glyburide	EHL 5–10h, PRC C, Lact ?
DiaBeta *Tab 2.5mg, 5mg* **Euglucon** *Tab 2.5mg, 5mg* **Gen-Glybe** *Tab 2.5mg, 5mg* **Generics** *Tab 2.5mg, 5mg*	**DM:** ini 2.5–5mg PO qd, maint 2.5–20mg PO qd or div bid; max 20mg/d

6.7.3 Oral Antidiabetics - α-Glucosidase Inhibitors

MA (acarbose): inhibition of glucosidase ⇒ intestinal glucose resorption ↓
AE (acarbose): diarrhea, abdominal pain, flatulence ; **CI** (acarbose): hypersensitivity to acarbose, DKA, inflammatory bowel diseases, colonic ulceration, partial obstruction

Acarbose	EHL 2h, PRC B, Lact ?
Glucobay *Tab 50mg, 100mg*	**DM:** ini 50mg PO qd, incr to 50mg PO bid, then tid at 1–2wk increments, max 300mg/d

6.7.4 Oral Antidiabetics - Meglitinides

MA/EF: stimul. insulin secret. via inhib. (closing) of ATP-sensitive potassium channels in beta cells (⇒ increases in beta-cell calcium influx); **AE:** hypoglycemia; **CI:** diabetic ketoacidosis, type 1 DM, hypersensitivity to repaglinide products

Nateglinide	EHL 1.5h, PRC C, Lact ?
Starlix *Tab 60mg, 120mg, 180mg*	**DM:** ini 120mg PO tid, maint 60–180mg PO tid
Repaglinide	EHL < 1h, PRC C, Lact ?
GlucoNorm *Tab 0.5mg, 1mg, 2mg*	**DM:** ini 0.5–2mg PO tid within 30min before a meal; max 16mg/d

6.7.5 Oral Antidiabetics - Biguanides

MA: cellular glucose uptake ↑, non-oxidative glucose metabolism ↑;
AE: lactic acidosis, N/V/D, flatulence, anorexia, complete blood count changes;
CI: type 1 DM, ren./hep./respir./cardiac insuff., Cr >136 umol/l in men or>124umol/l in women,CHF, sev.infect.,hypersens. to metformin, metabolic acidosis, concomitant useof iiodin.contrast media,DKA, ethanol abusus

Metformin	EHL 1.5–6.2h, PRC B, Lact ?
Glucophage *Tab 500mg, 850mg* **Generics** *Tab 500mg, 850mg*	**DM:** ini 500mg PO qd–bid, maint 500mg PO tid–qid or 850mg PO bid–tid, max 2550mg/d; DARF: contraind. in RF

6.7.6 Oral Antidiabetics - Thiazolidinediones

MA/EF: binding to peroxisome proliferator activated (PPA)-receptor in insulin target tissue ⇒ insulin effectiveness ↑ ⇒ cellular glucose uptake ↑, hepatic gluconeogenesis ↓
AE: edema, weight gain, anemia. Combination with metformin: anemia, hypo- and hyperglycemia, headache, diarrhea, stomachache, N, tiredness, edema. Combination with sulfonylureas: anemia, thrombopenia, hypo- and hyperglycemia, weight gain, edema
CI: acute heart failure, hepatic impairment, hypersensitivity to product ingredients

Pioglitazone	EHL 3-7h, PRC C, Lact ?
Actos *Tab 15mg, 30mg, 45mg*	**DM:** monotherapy or in combination with sulfonylureas, metformin, or insulin: ini 15-30mg PO qd, max 45mg/d; DARF: not req
Rosiglitazone	EHL 3-4h, PRC C, Lact -
Avandia *Tab 2mg, 4mg, 8mg*	**DM:** monotherapy or comb. with metformin or sulfonylureas: ini 4mg PO qd or 2mg bid, after 8-12wk to max 8mg/d; DARF: not req

6.7.7 Oral Antidiabetics - Combinations

AE (Avandamet): diarrhea, anemia, upper resp. tract infx, headache, fatigue;
CI (Avandamet): renal disease, congestive heart failure, acute or chronic metabolic acidosis

Glimepiride + Rosiglitazone	PRC C, Lact -
Avandaryl *Tab 1mg + 4mg, 2mg + 4mg, 4mg + 4mg*	**DM:** ini 1mg + 4mg PO qam, max 4mg + 8mg PO qam
Metformin + Rosiglitazone	PRC C, Lact -
Avandamet *Tab 500mg + 1mg, 500mg + 2mg, 500mg + 4mg, 1000mg + 2mg, 1000mg + 4mg*	**DM:** ini 500+1-2mg PO bid, max 2,000+ 8mg/d; DARF: contraind. in RF

6.8 Insulins

6.8.1 Short-Acting Insulins

MA/EF: glucose resorption in muscle and fat cells↑ ⇒ anabolic metabolism↑ (glycogen-, lipid- and protein synthesis), catabolic metabolism↓ (glycogenolysis, lipolysis, proteolysis)
MA/EF: faster resorption because of amino acid changes ⇒ shorter inject-eat-interval
AE: hypoglycemia, transient injection site reaction, pain at injection site, lipodystrophy, allergic reactions; **CI:** current hypoglycemic episode, systemic allergic reaction to insulin

Insulin Aspart	Duration: 3-5h, PRC no data, Lact ?
Novorapid *Inj 100 U/ml*	**DM:** individualized dosage SC 5-10min ac
Insulin Lispro	Duration: <6h, PRC B, Lact ?
Humalog *Inj 100 U/ml*	**DM:** indiv. dosage SC within 15min ac
Insulin Regular	Duration: 6-12h, PRC B, Lact +
Humulin R *Inj 100 U/ml* **Hypurin Regular** *Inj 100 U/10ml* **Novolin ge Toronto** *Inj 100 U/ml*	**DM:** individualized dosage SC 30min ac; **diabetic ketoacidosis:** ini 0.1 U/kg IV bolus, then 0.1 U/kg/h, decrease when blood glucose falls to < 250mg/dl

6.8.2 Intermediate- and Long-Acting Insulins

MA, EF, AE, CI see short-acting insulins →132

Insulin Detemir	Duration: 6–23h, PRC C, Lact ?
Levemir *Inj 100 U/ml*	**DM:** individualized dosage SC qd or bid
Insulin Lente	Duration: 18–26h, PRC B, Lact ?
Humulin L *Inj 100 U/ml* **Hypurin NPH** *Inj 100 U/10ml* **Novolin ge Lente** *Inj 100 U/ml*	**DM:** individualized dosage SC
Insulin NPH (isophane)	Duration: 10–24h, PRC B, Lact ?
Humulin N *Inj 100 U/ml* **Novolin ge NPH** *Inj 100 U/ml*	**DM:** individualized dosage SC
Insulin Ultralente	Duration: >36h, PRC B, Lact ?
Humulin U *Inj 100 U/ml* **Novolin ge Ultralente** *Inj 100 U/ml*	**DM:** individualized dosage SC

6.8.3 Insulin Glargine

MA/EF (insulin glargine): genetically changed insulin molecule, badly soluble in physiological pH-span ⇒ slow resorption ⇒ longer action; **AE:** hypoglycemia, injection site pain, lipodystrophy, pruritus, rash, allergic reactions, hypersensitivity
CI: hypoglycemia, prior hypersensitivity to any component of insulin glargine formulation

Insulin Glargine	Duration: 24h, PRC C, Lact ?
Lantus *Inj 100 U/ml*	**DM:** individualized dosage SC qd hs

6.8.4 Biphasic Insulins

Insulin Lispro + Insulin Lispro-protamine	
Humalog Mix 25 *Inj 25 + 75 U/ml*	**DM:** individualized dosage SC within 15min ac
Insulin Regular + Insulin NPH	
Humulin 10/90, 20/80, 30/70, 40/60, 50/50 *Inj 10 + 90 U/ml, 20 + 80 U/ml, 30 + 70 U/ml, 40 + 60 U/ml, 50 + 50 U/ml* **Novolin ge 10/90, 20/80, 30/70, 40/60, 50/50** *Inj 10 + 90 U/ml, 20 + 80 U/ml, 30 + 70 U/ml, 40 + 60 U/ml, 50 + 50 U/ml*	**DM:** individualized dosage

6.9 Antihypoglycemic Drugs

MA/EF (glucagon): cAMP mediated glycogenolysis in the liver ⇒ gluconeogenesis ↑ ⇒ blood glucose ↑
AE (dextrose): thrombophlebitis, rebound hypoglycemia, hypokalemia
AE (diazoxide): hypotension, tachycardia, aggravation of angina, N/V, hyperglycemia
AE (glucagon): N/V
CI (dextrose): anuria, diabetic coma + hyperglycemia, intracranial/intraspinal hemorrhage, delirium tremens in dehydrated patients, glucose-galactose malabsorption syndrome
CI (diazoxide): hypersensitivity to diazoxide or thiazide products, functional hypoglycemia;
CI (glucagon): pheochromocytoma, hypersensitivity to glucagon

Dextrose	EHL n/a
Generics *Sol (oral) 50g/bot, 75g/bot, 100g/bot, Inj 50mg/ml, 250mg/ml 2.5g/100ml, 5g/100ml, 10g/100ml, 20g/100ml, 30g/100ml, 40g/100ml, 50g/100ml, 60g/ 100ml, 70g/100ml*	**Hypoglycemia:** 10–25g IV; **hypoglycemia in conscious diabetics:** 10–20g of dextrose PO prn, may repeat prn q10–20min
Diazoxide	EHL 20–36h, PRC C, Lact ?
Proglycem *Cap 100mg*	**Hypoglycemia:** ini 3mg/kg/d PO div tid, maint 3–8mg/kg/ d div bid–tid
Glucagon	EHL 8–18min, PRC B, Lact ?
Generics *Inj 1mg/vial*	**Hypoglycemia:** 0.5–1mg IV/SC/IM, may rep. in 5–20min

6.10 Obesity Drugs

MA/EF (orlistat): inhibition of gastric and pancreatic lipase ⇒ hydrolysis of triglycerides into free fatty acids and monoglycerides ↓ ⇒ absorption ↓
MA/EF (phentermine): anorexigenic effect ⇒ loss of weight
MA/EF (sibutramine): central inhibition of neuronal reuptake of serotonin (and noradrenaline) ⇒ repletion ↑, body temperature ↑
AE (orlistat): stomachache, fatty stool, flatulence with stool excretion, tenesmus, headache, tiredness, resorption of fat soluble vitamins ↓
AE (phentermine): HTN, tachycardia, psychosis, nervousness, insomnia, dizziness
AE (sibutramine): appetite loss, constipation, dry mouth, sleeplessness, tachycardia, HTN, nausea, dizziness, headache, paresthesia, anxiety, vasodilation
CI (orlistat): chronic malabsorption syndrome, cholestasis
CI (phentermine): hypersensitivity to phentermine, hyperthyroidism, glaucoma, during or within 14d of MAO inhibitors, symptomatic CVS disease, advanced arteriosclerosis, mod-sev. HTN, pulmonary hypertension, history of drug abuse, alcoholism, agitated states, TCA
CI (sibutramine): anorexia nervosa or bulimia, psychiatric diseases, combined treatment with CNS- effective drugs, coronary heart disease, decompensated heart insufficiency, arrhythmia, arterial occlusive disease, CAD, CHF, during or within 14d of MAO inhibitors, poorly controlled HTN, arrythmias, cerebrovascular disease

Orlistat	EHL 1-2h, PRC B , Lact ?
Xenical *Cap 120mg*	**Obesity:** 120mg PO tid with meals; DARF: not req
Phentermine	EHL 20h, PRC C, Lact ?
Ionamin *Cap 15mg, 30mg*	**Obesity:** 15-30mg PO ac breakfast or qhs; DARF: see Prod Info
Sibutramine	EHL 1.1h, PRC C , Lact ?
Meridia *Cap 10mg, 15mg*	**Obesity:** 10mg PO qam, max15 mg/d; DARF: containdicated in severe RF

6.11 Thyroid Drugs

6.11.1 Iodine

AE: skin/mucous membrane irritation, headache, weakness, erythema
CI: hypersensitivity to iodine

Iodine (potassium iodine)	EHL no data, PRC D, Lact ?
Generics *Tab 3mg. Cap 0.22mg, Liq 0.15mg/0.04ml, 1mg/ml*	**Preparation of thyroidectomy:** 50-250mg PO 10-14d before surgery; **Thyroid blocking in radiation exposure:** 130mg PO qd x 3-7d or as directed by state health officials

6.11.2 Thyroid Hormones

MA/EF: growth, physical + mental development↑, protein synthesis↑, oxidative breakdown of fats and carbohydrates↑ (basal metabolism↑)
AE: tachycardia, extrasystoles, angina pectoris, weight loss, hyperthermia, diarrhea, nervousness, sleeplessness, tremors, muscle weakness
CI: thyrotoxicosis, acute MI, uncorrected adrenal insufficiency

Levothyroxine (T4)	EHL 5.3-9.5d, PRC A, Lact ?
Eltroxin *Tab 0.05mg, 0.1mg, 0.15mg, 0.2mg, 0.3mg* **Levo-T** *0.075mg, 0.125mg, 0.15mg, 0.3mg* **Synthroid** *Tab 0.025mg, 0.05mg, 0.075mg, 0.088mg, 0.1mg, 0.112mg, 0.125mg, 0.15mg, 0.175mg, , 0.2mg, 0.3mg, Inj 0.5mg/vial*	**Hypothyroidism:** ini 50mcg PO qd, incr by 25mcg q2-3wk, maint 100-200mcg PO qd; **CH** 0-3mo: 10-13mcg/kg/ d PO, 3-6mo: 8-10mcg/kg/d PO, 6-12mo: 6-8mcg/kg/d PO, 1-5y: 5-6mcg/kg/d PO, 6-12y: 4-5mcg/kg/d PO, >12y: 2-3mcg/kg/d PO, post-puberty: 1.6mcg/kg/d PO
Liothyronine (T3)	EHL 25h, PRC A, Lact ?
Cytomel *Tab 0.005mg, 0.025mg*	**Hypothyroidism:** ini 25mcg PO qd, incr by 12.5-25mcg q1-2wk, maint 25-75mcg PO qd; **goiter:** ini 5mcg PO qd, incr by 5-10mcg q1-2wk, maint 75mcg PO qd; **myxedema:** 5mcg PO qd, incr by 5-10mcg q1-2wk, maint 50-100mcg/d PO; **congenital hypothyroidism:** ini 5mcg PO qd, incr by 5mcg q3-4d until desired response is achieved

Thyroid - Dessicated	EHL 2-7d, PRC A, Lact ?
Thyroid hormone *Tab 30mg, 60mg, 125mg*	**Hypothyroidism:** ini 30mg PO qd, incr by 15mg q2-3wk to max180mg/d; **CH** 0-6 mo: 4.8-6mg/kg/d PO, 6-12mo: 3.6-4.8mg/kg/d PO, 1-5y: 3.0-3.6mg/kg/d PO **CH** 6-12y: 2.4-3.0mg/kg/d PO **CH** >12y: 1.2-1.8mg/kg/d PO

6.11.3 Antithyroid Drugs (Thioamides)

MA/EF: inhibition of thyroid hormone synthesis through inhibition of thyroidal peroxidase (J- → J). The incretion of already synthesized hormones is not inhibited.
Propylthiouracil: in addition partial inhibition of the conversion of T4 to T3.
AE: agranulocytosis, leukopenia, allergic skin reactions, development of goiter, GI DO, hepatitis, transient cholestasis;
AE (propylthiouracil): myelosuppression, lupus-like syndrome, drug fever, N/V, epigastric distress
AE (methimazole): N/V, rash/urticaria, epigastric distress, arthralgia, paresthesia
CI (methimazole): hypersensitivity to methimazole products, nursing
CI (propylthiouracil): hypersensitivity to antithyroid drugs, nursing

Methimazole	EHL 2-28h, PRC D, Lact ?
Tapazole *Tab 5mg, 10mg*	**Hyperthyroidism:** 5-20mg PO tid; maint 5-15mg/d; **thyrotoxic crisis:** 60-120mg/d PO div tid; **CH hyperthyroidism:** ini 0.4mg/kg/d PO div tid, maint 1/2 of ini dose; DARF: not req
Propylthiouracil	EHL 0.9-4.3h, PRC D, Lact ?
Propyl-Thyracil *Tab 50mg, 100mg*	**Hyperthyroidism:** ini 50-100mg PO tid, if >300mg/d div q4-6h, max 500mg/d; **CH:** ini 150mg/m2/d PO, 6-10y: 50-150mg div, maint 50mg PO bid, >10y: 150-300mg/d div div tid, maint 1/3-2/3 of ini dose DARF: CrCl <10ml/min: 50%, 10-50ml/min: 25%

6.12 Prolactin Inhibitors

MA: stimulation of hypophyseal dopamine receptors ⇒ inhibition of prolactin release
AE: N/V, GI disturbances, psychomotor- and extrapyramidal motor system DO, hypotension, bradycardia, peripheral vascular perfusion disturbances
AE (bromocriptine): hypotension, periph. vasoconstriction, dyskinesias, fatigue, N/V
AE (cabergoline): dizziness, headache, weakness, fatigue, orthostatic hypotension
CI: limited use in psychiatric DO, gastroduodenal ulcers, serious CVS diseases
CI (bromocriptine): hypersensitivity to bromocriptine products, HTN disorders of pregnancy, CAD, psychotic disorders
CI (cabergoline): hypersensitivity to ergot derivatives, uncontrolled HTN

Bromocriptine	EHL 50h, PRC C, Lact -
Parlodel *Tab 2.5mg, Cap 5mg* **Generics** *Tab 2.5mg, Cap 5mg*	**Hyperprolactinemia:** ini 1.25–2.5mg PO qhs, incr to 2.5mg PO bid in 2–3d, then incr to 2.5mg PO tid prn, max 20mg/d; **acromegaly:** ini 1.25–2.5mg PO qhs, incr to 10–20mg/d div qid over 2–4wks; **Parkinson's:** 1.25mg PO qhs, maint 2.5mg PO bib, incr 2.5mg/d q2–4wk, max 40mg/d; DARF: not req
Cabergoline	EHL 63–69h, PRC B, Lact ?
Dostinex *Tab 0.5mg*	**Hyperprolactinemia:** ini 0.25mg PO 2x/wk, incr by 0.25mg 2x/wk at 4wk intervals according to response, max 1mg 2x/wk
Quinagolide	EHL 17h, PRC C, Inhibits lactation
Norprolac *Tab 0.025mg, 0.05mg, 0.075mg, 0.15mg*	**Hyperprolactinemia:** ini 0.025mg PO qd x 3days, then 0.05mg PO qd x 3days, then 0.075mg PO qd, max 0.9mg/day

6.13 Anterior Pituitary Hormones

MA (cosyntropin): stimulation of adrenal cortex to secrete cortisol and adrenal steroids
MA (pegvisomant): growth hormone receptor antagonist
AE (pegvisomant): elevated liver enzymes, inj. site reaction
AE (somatropin): hyperglycemia, hypothyroidism, BP ↑, N/V, edema, retention of H_2O + natrium, developm. of antibodies;
CI (somatropin): active malignancy, acute critical illness (post open heart or abdominal surgery; multiple accidental trauma; acute respiratory failure), closed epiphyses, hypersensitivity to growth hormone or product ingredients;
CI (co-syntropin): Cushing's syndrome, active infection, pregnancy, lactation, CHF, PUD, acute psychosis

Clomiphene →296

Cosyntropin	EHL no data, PRC C, Lact ?
Cortrosyn *Inj 0.25mg/vial* **Synacthen Depot** *Inj 1mg/amp*	**Adrenal funct. screen. test:** 0.25mg IM/IV over 2min; **CH** <2y: 0.125mg IM/IV over 2min; **CH** >2y: see adults

Menotropins, FSH/LH, Follitropins, FSH, Chorionic Gonadotropins, hCG →296

Pegvisomant	EHL 6d, PRC B, Lact ?
Somavert *Inj 10mg/vial, 15mg/vial, 20mg/vial*	**Acromegaly:** ini 40mg SC x1, maint. 10mg SC qd, max 30mg/d

Somatropin (Growth Hormone)	EHL 18min, PRC C, Lact ?
Humatrope *Inj 5mg/vial; 6mg, 12mg, 24mg/cartridge* **Nutropin** *Inj 5mg/vial, 10mg/vial* **Saizen** *Inj 1.33mg/vial, 3.33mg/vial, 5mg/vial* **Serostim** *Inj 5mg/vial, 6mg/vial*	**GH deficiency:** ini 0.006mg/kg/d SC, max 0.0125mg/kg/d

6.14 Posterior Pituitary Hormones

MA (desmopressin): renal H_2O resorpt.↑,vasoconstr.;
AE(desmopressin): flushing, headache, nausea;
CI(desmopressin): hypersens. to desmopressin prod., CH< 3mo, Type II B v. Willebrand

Desmopressin	EHL IV 75.5min, PRC B, Lact ?
DDAVP *Tab 0.1, 0.2mg, Tab (dis) 60mcg, 120mcg, Spray (nasal) 0.01mg/Spray, Inj 0.004mg/ml* **DDAVP Rhinyle Nasal Sol.** *Spray 0.25mg/bot* **Minirin** *Tab 0.1mg* **Octostim** *Spray (nasal) 0.15mg/Spray, Inj 0.015mg/ml* **Generics** *Spray (nasal) 0.01mg/Spray, Tab 0.1mg, 0.2mg*	**Central diabetes insipidus:** 10–40mcg (0.1–0.4ml) intranasally qd or div bid–tid; 0.1–1.2mg/d PO qd or div bid–tid; 2-4mcg/d SC/IV div bid; **CH central diabetes insipidus:** 3mo–12y: 5–30mcg (0.05–0.3 ml) intranasally qd or div bid; 0.05mg PO bid; **Hemophilia A** →62 **enuresis** →286

7 Antimicrobials

G 0.1 Organism – Antibiotic

Organism	Penicillin G	Penicillin V	Dicloxacillin	Ampicillin	Piperacillin	Ampic.+Sulbact.	Cefadroxil	Cefuroxime	Cefotaxime	Imipenem	Doxycycline	Tigecycline	Clarithromycin	Gentamicin	Moxifloxacin	Ciprofloxacin	Cotrimoxazole	Metronidazole	Vancomycin	Linezolid
Streptococci A, B, C, G	■	■	L	E	E	E	□	□	E	E	L	■	□	–	□	L	L	–	E	□
Strept. viridans group	■	E	L	E	E	E	□	□	E	E	L	■	□	–	□	L	L	–	E	□
Strept. pneumoniae	□	E	E	E	E	E	□	□	□	E	E	■	□	–	■	L	L	–	□	□
Enterococcus	–	–	–	■	E	E	–	–	–	□	L	■	–	–	E	L	L	–	□	□
Staph. aureus (MSSA)	L	L	■	L	L	E	□	□	L	E	E	■	□	□	□	L	E	–	□	□
Staph. aureus (MRSA)	–	–	–	–	–	–	–	–	–	L	–	■	–	–	L	–	□	–	■	■
Corynebact. diphtheriae	■	E	L	E	E	E	L	–	–	L	L	–	■	L	E	–	L	–	E	□
Gonococci (Neiss. gonor.)	L	L	–	–	–	L	L	L	■	E	L	–	L	–	E	■	–	–	–	–
Meningococci (Neiss. men.)	■	–	–	E	E	E	L	E	□	E	–	–	–	–	E	□	□	–	–	–
Haemophilus influenzae	–	–	–	□	E	E	E	E	■	□	L	■	E	E	■	E	□	–	–	–
Escherichia coli	–	–	–	E	E	E	E	E	■	E	L	■	–	E	E	■	□	–	–	–
Klebsiella	–	–	–	–	L	L	E	E	■	E	L	■	–	E	E	■	□	–	–	–
Salmonella	–	–	–	L	E	E	L	L	E	E	L	□	–	E	E	■	E	–	–	–
Shigella	–	–	–	E	E	E	E	E	□	E	L	■	–	E	E	■	□	–	–	–
Proteus mirabilis	–	–	–	■	E	E	E	E	■	E	–	□	–	E	E	■	□	–	–	–
Proteus vulgaris	–	–	–	–	–	–	–	–	L	E	–	□	–	E	E	■	□	–	–	–
Enterobacter	–	–	–	–	L	–	–	–	□	■	–	■	–	E	L	■	L	–	–	–
Serratia	–	–	–	–	L	–	–	–	■	■	–	■	–	E	L	■	L	–	–	–
Pseudomonas aeruginosa	–	–	–	–	E	–	–	–	E	■	–	L	–	E	–	■	–	–	–	–
Borrelia	□	E	L	□	E	E	L	L	■	–	■	□	E	–	–	–	–	–	–	–
Legionella	–	–	–	–	–	–	–	–	–	–	■	■	■	L	□	□	L	–	–	–
Actinomyces	■	E	L	□	□	□	L	L	L	E	■	–	□	–	E	–	L	L	E	□
Clostridium (except Cl. diff.)	■	E	L	E	E	E	–	L	L	□	E	■	E	–	L	–	–	■	■	□
Bacteroides fragilis	–	–	–	L	L	E	–	–	L	■	–	□	–	–	L	–	–	■	–	–
Treponema	■	E	L	E	E	E	–	L	□	–	E	□	L	–	–	–	–	–	–	–
Chlamydia	–	–	–	–	–	–	–	–	–	–	■	□	□	–	□	□	–	–	–	–
Mycoplasma	–	–	–	–	–	–	–	–	–	–	■	■	■	–	□	L	–	–	–	–
Rickettsia	–	–	–	–	–	–	–	–	–	–	■	■	L	–	□	□	–	–	–	–

Key	
E	effective
L	low effectiveness
–	not recommended
■	first choice
□	alternative

from Antibiotics pocketcard 2008; Author: Hof H. Börm Bruckmeier Publishing

7.1 Penicillins

7.1.1 Penicillins - 1st Generation (Benzylpenicillins, Penicillinase-Sensitive)

S: Pneumo-, Strepto-, Meningo-, Staphylococcus, Actinomyces, Leptospira, C. diphtheria, Treponema, Borrelia, Past. multocida, Fusobacteria, Peptococcus, Clostridia
R: Enteric bacteria, Pseudomonas, B. fragilis, E. faecium, Nocardia, Mycoplasma, Chlamydia, beta-lactamase producing bacteria, Salmonella, V. cholerae
AE: allergic skin reactions, Lyell-syndrome, anaphylaxis, vasculitis, myoclonia, seizures, oral dryness, N/V, diarrhea, Herxheimer- reaction, complete blood count changes, hemolytic anemia, interstitial nephritis, superinfection by multiresistant bacteria or yeasts
CI: hypersensitivity to prod ingredients, penicillins (Pen G procaine: additional sulfites), hx of anaphylaxis, accelerated or serum sickness reaction to previous penicillin administration

Benzylpenicilloyl Polylysine	PRC C, Lact ?
Pre-Pen *Inj. 0.0006 M/amp*	**Penicillin sensitivity detection:** scratch test or 0.01–0.02ml intradermally

Penicillin G	EHL 20–50min, PRC B, Lact +
Crystapen *Inj 1,000,000 U/vial, 5,000,000 U/vial, 10,000,000 U/vial* **Penicillin G Potassium** *Inj 1,000,000 U/vial, 5,000,000 U/vial, 10,000,000 U/vial* **Penicillin G Sodium** *Inj 1,000,000 U/vial, 5,000,000 U/vial, 10,000,000 U/vial*	**Streptococcal, pneumococcal, meningococcal infx:** 1–5 mio U/d IV div q4–6h; **streptococcal or staphylococcal endocarditis:** 12–18 mio U/d IV div q4h; **enterococcal endocarditis:** 18–30 mio U/d continuous IV inf or div q4h with aminoglycoside; **meningococcal meningitis:** 20–40 mio U/d IV div q2–4h; **CH** <12y: 25,000–400,000 U/kg/d IV div q4–6h, neonates: see Prod Info

Penicillin G Benzathine	EHL 20–50min
Penicillin G *Inj 600,000 U/ml*	**Group A streptococcal upper respiratory infx:** 1.2 mio U IM x 1; **CH:** 25,000–50,000 U/kg IM x 1, max 1.2 mio U; **PRO of rheumatic fever:** 1.2 mio U IM q mo; **CH:** 25,000–50,000 U/kg IM q3–4wks, max 1.2 mio U/dose; **early syphilis:** 2.4 mio U IM x 1; **CH: early/congenital syphilis:** 50.000 U/kg IM x 1, max 2.4 mio U; **late syphilis:** 2.4 mio U IM qwk x 3 wk; **CH:** 50.000 U/kg IM qwk x 3wk, max 2.4 mio U

Penicillin G Procaine	EHL 20–30min
Generics *Inj 300,000 U/vial, 1,500,000 U/vial*	**Anthrax (postexposure PRO, inhal):** 1.2 mio U IM q12h, **CH:** 25,000U/kg IM q12h, max 1.2 mio U/dose, **cutaneous**: 600,000–1.2 mio U/d IM; **Streptococcal, staphylococcal infx:** 0.6–1.0 mio U IM qd for 7–10d **neurosyphilis:** 2.4 mio U IM qd + probenecid 500mg PO q6h for 10–14d; **CH:** 300.000 U IM qd; **congenital syphilis:** 50.000 U/kg IM qd for 10d; DARF: GFR (ml/min): 10–30: q8–12h, <10: q12–18h

Penicillin V	EHL 30–40min, PRC B, Lact +
Apo-Pen VK *Sol (oral) 125mg/5ml, 300mg/5ml, Tab 300mg* **Novo-Pen-VK** *Sol (oral) 300mg/5ml, Tab 300mg* **Nu-Pen-VK** *Tab 300mg* **Pen-Vee** *Sol (oral) 180mg/5ml, 300mg/5ml, Tab 300mg* **Generics** *Tab 300mg*	**Infection:** 125–500mg PO q6–8h; **CH** <12y: 25mg–50mg/kg/d PO div q6–8h, max 3g/d; **PRO of recurrent rheumatic fever/pneumococcal infections:** 250mg PO bid; **CH** <5y: 125mg PO bid; **CH** ≥5y: 250mg PO bid; DARF: CrCl (ml/min): 10–15: q8–12h, <10: q 12–16h

7.1.2 Penicillins - 2nd Generation (Penicillinase-Resistant)

S/R: highly effective against beta-lactamase producing S. aureus; otherwise very narrow spectrum + lower activity against all other gram-positive bacteria than penicillin G
AE/CI: see benzylpenicillins →142
AE (cloxacillin): fever, rash, N/V, diarrhea, hepatotoxicity; **CI:** hypersensitivity to product ingredients/penicillins

Cloxacillin	EHL 0.5–1h, PRC B, Lact ?
Apo-Cloxi *Cap 250mg, 500mg, Sol (Oral) 125mg/5ml* **Novo-Cloxin** *Cap 250mg, 500mg, Sol (Oral) 125mg/5ml* **Nu-Cloxi** *Cap 250mg, 500mg, Sol (Oral) 125mg/5ml* **Cloxacillin sodium** *Inj 500mg/vial, 1000mg/vial, 2000mg/vial*	**Staphylococcal infx:** 250–500mg PO q6h; 250–250mg IV/IM q4–6h, severe infections: upto 2g IV/IM q4h **CH** 50–100mg/kg/d PO/IV/IM div q6h, max 4g/d; severe infections: 150–200mg/kg/d IV/IM div q6h, max 12g/d DARF: not req

7.1.3 Penicillins - 3rd Generation (Aminopenicillins)

S: compared to penicillin G additional action against Enterococcus, H. influenza, E. coli, Listeria, P. mirabilis, Salmonella, Shigella
R: B. fragilis, Pseudomonas, E. faecium, Nocardia, Mycoplasma, Chlamydia, beta-lactamase producing bacteria, Klebsiella, Yersinia
AE/CI: see benzylpenicillins →142 ; **CI:** history of allergy to penicillins

Amoxicillin	EHL 1-2h, PRC B, Lact +
Apo-Amoxi *Cap 250mg, 500mg, Sol (oral) 125mg/5ml, 250mg/5ml* **Lin-Amox** *Cap 250mg, 500mg, Sol (oral) 125mg/5ml, 250mg/5ml* **Novamoxin** *Cap 250mg, 500mg, Sol (oral) 125mg/5ml, 250mg/5ml, Tab (chew) 125mg, 250mg* **Nu-Amoxi** *Cap 250mg, 500mg, Sol (oral) 125mg/5ml, 250mg/5ml* **Generics** *Cap 250mg, 500mg, Sol (oral) 125mg/5ml, 250mg/5ml*	**Respiratory tract, ENT, genitourinary tract, skin, infx:** 250-500mg PO q8h or 500-875mg PO q12h, max 2-3g/d; **CH** <20kg: 20-40mg/kg/d PO div q8h; **endocarditis PRO:** 2g PO 1h before the procedure; **CH:** 50mg/kg PO 1h before the procedure, max 2g; DARF: GFR (ml/ min) 10-50: q8-12h, <10: q12-24h
Ampicillin	EHL 1-1.8 h and 15-20 h, PRC B, Lact +
Nu-Ampi *Cap 250mg, 500mg, Susp (oral) 125mg/5ml, 250mg/5ml* **Generics** *Cap 250mg, 500mg, Susp (oral) 125mg/5ml, 50mg/5ml Inj 250mg/vial, 500mg/vial, 1g/vial, 2g/vial*	**Respirat. tract, GI infx, UTI:** 250-500mg PO/IV/IM q6h; **CH** <40kg 25-50mg/kg/d IV/ IM div q6h; <20kg 50-100mg/kg/d PO div q6-8h; **meningitis or septicemia:** 8-14g/d IV div q3-4h; **CH** <40kg 100-200mg/kg/d IV/IM div q3-4h; **endocarditis PRO:** 2g IM/IV 30min before procedure **CH:** 50mg/kg IV/IM 30min before procedure; **endocard. Tx**: 12g/d IV contin. or div q4h;DARF: GFR (ml/min)>50: q6h, 10-50:q6-12h, <10: q12-24h
Pivampicillin	EHL 1h, PRC B, Lact ?
Pondocillin *Sol (oral) 175mg/5ml, Tab 500mg*	**Respirat. tract, ENT, gyne, urinary tract infect.:** 500mg PO bid, 15-30ml (525-1050mg) PO bid; **CH** 7-10y: 10ml (350mg) PO bid, 4-6y 7.5ml (262.5mg) PO bid, 1-3y 5ml (175mg)PObid, max 500mg PO bid; **gonoc. urethr.:** 1.5g single dose with 1g probenecid

7.1.4 Penicillins - 4th Generation (Extended Spectrum, Antipseudomonal)

S/R: similar to aminopenicillins, but highly effective against Ps. aeroginosa
AE/CI: see benzylpenicillins →142
AE (piperacillin): fever, headache, rash **CI:** hypersensitivity to piperacillin

Piperacillin	EHL 3.33h, PRC B, Lact +
Generics *Inj 2g/vial, 3g/vial, 4g/vial*	**Sepsis, nosocomial pneumonia, intra-abdominal, urinary tract, skin and soft tissue infx:** 2–3g IM q6–12h; 3–4g IV q4–6h, max 24g/d; **CH:** 200–300mg/kg/d div q4–6h; DARF: GFR (ml/min): 10–50: q6–8h, <10: q8h

7.1.5 Penicillin + β-Lactamase Inhibitor

AE (amoxicillin + clavulanate): headache, rash, N/V, diarrhea
AE (piperacillin + tazobactam): rash, diarrhea, headache, N/V
AE (ticarcillin + clavulanate): hypersensitivity reactions, headache, seizures, pseudomembranous colitis, thrombophlebitis
CI (amoxicillin + clavulanate, piperacillin + tazobactam): hypersensitivity to penicillins + product ingredients, (amoxicillin + clavulanate): suspected or confirmed mononucleosis

Amoxicillin + Clavulanate	PRC B, Lact +
Apo-Amoxi-Clav *Tab 250mg + 125mg, 500mg + 125mg, 875mg + 125mg, Susp (oral) 125mg + 31.25mg/5ml, 250mg + 62.5mg/5ml* **Clavulin** *Tab 250mg + 125mg, 500mg + 125mg, 875mg + 125mg, Susp (oral) 125mg/5ml + 31.25mg/ 5ml, 200mg/5ml + 28.5mg/5ml, 250mg/5ml + 62.5mg/ 5ml, 400mg/5ml + 57mg/5ml* **Novo-Clavamoxin** *Tab 875mg + 125mg* **Ratio-Aclavulanate** *Tab 250mg + 125mg, 500mg + 125mg, 875mg + 125mg, Susp (oral) 125mg + 31.25mg/5ml, 250mg + 62.5mg/5ml*	**UTI, respiratory tract, skin infx, sinusitis, otitis media:** 500–875 + 125mg PO q12h or 250–500 +125mg PO q8h; **CH:** (amoxicillin component) 25–45mg/kg/d PO div q12h or 20–40mg/kg/d PO div q8h; DARF: GFR (ml/min): 10–30: 250–500 + 125mg q12h; <10: 250–500 + 125mg PO q24h

Piperacillin + Tazobactam	PRC B, Lact +
Tazocin *Inj 2g/vial + 0.25g/vial, 3g/vial + 0.375g/vial, 4g/vial + 0.5g/vial*	**Intra-abdominal, skin infx, community-acquired pneumonia, febrile neutropenia:** 3 + 0.375g IV q6h; DARF: GFR (ml/min): 20–40: 2 + 0.25g IV q6h; <20: 2 + 0.25g IV q8h
Ticarcillin + Clavulanate	PRC B, Lact +
Timentin *Inj 3g/vial + 0.1g/vial, 30g/vial + 1g/vial*	**Systemic infx, UTI:** 3 + 0.1g IV q4–6h; **CH:** 300mg/kg/d ticarcillin component IV div q6h; DARF: ini 3.1g, then GFR (ml/min): 30–60: 2g IV q4h; 10–30: 2g IV q8h; <10: 2g IV q12h; <10 with hepatic dysfunction: 2g IV q24h

7.2 Cephalosporins

7.2.1 Cephalosporins - 1st Generation

S: act as penicillin G substitutes, but resistant to staphylococcal penicillinase; also activity against Proteus mirabilis, E. coli + Klebsiella pneumoniae; cefazolin-group: Staphylo-, Strepto-, Pneumococcus, N. meningitis, E. coli, Klebsiella, Prot. mirabilis, H. influenza
R (cefazolin-group): Enterococcus, Pseudomonas, Acinetobact., Listeria, Chlamydia, Mycoplasma, gram-neg. ß-lactamase- producing bacteria
AE (cephalosporins): allergic skin reactions, Lyell-syndrome, anaphylaxis, N/V, diarrhea, transaminases↑, cholestasis, interstitial pneumonia, complete blood count changes, hemolytic anemia, creatinine↑, interstitial nephritis, superinfection by bacteria or yeasts
CI (cephalosporins): hypersensitivity to cephalosporins

Cefazolin	EHL 1.5–2.5h, PRC B, Lact +
Generics *Inj 500mg/vial, 1g/vial, 10g/vial*	**Pneumonia:** 500mg IV/IM q12h, **mild infx from gram pos. cocci:** 250–500mg IV/IM q8h, **uncomplicated UTI:** 1g IV/IM q12h **mod-severe infections:** 500mg–1g IV/IM q6–8h, **surgical PRO:** 1g IM/IV 30–60min preop, 0.5–1g during surgery >2h, 0.5–1g q6–8h for 24h postop; **CH:** 25–50mg/kg/d IM/IV div q6–12h; 100mg/kg/d for severe infx; DARF: GFR (ml/min): >55: 100%, 35–54: 100% at least q8h, 11–34: 50% q12h, 0–10: 50% q18–24h

7.2.2 Cephalosporins - 1st Generation - Oral Cephalosporins

S: similar spectrum to cefazolin-group, highly effective against gram-positive bacteria, low effectiveness against gram-negative bacteria
R: Pseudomonas, Enterococcus, Prot. vulgaris, Morganella, Citrobacter, Serratia, enteric bacteria, Acinetobact., B. fragilis, Listeria, Chlamydia, Mycoplasma
AE/CI: see Cephalosporins - 1st Generation →146

Cefadroxil	EHL 1.2–1.7h , PRC B, Lact +
Duricef *Cap 500mg* **Generics** *Cap 500mg*	**UTI:** 1–2g/d PO qd or div bid; **skin and soft tissue infx, pharyngitis, tonsillitis:** 1g/d PO qd or div bid for 10d; **CH:** 30mg/kg/d PO div bid; DARF: ini 1g, then: GFR (ml/min): 26–50: 0.5g q12h; 10–25: 0.5g q24h; 0–10: 0.5g q36h
Cephalexin	EHL 0.9h, PRC B, Lact +
Apo-Cephalex *Tab 250mg, 500mg* **Novo-Lexin** *Cap 250mg, 500mg, Susp (oral) 125mg/5ml, 250mg/5ml, Tab 250mg, 500mg* **Nu-Cephalex** *Tab 250mg, 500mg*	**Pneumonia, skin infx, UTI:** 250–500mg PO q6h, max 4g/ d; **CH:** 25–50mg/kg/d PO div q6h, max 4g/d; **acute osteomyelitis:** (after IV therapy) 500mg–1g PO q6h, **CH:** 100–150mg/kg/d div q6h; DARF: GFR (ml/min) >50: 100%, <50: 250–500mg q12h

7.2.3 Cephalosporins - 2nd Generation

S (cephalosporins - 2nd generation): greater activity against three additional gram-negative organisms, H. influenzae, some Enterbacter aerogenes and some Neisseria species, whereas activity against gram-positive organisms is weaker; cefuroxim group: see Cephalosporins - 1st Generation →146, higher effectiveness against E. coli, Klebsiella, Prot. mirabilis, H. influenza, ß- lactamase producing bacteria; cephamycins/cefoxitin group (S/R): highly effective against ß-lactamase-producing anaerobic bacteria (for example Bacteroides)
R (cefuroxime-group): Enterococcus, Pseudomonas, Acinetobact., Listeria, Chlamydia, Mycoplasma
AE/CI: see Cephalosporins - 1st Generation →146

Cefoxitin	EHL 0.8–1h, PRC B, Lact +
Generics *Inj 1g/vial, 2g/vial, 10g/vial*	**Pneumonia, genitourinary and gynecologic infx, sepsis, intra-abdominal, skin, bone and joint infx:** 1–2g IV q6–8h; **CH:** 80–160mg/kg/d IV div q4–6h, max 12g/d; DARF: ini: 1–2g IV, then GFR (ml/min) 30–50: 1–2g IV q8–12h 10–29: 1–2g IV q12–24h, 5–9: 0.5–1g IV q12–24h, <5: 0.5g IV q24–48h

Cefuroxime Sodium	EHL no data, PRC B, Lact +
Zinacef *Inj 750mg/vial, 1.5g/vial, 7.5g/vial* **Generics** *Inj 750mg/vial, 1.5g/vial, 7.5g/vial*	**Uncomplicated infections/UTI/soft tissue/ pneumonia:** 750mg IV/IM q8h; **CH:** 30–100mg/kg/d div tid-qid; **Bone + joint infx, severe infection, gram neg. pneumonia:** 1.5g IV/IM q8h; **CH:** 70–150mg/kg/d IV div q8h; **meningitis:** 3gIV q8h; **CH:** 200–240mg/kg/d IV div tid–qid; **gonorrhea:** 1.5g IM as single dose together with 1g Probenecid PO; DARF: GFR (ml/min): >20: 750–1500mg q8h; 10–20: 750mg q12h; <20: 750mg q24h

7.2.4 Cephalosporins - 2nd Generation - Oralcephalosporins

S/R (oral cephalosporins 2nd generation): see cefuroxime-group →147
AE/CI: see Cephalosporins - 1st Generation →146

Cefaclor	EHL 30–60min, PRC B, Lact +
Ceclor *Cap 250mg, 500mg, Susp (oral) 125mg/5ml, 250mg/5ml, 375mg/5ml* **Generics** *Cap 250mg, 500mg, Susp (oral) 125mg/5ml, 250mg/5ml, 375mg/5ml*	**Respiratory tract infx, otitis media, UTI, skin infx, bone and joint infx:** 250–500mg PO tid; **CH:** 20–40mg/kg/d PO div q8–12h, max 2g/d; DARF: GFR (ml/min): <50: 50%

Cefprozil	EHL 1–2h, PRC B, Lact +
Cefzil *Tab 250mg, 500mg, Susp (oral) 125mg/5ml, 250mg/5ml* **Generics** *Tab 250mg, 500mg, Susp (oral) 125mg/5ml, 250mg/5ml*	**Pharyngitis, tonsillitis, UTI:** 500mg PO qd; **sinusitis:** 250–500mg PO bid; **skin infx:** 250mg PO bid or 500mg PO qd; **CH:** 6mo–12y: 7.5–15mg/kg PO q12h; DARF: GFR (ml/min) <30: 50%

Cefuroxime-Axetil	EHL 1.1–1.3h , PRC B, Lact +
Ceftin *Tab 250mg, 500mg, Susp (oral) 125mg/5ml, 250mg/5ml* **Generics** *Tab 250mg, 500mg*	**Early lyme disease:** 500mg PO bid for 20d; **bronchitis, tonsillitis, pharyngitis, sinusitis, skin infx:** 250mg PO bid; **pneumonia:** 500mg PO bid; **gonorrhea:** 1g PO x 1; **UTI:** 125–250mg PO bid for 7–10d; **CH** >3mo: 10–15mg/kg PO bid, max 1g/d

7.2.5 Cephalosporins - 3rd Generation

S (cephalosporins - 3rd generation): inferior to first generation cephalosporins against gram-positive cocci, but enhanced activity against gram-negative bacilli (see 2nd generation cephalosporins →147 plus most other enteric organisms) and Serratia marcescens. (ceftriaxone or cefotaxime: agents of choice in Tx of meningitis; ceftazidime: activity against Ps. aeruginosa); cefotaxime sodium-group: higher bactericidal effect against gram-negative germs (i.e. Klebsiella, H. influenza)
R: cefotaxime sodium-group: Enterococcus, Legionella, Chlamydia, Mycoplasma, Listeria, Clostridium diff.;
AE/CI: see Cephalosporins - 1st Generation →146

Cefotaxime	EHL 0.8–1.4h, PRC B, Lact +
Claforan *Inj 500mg/vial, 1g/vial, 2g/vial*	**Pneumonia, UTI, gynecologic, skin, intra-abdom., bone, joint, CNS infx, uncomplicated:** 1g IM/IV q12h; **moderate/severe:** 1–2g IM/IV q8h; **severe:** 2g IV q6–8h. **life-threatening:** 2g IV q4h, max 12g/d; **neonates** 1–4 wk: 50mg/kg IV q8h, **CH:** 1mo–12y: 50–180mg/kg/d IM/IV div q4–6h; DARF: GFR (ml/min): <20: 50%

Ceftazidime	EHL 1.6–2h, PRC B, Lact +
Fortaz *Inj 1g/vial, 2g/vial, 6g/vial* **Generics** *Inj 1g/vial, 2g/vial, 6g/vial*	**Unomplic. UTI:** 250mg IM/IV q12h; **skin infx, uncomplicated pneumonia:** 500mg–1g IM/IV q8h; **complicated UTI:** 500mg IM/IV q8–12h; **bone inx:** 2g IV q12h; **life-threatening infx:** 2g IV q8h; **CH** 1–2m 12.5–25mg/kg IV q12h; 2m–12y 10–33mg/kg IV q8h; **cystic fibrosis with pseudomonas infx:** 50–75mg/kg IV q8h; DARF: GFR (ml/min): 31–50: 1g IV q12h, 16–30: 1g IV q24h; 6–15: 500mg IV q24h, <5: 500mg IV q48h
Ceftriaxone	EHL 5–9h, PRC B, Lact +
Rocephin *Inj 250mg/vial, 1g/vial, 2g/vial, 10g/vial*	**UTI, respir. tract, intra-abdom. infx, sepsis, endocarditis, meningitis, lyme disease**: 1–2g IM/IV q24h or div q12h, max 4g/d; **gonorrhea:** 250mg IM x 1; **CH** 50–75mg/kg/d IM/IV div q12–24h, max 2g/d; **CH meningitis:** 100mg/kg/d div q12h, max 4g/d; DARF: not req

7.2.6 Cephalosporins - 3rd Generation - Oralcephalosporins

S/R (oral cephalosporins 3rd gen.): more effective and broader spectrum then 2nd gen. cephalosporins against gram-neg. bacteria; less effective against gram-positive bacteria
AE/CI: see Cephalosporins - 1st Generation →146

Cefixime	EHL 3–4h, PRC B, Lact ?
Suprax *Tab 400mg, Susp (oral) 100mg/5ml*	**Respiratory tract infx, UTI, pharyngitis, tonsillitis:** 400mg PO qd; **gonorrhea:** 400mg PO as single dose; **CH** >6mo: 8mg/kg/d qd or div bid; DARF: GFR (ml/min): >60: 100%, 21–60: 75%, <20: 50%

7.2.7 Cephalosporins - 4th Generation

S: wide antibacterial spectrum, Strepto- and Staphylococci (only methicillin susceptible ones); also aerobic gram-negatives like Enterobacter, E. coli, Klebsiella pneumoniae, Proteus mirabilis and Ps. aeruginosa
see Cephalosporins - 1st Generation →146

Cefepime	EHL 2h, PRC B, Lact ?
Maxipime *Inj 1g/vial, 2g/vial*	**Uncompl or complicated UTI, skin infx, mild-mod. pneumonia:** 0.5–1g IM/IV q12h; **intra-abdominal, severe pneumonia**: 2g IV q12h; **febrile neutropenia:** 2g IV q8h; **CH** 2mo–12y: 50mg/kg IV q12h; DARF: GFR (ml/ min): <11: 0.25–1g q24h, 11–29: 0.5–2g q24h

7.3 Carbapenems

S: almost all gram-positive and gram-negative bacteria
R: Mycoplasma, Chlamydia, Legionella, Ps. cepacia, Xanthonomas maltophilia, E. faecium
AE: N/V, diarrhea, liver enz.m, allergic reactions, complete blood count changes, CNS DO
CI: hypersensitivity to product ingredients, penicillins, cephalosporins, and other beta lactams

Ertapenem	EHL 4h, PRC B, Lact ?
Invanz *Inj 1g/vial*	**Abdominal, skin, lung infx:** 1g IM/IV qd x 5–14d; **CH** 3mo–12yo: 25mg/kg/d IM/IV div bid x 5–14d; >13yo: 1g IM/IV qd x 5–14d; DARF: GFR (ml/min) <30: 500mg qd; HD: 150mg suppl. if maint. given <6h prior to HD
Imipenem-Cilastatin	EHL 1h, PRC C, Lact ?
Primaxin *Inj 250mg/vial, 500mg/vial*	**Mild infx:** 250mg IV q6h; **moderate:** 500mg IV q8h; **severe:** 500mg q6h; **life threatening:** 1g IV q6–8h; max 4g/d; **CH** >3mo: 15–25mg/kg IV q6h; DARF: GFR (ml/min) 31–70 max 2g q6h, 21–30 max 1.5g q8h, 0–20 max 1g q12h

Meropenem	EHL 1h, PRC B, Lact ?
Merrem *Inj 500mg/vial, 1g/vial*	**Complicated UTI, skin infx, gyne infx, PID, comm. aquired pneumonia:** 500mg IV q8h; **nosocomial pneumonia, intra-abdominal infx, septicemia:** 1g IV q8h; **meningitis:** 2g IV q8h; **CH** 3–12y: 20–40mg/kg tid; DARF: GFR (ml/min) 26–50: 0.5–2g q12h; 10–25: 50% q12h; <10: 50% q24h

7.4 Glycopeptides

S: aerobic and anaerobic gram-positive bacteria, methicillin resistant S. aureus (MRSA)
R: all gram-negative Bacteria, Mycoplasma, Chlamydia
AE: allergic reactions, thrombophlebitis, ototoxicity, nephrotoxicity, complete blood count changes, red man/neck syndrome, N/ V; **CI:** hypersensitivity to product ingredients

Vancomycin	EHL 4–6h, PRC C, Lact + serum-lev. (mcg/ml): peak 30–40; trough 5–10
Vancocin *Cap 125mg, 250mg, Inj 500mg/vial, 1g/vial, 10g/vial* **Generics** *Inj 500mg/vial, 1g/vial*	**MRSA infx, other staphylococcal or streptococcal infx, endocarditis:** 500mg IV q6h or 1g IV q12h or 30mg/kg/d IV div q12; **CH** >1mo: 40mg/kg/d IV div q6h; **clostridium difficile diarrhea:** 125–500mg PO q6–8h for 7–10d; **CH:** 40mg/kg/d PO div tid–qid; DARF: GFR (ml/min): >50: 500mg IV q12h, 10–50: 500mg IV q24–48h, <10: 500mg IV q48–96h

7.5 Tetracyclines

S: many gram-pos. + gram-neg. bacteria, e.g. Chlamydia, Mycoplasma, Rickettsia, Yersinia, Borrelia, Leptospira, Treponema, Actinomyces
R: P. aeruginosa, Providencia, Serratia, Proteus, Morganella
AE: allergic skin reactions, phototoxic reactions, N/V/D, diziness, reversible irregularities in bone growth (children < 8y), irreversible tooth staining + crown deformation (**CH** < 8y), intracranial pressure ↑, complete blood count changes, superinfection by bacteria or yeasts
CI: hypersensitivity to tetracyclines, severe hepatic or renal dysfunction, children < 8y, pregnancy, lactation **CI** (doxycycline) myasthenia gravis

Demeclocycline	EHL 10–17h, PRC D, Lact +
Declomycin *Tab 150mg, 300mg*	**Infx general:** 150mg PO qid or 300mg PO bid; **SIADH:** 3.25–3.75mg/kg PO q6h; **CH** >8y: 8–12mg/kg/d PO div q6–12h; DARF: avoid
Doxycycline	EHL 12–24h, PRC D, Lact ?
Apo-Doxy *Cap 100mg, Tab 100mg* **Doxycin** *Cap 100mg, Tab 100mg* **Novo-Doxylin** *Cap 100mg, Tab 100mg* **Vibra-Tabs** *Cap 100mg, Tab 100mg* **Generics** *Cap 100mg, Tab 100mg*	**Infx general:** d1 100mg PO bid, then 100mg qd; upto 200mg PO qd or bid for severe infections; **acne, rosacea:** 100mg PO qd; **nongonococcal urethritis and chlamydial infx:** 100mg PO bid for 7d; **lyme disease:** 100mg PO bid for 14–21d; **PRO malaria:** 100mg PO qd, start 1–2d before travel, continue for 4wks after return; **early syphilis:** 100mg PO bid x 14d; DARF: not req
Minocycline	EHL 11–22h, PRC D, Lact +
Minocin *Cap 50mg, 100mg* **Generics** *Cap 50mg, 100mg*	**Infx general:** d1 200mg PO, then 100mg PO q12h; **CH** >8y: d1 4mg/kg PO, then 2mg/kg bid; **acne vulgaris:** d1 100mg PO, then 50mg PO qd, **rosacea:** 50–100mg PO qd x 6–8wks
Tetracycline	EHL 8–10h, PRC D, Lact +
Apo-Tetra *Cap 250mg* **Nu-Tetra** *Cap 250mg*	**Infx general:** 250–500mg PO qid; **CH** >8y: 25–50mg/kg/d PO div bid–qid, max 3g/d; **acne vulgaris:** ini 500mg PO bid, maint 250–500mg PO qd; **rosacea:** 500mg PO bid x 2wks, then 500mg PO qd until controlled, then 250mg Po qd x 3–4wks; **brucellosis:** 500mg PO q6h x 3wks with streptomycin; **early syphilis:** 500mg PO qid x 14d; **nongonococc. STD:**500mg PO qd x7d **lyme disease:** 500mg PO qid, DARF: GFR (ml/min) >50: q8–12h, 10–50: q12–24h, <10: q24h

Tigecycline	PRC D, Lact ?
Tygacil *Inj 50mg/5ml*	**Abdominal, skin infx:** ini 100mg IV then 50mg IV q12h x 5–14d qid; Liver disease class C Child-Pugh: decr. maint. by 50%

7.6 Macrolides

S: Streptococcus, Pneumoccous, Chlamydia, Legionella, Mycoplasma pneumoniae, Listeria, Actinomyces, Campylobacter, H. pylori, M. avium intracellulare (MAC)
R: Brucella, enteric bacteria, Nocardia, Mycoplasma hominis, B. fragilis, Fusobacteria, Pseudomonas;
MA/EF: (daptomycin) cyclic lipopeptide, binds Gram-positive bacterial membranes/ calcium-dependant manner, causes rapid depolarization of membrane potential, inhibition of protein, DNA, and RNA synthesis;
AE: allergic skin reactions, N/V/D, abdominal pain, cholestasis, headache
CI: hypersensitivity to product,
CI: (erythromycin estolate) liver disease, pregnancy
CI: (clarithromycin, erythromycin): use with astemizole, terfenadine, cisapride, pimozide

Azithromycin	EHL 11–57h, PRC B, Lact ?
Z-Pak *Tab 250mg* **Zithromax** *Tab 250mg, 600mg, Susp 100mg/5ml, 200mg/5ml, Inj 500mg/vial* **Generics** *Tab 250mg, 600mg, Susp 100mg/5ml, 200mg/5ml*	**upper/lower respiratory infection, skin infx, community-acquired pneumonia:** PO: 500mg PO on 1st day, then 250mg PO qd for 5d total; IV: 500mg IV qd for 2d, then 500mg PO qd for 7–10d total; **PID:** 500mg IV for 1day then 250mg PO qd for total 7days; **genitourin. infx, chlamydial infx:** 1g PO as single dose; **gonorrhea:** 2g PO as single dose; **PRO of M. avium complex:** 1.2g PO qwk; **CH otitis media:** 30mg/kg PO single dose or 10mg/kg PO qd for 3days; **CH comm. acq. pneumonia:** 10mg/kg PO as single dose then 5mg/kg/d for days 2–5, **CH pharyngits:** 12mg/kg PO qd for 5days, max 500mg/d; DARF: not req

Clarithromycin	EHL 3-7h, PRC C, Lact ?
Biaxin *Tab 250mg, 500mg, Susp (oral) 125mg/5ml, 250mg/5ml* **Biaxin XL** *Tab ext. release 500mg* **Generics** *Tab 250mg, 500mg*	**Upper/lower respiratiry infx, exacerbation of chronic bronchitis:** 250-500mg PO bid or 1g ext rel. PO qd for 7d; **pharyngitis/tonsilitis:** 250mg PO bid for 10d; **pneumonia, sinusitis:** 500mg PO bid or 1g ext. rel. PO qd for 14d; **uncomplicated skin infx:** 250mg PO bid; **PRO/Tx of mycobacterium avium complex:** 500mg PO bid in combination with **antimyco-bacterial drugs; h. pylori triple Tx:** 500mg PO bid with omeprazole 20mg bid and amoxicillin 1g bid for 10d; **CH** >6mo: 7.5mg/kg PO bid; DARF: GFR (ml/min) <30: 50%
Daptomycin	EHL 7.7-8.3h, PRC B, Lact ?
Cubicin *Inj 500mg/via*	**Complicated skin and skin structure infections:** 4 mg/kg IV qd x 7-14 days; **S. aureus bloodstream infections:** 6 mg/kg IV qd x 10-42 days DARF: GFR (ml/min) <30: q48h
Erythromycin Base	EHL no data, PRC B, Lact ?
Apo-Erythro Base *Tab 250mg* **Apo-Erythro E-C** *Cap 250mg, 333mg* **Erybid** *Tab ext. rel. 500mg* **Eryc** *Cap ext.rel. 250mg, 333mg* **PCE** *Tab 333mg*	**Respiratory, campylobacter jejuni, chlamydia, mycoplasma pneumoniae infx, nongonococcal urethritis, legionnaire's disease:** 250mg PO q6h or 333mg PO q8h or 500mg bid, max 4g/d; **CH:** 7.5-25mg/kg PO q6h or 15-25mg PO q12h; DARF: GFR (ml/min): <10: 50-75%, max 2g/d
Erythromycin Estolate	EHL no data, PRC B, Lact +
Generics *Cap 250mg*	250mg PO q6h or 333mg PO q8h or 500mg bid, max 4g/d; **CH:** 7.5-25mg/kg PO q6h or 15-25mg PO q12h DARF: GFR (ml/min): <10: 50-75%, max 2g/d

Erythromycin Ethylsuccinate	EHL no data, PRC B, Lact +
Apo-Erythro-ES *Tab 600mg* **E.E.S.** *Tab 600mg, Gran (oral) 200mg/5ml, Susp (oral) 200mg/5ml, 400mg/5ml* **Novo-Rythro ethylsuccinate** *Susp (oral) 200mg/5ml, 400mg/5ml*	400mg PO q6h, max 4g/d, **CH:** 12–40mg/kg PO q6h; DARF: GFR (ml/min): <10: 50–75%, max 2g/d
Erythromycin Ethylsuccinate + Sulfisoxazole	PRC C, Lact ?
Pediazole *Susp (oral) 200 + 600mg/5ml*	**CH >2m otitis media:** 50mg/kg/d erythromycin + 150mg/kg/d sulfisoxazole div tid–qid for 10d
Erythromycin Lactobionate	EHL no data, PRC B, Lact +
Generics *Inj 500mg/vial, 1g/vial*	**Infx:** 250–500mg IV q6h, or 15–20mg/kg/d IV div q6h, max 4g/d, **CH:** 20–40mg/kg/d IV div q6h, max 4g/d; DARF: GFR (ml/min): <10: 50–75%, max. 2g/d
Erythromycin Stearate	EHL no data, PRC B, Lact +
Apo-Erythro-S *Tab 250mg* **Generics** *Tab 250mg*	**Infx:** 250–500mg PO q6–12h
Spiramycin	EHL no data, PRC B, Lact +
Rovamycine *Cap 750,000U*	**Lung, oral, skin Infx:** 3,000,000–4,500,000 U PO bid; **Severe infection:** 6,000,000 to 7,500,000 U PO bid; **Gonorrhea:** 12,000,000 –13,500,000 U PO x 1; **CH:** 150,000 U/kg/d PO div bid–tid

7.7 Aminoglycosides

S: enteric bacteria, Pseudomonas, Staphylococcus, Serratia, Yersinia, Pasteurella, Brucella
R: Enterococcus, Anaerobic bacteria, Streptococcus, Pneumococcus
AE: nephrotoxicity, ototoxicity, neurotoxicity, neuromuscular blockage, paresthesia, renal damage, complete blood count changes, allergic reactions, N/V/D, diziness
CI: hypersensitivity to product ingredients
CI (paromomycin) intestinal obsruction

Amikacin	EHL no data, PRC D, Lact + serum-lev. (mcg/ml): peak: 30; trough: 5–10
Amikin *Inj 250mg/ml* **Generics** *Inj 250mg/ml*	**Gram-negative infx:** 15mg/kg/d IV/IM div bid, max 1.5g/d, max 15g total course; **neonates:** ini 10mg/kg, then 7.5mg/kg IM/IV q12h; DARF: GFR (ml/min) >50: 60–90% q12h, 10–50: 30–70% q12–18h, <10: 20–30% q24–48h
Gentamicin	EHL 2h, PRC C, Lact ? serum-level (mcg/ml): peak 5–10; trough <2
Garamycin *Inj 10mg/ml, 40mg/ml* **Generics** *Inj 0.8mg/ml, 1mg/ml, 1.2mg/ml, 1.6mg/ml, 10mg/ml, 40mg/ml*	**Gram-negative infx:** 3–6mg/kg/d IV/IM div tid, **neonates:** 2.5–3mg/kg IM/IV q12h; **CH:** 5–6mg/kg/d IM/IV div q8h; DARF: GFR (ml/min) 35–70: q12h, 24–34: q18h,16–23: q24; 10–15: q36h; 5–9: q48h
Paromomycin	PRC ?, Lact ?
Humatin *Cap 250mg*	**Intestinal amebiasis:** 25–35mg/kg/d div tid for 5–10days
Streptomycin	EHL 2.5h, PRC D, Lact +
Generics *Inj 1g/vial*	**Streptococcal endocarditis:** 1g IM/IV bid for 1wk, then 0.5g bid for 1wk; **TB:** 15mg/kg IM qd, max 1g/d, can reduce to 25mg/kg IM 2–3x/wk; **tularemia:** 1–2g/d div doses for 7–14dorafebrile for 5–7d; **plague:** 2–4g/d div doese until afebrile for 3days; **CH TB:** 20–40mg/kg IM qd, max 1g/d; DARF: GFR (ml/min) >50: 7.5mg/kg q24h, 10–50: 7.5mg/kg q24–72h, <10: 7.5mg/kg q72–96h
Tobramycin	EHL 2h, PRC D, Lact + serum-level (mcg/ml): peak 5–10; trough <2.
TOBI*Sol (inhal) 300mg/amp* **Generics***Inj 10mg/ml, 40mg/ml*	**Infx:** 3–5mg/kg/d IV/IM div tid; **cystic fibrosis/chronic P. aeruginosa:** 300mg inhal nedulizer bid for 28d, then 28d off, **neonates:** 4mg/kg/d IV div bid; **CH**: 6–7.5mg/kg/d IV/IM div tid–qid; ; DARF: GFR (ml/min): ini 1mg/kg IM/IV, >50: 60–90% q8–12h; 10–50:30–70%q12h–24,<10:20–30% q24– 48h

7.8 Lincosamides

S: Pneumo-, Staphylo-, Streptococcus, C. diphtheria, anaerobics, B. fragilis, Cl. perfringens
R: Enteric bacteria, P. aeruginosa, Entero-, Gono-, Meningococcus, H. influenza, Mycoplasma, Listeria; **AE:** N/V, diarrhea, pseudomembranous enterokolitis, allergic skin reactions, LFT↑, erythema exsudativum, thrombophlebitis (when used iv)
CI: caution with Myasthenia gravis, hypersensitivity to product ingredients, newborn
CI: (lincomycin) monilial infection

Clindamycin	EHL 1.5–5h, PRC B, Lact ?
Dalacin C *Cap 150mg, 300mg, Sol (oral) 75mg/5ml, Inj 150mg/ml* **Generics** *Cap 150mg, 300mg*	**Anaerobic and other infx:** 1.2–1.8g/d IV/IM div bid–qid, max 4.8g/d or 150–450mg PO qid; **CH** > 1mo: 20–40mg/kg/d IV div q6–8h or 8–20mg/kg/d PO div tid–qid; DARF: not req, reduce dose with hep. impairment

Lincomycin	PRC A, Lact ?
Lincocin *Inj 300mg/ml*	**Gram positive infection:** 600mg IM q12–24h, 600mg IV q8–12h, **CH:** 10mg/kg IM q12–24h, 10–20mg/kg/d IV div q8–12h

7.9 Chloramphenicol

S: wide range of gram-positive and gram-negative organisms (note: because of its toxicity limited clinical use)
AE: N/V, irreversible aplastic anemia, rash, myelosuppression, gray baby syndrom
CI: hypersensitivity to chloramphenicol products

Chloramphenicol	EHL 1.6–3.3h, PRC C, Lact -
Generic *Inj 1g/vial*	**Infx:** 50mg/kg/d IV div q6h, max 100mg/kg/d; **CH** >4wk: 50mg/kg/d IV div q6h, upto 100mg/kg/d IV div q6h, DARF: not req

7.10 Quinolones

7.10.1 Fluoroquinolones 1st Group

Group I: indicated almost exclusively for UTI; **S:** enteric bacteria, Campylobacter, Salmonella, Shigella, Gonococcus; **R:** Anaerobic bacteria, Chlamydia, Mycoplasma, E. faecium, Ureaplasma; **AE** (quinolones): allergic skin reactions, phototoxicity, muscle weakness, muscle pain, tachycardia, BP↓, CNS disturbances, cholestasis, hepatitis, cristalluria; **AE** (norfloxacin): dizziness, nausea, headache, abdominal cramping; **CI** (norfloxacin): hypersensitivity to norfloxacin or other fluoroquinolones

Norfloxacin	EHL 2–4h, PRC C, Lact ?
Apo-Norflox *Tab 400mg* **Generics** *Tab 400mg*	**Simple UTI:** 400mg PO bid for 3d; **complicated UTI:** 400mg PO bid for 10–21d; **traveler's diarrhea:** 400mg PO bid for 3d; **gonorrhea:** 800mg PO as single dose; DARF: GFR (ml/min) <30: 400mg PO qd

7.10.2 Fluoroquinolones - 2nd Group

S: high activity vs. gram-negatives like enterobacteria + H. influenzae, different activity vs. pseudomonas, low activity vs. Staphylo-, Pneumo-, Enterococcus, Mycoplasma, Chlamydia AE/**CI** (quinolones): see Fluoroquinolones - 1st Group →159; **AE** (ciprofloxacin): dizziness, headache, diarrhea; **AE** (ofloxacin): nausea, insomnia, headache, dizziness, diarrhea; **CI** (ciproflox., oflox.): hypersensitivity to product ingredients/quinolones

Ciprofloxacin	EHL 3–6h, PRC C, Lact -
Apo-Ciproflox *Tab 100mg, 250mg, 500mg, 750mg* **Cipro** *Tab 250mg, 500mg, 750mg, Susp (oral) 500mg/5ml, Inj 2mg/ml, 10mg/ml* **Cipro XL** *Tab ext. rel. 500mg, 1,000mg* **Generics** *Tab 250mg, 500mg, 750mg*	**Simple UTI:** 250mg PO bid for 3d or ext. rel. 500mg PO qd x 3d; **UTI, bone and joint infx:** 250–500mg PO bid or 400v1200mg IV/d div bid–tid; **chronic bacterial prostatitis:** 500mg PO bid for 28d; **traveler's diarrhea:** 500mg PO bid for 5–7d; **typhoid fever:** 500mg PO bid for 10d; DARF: GFR (ml/min) 30–50: 250–500mg PO q12h; 5–29: 250–500mg PO q18h or 200–400mg IV q18–24h

Ofloxacin	EHL 5–7.5h, PRC C, Lact -
Apo-Oflox *Tab 200mg, 300mg, 400mg* **Floxin** *Tab 300mg, 400mg*	**Infx:** 300–400mg PO bid for 7–14d; **prostatitis:** 300–400mg PO bid for 6wk; DARF: GFR (ml/min): 20–50: 100% q24h, <20: 50% q24h

7.10.3 Fluoroquinolones - 3rd Group

S: additional activity Staphylo-, Pneumo-, Streptococcus, Chlamydia, Mycoplasma
AE, CI (quinolones): see Fluoroquinolones - 1st Group →159
AE (levofloxacin): N/V, diarrhea, headache
CI (levofloxacin): hypersensitivity to levofloxacin products/quinolones

Levofloxacin	EHL 6–8h, PRC C, Lact -
Levaquin *Tab 250mg, 500mg, 750mg Inj 5mg/ml, 25mg/ml*	**Infx:** 250–500mg PO/IV qd for 3–14d; **Complicated skin infx.:** 500mg PO/IV bid for 10–14d; DARF: ini 250– 500mg PO/IV, then GFR (ml/min): 20–49: 250mg q24h; 10–19: 250mg q48h; <10, dialysis: 250mg q48h

7.10.4 Fluoroquinolones - 4th Group

S: additional activity against anaerobic bacteria
AE, CI (quinolones): see Fluoroquinolones - 1st Group →159
AE (gemifloxacin): diarrhea, rash, nausea, headache, abdominal pain
AE (moxifloxacin): nausea, diarrhea, headache, dizziness
CI (gemifloxacin, moxifloxacin): hypersensitivity to product ingredients/quinolones

Gemifloxacin	EHL 8-15h, PRC C
Factive *Tab 320mg*	**Infx:** 320mg PO qd for 5d; DARF: CrCl <40ml/min: 160mg PO qd
Moxifloxacin	EHL 9–16h, PRC C
Avelox *Tab 400mg, Inj 400mg/250ml*	**Infx:** 400mg PO qd for 5–10d; DARF: not req

7.11 Urinary Tract Antiseptics

AE (methenamine): N/V, diarrhea, cramping; **AE** (nitrofurantoin): pulmonary hypersensitivity, hemolytic anemia, peripheral neuropathy, N/V/D
CI (methenamine): severe dehydration, renal or hepatic insufficiency, use of sulfonamides, hypersensitivity to methenamine**CI** (nitrofurantoin): anuria, CrCl <60ml/min, pregnant patients (38–42wk gestation), neonates, hypersensitivity to nitrofurantoin

Methenamine Mandelate	EHL 4.3h, PRC C, Lact +
Mandelamine *Tab 500mg*	**Tx/PRO of recurrent or chronic UTI:** 1g PO qid; **CH** 6–12y: 50–75mg/kg/d div qid; DARF: GFR (ml/min): >50: 100%; <50: not rated

Nitrofurantoin	EHL 20min–1h, PRC B, Lact
Macrobid *Cap100mg* **Macrodantin** *Cap 50mg, 100mg* **Novo-Furantoin** *Cap 50mg, 100mg* **Generics** *Cap 50mg, 100mg*	**UTI:** 50–100mg PO qid for 7d or at least 3d after sterile urine; **CH** >1mo: 5–7mg/kg/d PO div qid for 7d or at least 3d after sterile urine; DARF: GFR (ml/min): >50: 100%; <50: not rated

7.12 Folate Antagonists

7.12.1 Sulfonamides

S (sulfonamids, including co-trimoxazole): active against selected enterobacteria, chlamydia, Pneumocystis, nocardia
AE (sulfonamids): N/V, allergic reactions, erythema exudativum multiforme, photosensitivity, renal damage, complete blood count changes; **AE** (sulfadiazine): crystalluria, RF; **AE** (sulfamethoxazole): crystalluria, blood dyscrasias
AE (sulfisoxazole): N/V, diarrhea, blood dyscrasias
CI: hypersensitivity to sulfonamides, previous erythema exudativum, severe hepatic + renal dysfunction, newborns, infants < 2mo, patients receiving methenamine

Sulfamethoxazole	EHL 10h, PRC C, Lact ?
Generics *Tab 500mg*	**UTI:** ini 2g, then 1g PO bid–tid; **CH** > 2mo: ini 50–60mg/kg, then 25–30mg/kg PO bid, max 75mg/kg/d

Sulfisoxazole	EHL 7h, PRC C, Lact ?
Sulfizole *Tab 500mg* **Generics** *Tab 500mg*	**UTI:** ini 2–4g, then 4–8g/d PO div q4–6h; **CH** >2mo: ini 75mg/kg, then 150mg/kg/d PO div q4–6h; DARF: GFR (ml/min): >50: q6h; 10–49: q8–12h; <10: q12–24h

7.12.2 Trimethoprim

AE: rash, pruritus, effects of folate deficiency (megaloblastic anemia, leukopenia, granulozytopenia)
CI: hypersensitivity to trimethoprim products, megaloblastic anemia (folate deficiency)

Trimethoprim	EHL 5–17h, PRC C, Lact +
Generics *Tab 100mg, 200mg*	**Uncomplicated UTI:** 100mg PO q12h or 200mg PO q24h; DARF: GFR (ml/min): 15–30: 50mg PO q12h; <15: not rated

7.12.3 Co-trimoxazole

S: almost all aerobic bacteria, Pneumocystis carinii; **R:** P. aeruginosa, Treponema, Clostridium, Leptospiria, Rickettsia, Chlamydia psittaci, Mycoplasma
AE: exanthema, photodermatosis, Lyell-Syndrome, complete blood count changes, hemolytic anemia, N/V, rash, urticaria
CI: hypersensitivity to sulfonamides or trimethoprim, glucose-6-phosphat-dehydrogenase deficiency, severe complete blood count change, severe renal insufficiency, infants < 2mo

Sulfamethoxazole + Trimethoprim (Co-trimoxazole)	PRC C, Lact ?
Apo-Sulfatrim *Tab 100+20mg, 400+ 80mg, 800+160mg, Susp 200+40mg/5ml* **Novo-Trimel** *Tab 400+80mg, 800+160mg Susp 200+40mg/5ml* **Nu-Cotrimox** *Tab 400+80mg, 800+160mg Susp 200+40mg/5ml* **Protrin** *Tab 400+80mg, 800+160mg* **Septra** *Inj 400+80mg/5ml* **Trisulfa** *Tab 400+80mg*	**UTI:** 800mg + 160mg PO q12h for 3–7d; **exacerbation of chronic bronchitis:** 800mg + 160mg PO q12h for 14d; **travelers' diarrhea:** 800mg + 160mg PO q12h for 5d; **pneumocystis Tx:** 15–20 (TMP) + 75–100 (SMZ) mg/kg/ d IV div q6–8h or PO div q6h for 14–21d; **pneumocystis PRO:** 800mg + 160mg PO qd; **CH:** 40–100mg/kg + 8–20mg/kg PO/IV; DARF: GFR (ml/min): > 30: 100%; 15–30: 50%, <30: not rated

7.13 Nitroimidazoles

S: obligate anaerobic bacteria (i.e. Bacteroides, Clostridium), Campylobacter, H. pylori, Gardnerella vaginalis, Trichomonas vaginalis, Giardia lamblia, Entamoeba histolytica
R: all aerobic and facultative anaerobic bacteria, Actinomyces, Propionibacteria
AE: GI disturbances, bitter/metallic taste, CNS-disturbances, seizures, allergic skin reactions, alcohol intolerance; **CI:** hypersensitivity to metronidazole

Metronidazole	EHL 6–11h, PRC B, Lact ?
Flagyl *Cap 500mg* **Florazole ER** *Tab ext. release 750mg* **Generics** *Tab 250mg* *Inj 5mg/ml*	**Anaerobic bacterial infx:** 500mg PO/IV q8h or 1.5g IV q24h; **Bacterial vaginosis:** 500mg PO bid x 7d; **Trichomoniasis:** 2g PO x 1 or 250mg PO bid x 10d; **Amebiasis:** 750mg PO q8h x 5–7d; **Giardiasis:** 250mg PO bid x 5–7d; **pseudomembranous colitis:** 500mg PO tid; tri; **CH anaerobic bacterial infx:** ini 15mg/kg IV, then 7.5mg/kg IV bid or 30mg/kg/d PO div qid; DARF: GFR (ml/min) >10: 100%, <10: 50%

7.14 Streptogramines

S: all gram-positive cocci, incl. MRSA, E. faecium, penicillin-G-resistent Pneumococcus, Mor. catarrhalis, Legionella, Mycoplasma pneumoniae, Chlamydia, Prevotella, Fusobacteria, Peptostreptococcus, Clostridia; **R:** H. influenza, E. faecalis, B. fragilis
AE: vein irritation, pruritus, erythema and burning on the face and upper body, N/V, arthralgia, myalgia, transaminases↑, bilirubin↑, alkaline phosphatase↑
CI: severe hepatic insufficiency, combination with drugs that prolong QT interval, hypersensitivity to dalfopristin/quinupristin/ streptogramins

Dalfopristin + Quinupristin PRC B, Lact ?

Synercid *Inj 350mg/vial + 150mg/vial*	**Vancomycin-resistant E. faecium infx:** 7.5mg/kg IV q8h; **complicated staphyl. skin infx:** 7.5mg/kg IV q12h; DARF: not req

7.15 Other Antimicrobials

AE (fosfomycin): diarrhea, headache, N/V; **AE** (linezolid): diarrhea, headache, nausea
CI (fosfomycin, linezolid): hypersensitivity to product ingredients

Fosfomycin EHL 5.7 (+/- 2.8)h, PRC B, Lact ?

Monurol *Susp 3g/pkt*	**UTI:** 3g PO as single dose

Linezolid EHL 5h, PRC N, Lact ?

Zyvoxam *Tab 600mg, Inj 2mg/ml*	**MRSA, vancomycin-resistant E. faecium infx:** 600mg IV/PO q12h for 14–28 d; **complicated skin infx, pneumonia**: 600mg IV/PO q12h for 10–14d; **uncompl. skin infx:** 400mg PO q12h for 10–14d; DARF: not req

7.16 Antimycobacterials

7.16.1 Antituberculosis Drugs - Single Ingredient Drugs

S (ethambutol): M. tuberculosis, M. kansasii, M. avium-intracellulare
S (isoniazid): M. tuberculosis, M. kansasii
S (pyrazinamide): M. tuberculosis
S (rifampicin): M. tuberculosis, gram-positive cocci, Legionella, Chlamydia, M. lepra, Meningococcus, Gonococcus, H. influenza, Bacteroides
S (streptomycin): M.tuberculosis, Brucella, Yersinia pestis, Francisella tularensis

AE (ethambutol): optic neuritis, transaminases↑, allergic reactions;
AE (isoniazid): peripheral neuropathy, transaminases↑, hepatotoxicity, acne, leukopenia, microhematuria;
AE (pyrazinamide): hyperuricemia, vomiting, transaminases↑, liver toxicity, disturbances of hematopoiesis, mild nausea + anorexia, arthralgia;
AE (rifampicin): transaminases↑, cholestasis, red discoloration of the urine, neutropenia, thrombopenia, RF
AE (streptomycin): nephrotoxicity, neurotoxicity, hypersensitivity, ototoxicity
CI (ethambutol): optic neuritis, hypersensitivity to ethambutol products
CI (isoniazid): acute liver disease, previous isoniazid-associated hepatitis
CI (pyrazinamide): severe hepatic dysfunction, hypersensitivity to pyrazinamide products, acute gout
CI (rifampicin): severe hepatic dysfunction
CI (streptomycin): severe renal insufficiency, inner ear damage, hypersensitivity to streptomycin/aminoglycosides

Ethambutol	EHL 2.5–4h, PRC B, Lact +
Etibi *Tab 100mg, 400mg*	**TB:** 15–25mg/kg PO qd **mycobacterium avium complex:** 15–25mg/kg PO qd, **CH** see adults; DARF: GFR (ml/min) 10–50: q24–36h, <10: q48h
Isoniazid	EHL 0.7–4h, PRC C, Lact +
Isotamine *Tab 300mg Syr 50mg/5ml* **Generics** *Tab 50mg,100mg, 300mg, Syr 50mg/5ml*	**TB Tx:** 5–10mg/kg PO/IM qd, max 300mg/d PO or 15mg/kg, max 900mg 2x/wk, **CH:** 10–20mg/kg/d PO, max 300mg; **TB PRO:** 300mg PO qd, **CH:** 10–15mg/kg/d PO, max 300mg; DARF: GFR (ml/min) >10: 100%, <10: 50%
Pyrazinamide	EHL 9–23h, PRC C, Lact ?
Tebrazid *Tab 500mg*	**TB Tx:** 15–30mg/kg PO qd, max 2g/d or 50–70mg/dose, max 4g/dose 2x/wk; **CH** see adults; DARF: endstage RF: 12–20mg/kg/d
Rifampin	EHL 3h, PRC C, Lact +
Rifadin *Cap 150mg, 300mg* **Rofact** *Cap 150mg, 300mg*	**TB:** 10mg/kg PO qd, max 600mg/d, **meningococcal PRO:** 600mg PO bid for 2d, **CH TB:** 10–20mg/kg PO/IV qd, max 600mg/d; **CH meningococcal PRO:** 10mg/kg PO bid for 2d

Streptomycin	EHL 2.5h, PRC D, Lact +
Generics *Inj 1g/vial*	**TB:** 15mg/kg IM qd, max 1g/d or 25–30mg/kg IM max 1.5g/d biw–tiw; **CH TB:** 20–40mg/kg IM qd, max 1g/d; DARF: GFR (ml/min) >50: 100% q24h, 10–50: 100% q24–72h, <10: 100% q72–96h

7.16.2 Antituberculosis Drugs - Combinations

Isoniazid + Pyrazinamide + Rifampin	
Rifater *Tab 50mg + 300mg + 120mg*	**TB:** > 55kg: 6 Tab PO qd; 45–54kg: 5 Tab PO qd, < 44kg: 4 Tab PO qd

7.16.3 Other Antimycobacterials

S (dapsone): M. tuberculosis, M. leprae, Pneumocystis carinii
S (rifabutin): M. tuberculosis, M. marinum, M. kansasii, M. leprae, M. avium-intracellulare, gram-positive cocci, Legionella, Chlamydia, Gonococcus
AE (dapsone): dose-related hemolysis, methemoglobinemia, peripheral neuropathy, N/V
AE (rifabutin): red-orange discoloration of urine, N/V, liver enzymesm, jaundice, anemia, leukopenia, eosinophilia, neutropenia, thrombopenia, fever, skin discoloration, reversible uveitis, rash
CI (dapsone): hypersensitivity to dapsone products
CI (rifabutin): hypersensitivity to other rifamycins

Dapsone	EHL 10–50h, PRC C, Lact -
Generics *Tab 100mg*	**Leprosy:** 50–100mg PO qd with other anti-leprosy drugs; **CH:** 1–2mg/kg/d PO, max 100mg/d; **pneumocystis PRO:** 100mg PO qd; **pneumocystis Tx:** 100mg PO qd; **CH:** 2mg/kg/d PO, max 100mg/d
Rifabutin	EHL 45h, PRC B, Lact ?
Mycobutin *Cap 150mg*	**Mycobacterium avium PRO:** 300mg PO qd or 150mg PO bid; **mycobacterium avium Tx:** 300mg PO qd in combination with a macrolide

7.17 Antivirals

7.17.1 Anti-CMV Drugs

MA/Ind (ganciclovir, valgancicl.): nucleoside analogue, inhibition of DNA synthesis of CMV
AE (ganciclovir): neutropenia, thrombopenia, fever, headache, nausea
AE (valganciclovir): diarrhea, neutropenia, thrombocytopenia, anemia, fever, headache, nausea, abdominal pain, insomnia, peripheral neuropathy
CI (ganciclovir): severe leuko- or thrombopenia, children and adolescents < 18
CI (valganciclovir): hypersensitivity to valganciclovir or ganciclovir

Ganciclovir	EHL 2.5–5h, PRC C, Lact ?
Cytovene *Cap 250mg, 500mg, Inj 500mg/vial*	**CMV retinitis:** 5 mg/kg IV bid for 14–21 d, then 5mg/kg IV qd or 1g PO tid; **CMV PRO in AIDS:** 1g PO tid; DARF: see Prod Info
Valganciclovir	EHL 4h, PRC C, Lact -
Valcyte *Tab 450mg*	**CMV retinitis**: ini 900mg PO bid for 21d, then 900mg qd; DARF: GFR (ml/min): >60: 100%; 40–59: ini 450mg bid, then 450mg qd; 25–39: ini 450mg qd, then 450mg qod; 10–24: ini 450mg qod, then 450mg biw

7.17.2 Anti-Herpetic Drugs

MA/Ind (acyclovir): inhibition of the viral DNA-polymerase; herpes simplex, varicella zoster
MA/Ind (famciclovir): inhibition of the DNA-Polymerase; herpes genitalis, varicella zoster
MA/Ind (valacyclovir): better resorption than acyclovir, varicella zoster infx
AE (acyclovir): renal dysfunction, exanthema, complete blood count changes, N/V headache, rash, phlebitis;
AE (famciclovir): headache, dizziness, diarrhea;
AE (valacyclovir): headache, N/V
CI (famciclovir): hypersensitivity to famciclovir or penciclovir;
CI (acyclovir): hypersensitivity to acyclovir;
CI (valacyclovir): hypersensitivity to valacyclovir or acyclovir

Acyclovir	EHL 3h, PRC B, Lact ?
Zovirax *Tab 200mg, 400mg, 800mg, Susp 200mg/5ml* **Generics** *Tab 200mg, 400mg, 800mg, Inj 500mg/vial*	**CMV infx:** 500mg/square meter IV q8h; **herpes simplex encephalitis:** 10mg/kg IV q8h for 10d; **mucocutaneous herpes:** 5–10mg/kg IV q8h for 5–7d; **varicella zoster in immunocompromised patients:** 10–12mg/kg IV q8h for 7–14d; **varicella zoster in immunocompetent patients:** 5mg/kg IV q8h for 5–7d or 800mg PO q4h for7–10d; **ini herpes genitalis:** 200mg PO 5 x/d for 7–10d; **recurrent herpes genitalis:** 400mg PO bid for up to 12 mo; **chickenpox:** 800mg PO qid for 5d; DARF: GFR (ml/ min): >50: 100% q8h (IV), 25–50: 100% q12h (IV), 10–25: 100% q24h (IV), 0–10: 50% q24h (IV)

Famciclovir	EHL 2–2.3h, PRC B, Lact ?
Famvir *Tab 125mg, 250mg, 500mg* **Generics** *Tab 125mg, 250mg, 500mg*	**Herpes simplex in AIDS:** 500mg PO bid for 7d; **recurrent genital herpes:** 125mg PO bid for 5d; **herpes PRO:** 250 mg PO bid; **herpes zoster:** 500mg PO q8h for7d; DARF: see Prod Info

Valacyclovir	EHL 2.5–3.6h, PRC B, Lact -
Valtrex *Tab 500mg*	**Herpes zoster:** 1g PO tid for 7 d; **ini. genital herpes:** 1g PO bid for 10 d; **recurrent genital herpes:** 500mg PO bid for 5d; **herpes PRO:** 500–1,000 mg PO qd; DARF: see Prod Info

7.17.3 Anti-Influenza Drugs

MA/Ind (amantadine): prevents uncoating and maturation of influenza viruses
MA/Ind (zanamivir): inhibition of the viral neuraminidase, inhibition of the release of newly built influenza A + B viruses;
AE (amantadine): nausea, dizziness, insomnia;
AE (oseltamivir): N/V, bronchitis, insomnia, vertigo;
AE (zanamivir): respiratory symptoms, thrombotic thrombocytopenic purpura, hemolytic uremic syndrome
CI (amantadine, oseltamivir, zanamivir): hypersensitivity to product ingredients

Amantadine	EHL 10–14h, PRC C, Lact -
Endantadine *Cap 100mg* **Symmetrel** *Cap 100mg, Syr 50mg/5ml* **Generics** *Cap 100mg*	**Influenza A:** 100mg PO bid; **CH** 1–9 yr or <40kg: 5mg/kg/ d PO, max. 150mg/d div bid, 10 yr and older: 100mg PO bid; **Parkinsonism**; DARF: ini 200mg, then GFR (ml/ min) 30–50: 100mg qd, 15–29: 100mg qod, <15: 200mg q7d,

Oseltamivir	EHL 1–3h, PRC C, Lact ?
Tamiflu *Cap 75mg, Susp (oral) 12mg/ml*	**Influenza A, B Tx:** 75mg PO bid for 5d; **Influenza A, B PRO:** 75mg PO qd; DARF: GFR (ml/min) <30: 75mg qd

Zanamivir	EHL 1.6–5.1h, PRC B, Lact ?
Relenza *Cap (inhal) 5mg*	**Influenza A, B Tx:** 2 inhal bid for 5d; **CH** >7 yr: see adults; DARF: not req

7.17.4 Interferons

MA/EF: antiviral, growth inhibiting and immune regulatory effects
AE: fever, sweating, chills, tiredness, joint and soft-tissue pains, complete blood count changes, cardiac arrhythmias, depression, tremors, convulsions, paresthesia, GI disturbances, hair loss, exanthema, pruritus; **AE** (interferon alfacon-1): flu like symptoms, depression, N/V, granulocytopenia; **AE** (interferon alfa-2b + Ribavirin): anemia, insomnia, irritability, depression, headache, nausea
CI: coronary diseases, CNS DO, severe hepatic dysfunction, RF, severe bone marrow damage
CI (interferon alfacon-1): hypersensitivity to alfa interferons/E. coli derived products
CI (interferon alfa-2b + Ribavirin): hypersensitivity to ribavirin or alfa interferon, autoimmune hepatitis

Interferon alfa 2a	EHL 3.7–8.5 h
Roferon A *Inj 3, 9, 18 million U/vial*	**Chronic hepatitis C:** 3 mio U 3x/wk SC/IM
Interferon alfa 2b	EHL 2–3 h
Intron A *Inj 3,10,18, 30, 60 million U/vial*	**Chronic hepatitis B:** 5 mio U qd or 10 mio U 3x/wk SC/ IM for 16 wk; **chronic hepatitis C:** 3 mio U SC/IM 3x/wk upto 18months
Interferon alfacon-1	EHL 0.5–7h, PRC C, Lact ?
Infergen *Inj 0.03mg/ml*	**Chronic hepatitis C:** 9mcg SC 3x/wk for 24 wk; 15mcg SC 3x/wk for 24 wk for relapse or no response-9mcg dose
Interferon beta 1a	EHL 69h, PRC C, Lact ?
Avonex *Inj 33mcg/vial* **Rebif** *Syr 22mcg/0.5ml, 44mcg/0.5ml* *Inj 11mcq/vial, 44mcg/vial*	**Relapsing form of multiple sclerosis:** (Avenox): 30mcg IM qwk; (Rebif): 22–44mcg SC tiw
Interferon beta 1b	PRC C , Lact ?
Betaseron *Inj 0.3mg/vial*	**Relapsing form of multiple sclerosis:** ini 0.25mg sc qod
Peginterferon alfa 2a	EHL 60h, PRC C, Lact ?
Pegasys *Syr 180mcg/0.5ml, Inj 180mcg/ml*	**Chronic hepatitis C:** 180mcg SC qwk

Peginterferon alfa-2a + Ribavirin	PRC X, Lact ?
Pegasys RBV *Syr 180mcg/0.5ml, Inj 180mcg/ml, Cap 200mg*	**Chronic hepatitis C:** (Genotype 1, 4): 180 µg SC qwk (Pegasys) and Ribavirin 1000mg (<75kg) or 1200mg (>75kg) PO daily div bid for 48 weeks; (Genotype 2, 3): 180 µg SC qwk (Pegasys) and Ribavirin 800mg PO daily div bid for 24 weeks
Peginterferon alfa 2b	EHL 40h, PRC C, Lact ?
Unitron PEG *Inj 74mcg/vial, 118.4mcg/vial, 177.6mcg/vial, 222mcg/vial*	**Chronic hepatitis C:** 1mcg/kg/wk SC;
Peginterferon alfa 2b + Ribavirin	PRC X, Lact ?
Pegetron *Inj 74mcg/vial, 118.4mcg/vial, 177.6mcg/vial, 222mcg/vial, + Cap 200mg*	**Chronic hepatitis C:** 1.5 mcg/kg SC qwk (Peginterferon alfa-2b) and Ribavirin 800 mg (<64kg), 1000mg (64-85kg), or 1200mg (>85kg) PO daily div bid

7.17.5 Anti-Respiratory-Syncytial-Virus Drugs

MA/Ind (ribavirin): guanosine analogue, inhibition of the RNA polymerase of HCV
AE (palivizumab): rash, rhinitis, upper respiratory tract infx;
AE (ribavirin): rash, respiratory dysfunction, conjunctivitis;
CI (ribavirin): hypersensitivity to ribavirin products
CI (palivizumab): hypersensitivity to palivizumab products

Palivizumab	EHL 20d (age<24m), 18d (adults), PRC C
Synagis *Inj 50mg/vial, 100mg/vial*	**Prevention of severe respiratory syncytial virus infx:** 15mg/kg IM
Ribavirin	EHL Inhal 9.5h, IV/PO 24–36h, PRC X, Lact ?
Virazole *Sol (inhal) 6g/vial*	**Severe respiratory syncytial virus infx:** aerosol 12h/d for 3d; **CH** see adults

7.17.6 Anti-Hepatitis B Drug

MA (entecavir): guanosine nucleoside analogue, inhibits all three functional activities of the HBV polymerase; (adefovir): nucleoside phosphonate analog of adenosine monophosphate, results in DNA chain termination.; (telbivudine): synthetic thymidine nucleoside analogue, activity against HBV DNA polymerase
AE (adefovir): asthenia, headache, and abdominal pain, nephrotoxicity; (entecavir): headache, fatigue, dizziness, nausea; (telbivudine): CK elevation, upper respiratory tract infection, nasopharyngitis, fatigue, headache, dizziness, myalgia
CI: hypersensitivity to product

Adefovir	EHL 7.5h, PRC C, Lact ?
Hepsera *Tab 10mg*	**HBV infx**: 10mg PO qd; DARF: CrCL 20–49: give q48h; 10–19: give q72h; HD: give q7d after HD
Entecavir	EHL 128–149h, PRC C, Lact +
Baraclude *Tab 0.5mg, Sol (oral) 0.05mg/ml*	**HBV infx:** nucleoside-naive: 0.5mg PO qd; DARF: CrCl 30–50: 0.25mg qd, 10–30: 0.15mg qd; <10: 0.05mg qd; HD: 0.05mg qd after HD; lamivudine-refractory: 1mg PO qd; DARF: CrCl 30–50: 0.5mg qd, 10–30: 0.3mg qd; <10: 0.1mg qd; HD: 0.1mg qd after HD
Lamivudine (3TC)	EHL 3–7h, PRC C Lact ?
3TC *Tab 150mg, Sol (oral) 10mg/ml* **Heptovir** *Tab 100mg, Sol (oral) 5mg/ml*	**HBV infx:** 100mg PO qd, **CH** 3 mo–16 yr: DARF: CrCl: 30-50: ini 100mg then 50mg qd; 15-30: ini 100mg then 25mg qd; 5-15: ini 35mg then 15mg qd; <5: ini 35mg then 10mg qd
Telbivudine	EHL 40-49h, PRC B, Lact ?
Sebivo *Tab 600mg*	**HBV infx:** 600mg PO qd; DARF: CrCl >50: 600mg qd; 30–49: 600mg q48h; <30 (not requiring dialysis) 600 mg q72h; ESRD: 600mg q96h

7.17.7 Anti-HIV Drugs: Nucleoside Reverse Transcriptase Inhibitors

MA/Ind (nucleoside analogues): blockage of the transformation of RNA into DNA through chemically altered nucleosides in HIV-infx; **MA** (emtricitabine): nucleotide/nucleoside reverse transcriptase inhibitor; **AE** (abacavir): N/V, fatigue, fever, headache, diarrhea, loss of appetite, lactic acidosis/severe hepatomegaly with steatosis, hypersensitivity reactions (some fatal); **AE** (didanosine, stavudine): polyneuropathy, pancreatitis, diarrhea, exanthema; **AE** (lamivudine): headache, N/V, pancreatitis, lactic acidosis/hepatomegaly, fatigue; **AE** (zalcitabine): polyneuropathy, dermatitis, mucositis, pancreatitis, granulocytopenia, anemia; **AE** (zidovudine): anemia, leukopenia, myopathy, nausea, headache; **CI** (abacavir): severe hepatic dysfunction, hypersensitivity to abacavir products **CI** (didanosine): acute pancreatitis, combination with rifampicin, hypersensitivity to product ingredients; **CI** (lamivudine): hypersensitivity; **CI** (stavudine): hypersensitivity to product ingredients; **CI** (zalcitabine): polyneuropathy, pancreatitis, hypersensitivity to product ingredients; **CI** (zidovudine): leukopenia<750/µl, Hb<7.5g/dl, hypersensitivity

Abacavir (ABC)	EHL 1–2h, PRC C, Lact -
Ziagen *Tab 300mg, Sol (oral) 20mg/ml*	**HIV infx:** 300mg PO bid in combination with other antiretroviral drugs; **CH** 3 mo–16 yr: 8mg/kg PO bid, max. 300mg PO bid; DARF: not req
Abacavir + Lamivudine + Zidovudine	PRC C, Lact +
Trizivir *Tab 300 + 150 + 300mg*	**HIV infx**: 1 tab PO bid; DARF: see indiv drugs
Didanosine (ddI)	EHL 1.3–1.5h, PRC B, Lact ?
Videx *Tab (chew) 25mg, 50mg, 100mg, 150mg, Sol (oral) 4g/240ml, Tab ent. coated 125mg, 200mg, 250mg, 400mg*	**HIV infx:** >60kg: 400mg PO qd or 200mg PO bid as Tab or 250mg PO bid buffered powder; <60kg: 250mg PO qd or 125mg PO bid as Tab or 167mg PO bid buffered powder in combination with other antiretroviral drugs; **CH:** 120mg/square meter PO bid; DARF: see Prod Info
Emtricitabine	EHL 10h, PRC B, Lact +
Emtriva *Tab 200mg*	**HIV infx:** 200mg PO qd; DARF: CrCl (ml/min): 30–49: give q48h; 15–29: give q72h; <15: give q96h; **CH** <3mo: 3mg/kg PO qd; 3mo–17yo: 6mg/kgPO qd
Emtricitabine + Tenofovir	PRC B, Lact +
Truvada *Tab 200mg + 300mg*	**HIV infx:** 1 tab PO qd; DARF: CrCL (ml/min): 30–49: give q48h, <30: contraindicated

Lamivudine (3TC)	EHL 3–7h, PRC C Lact ?
3TC *Tab 150mg, Sol (oral) 10mg/ml* **Heptovir** *Tab 100mg, Sol (oral) 5mg/ml*	**HIV infx:** 150mg PO bid in combination with other antiretroviral drugs; **chronic hepatitis B:** 100mg PO qd; **CH** 3 mo–16 yr: **HIV infx:** 4mg/kg, max. 150mg PO bid DARF: **HIV-Tx** GFR (ml/min): >50: 150mg bid, 30–49: 150mg qd, 15–29:ini. 150mg, then 100mg qd, 5–14: ini. 150mg, then 50mg qd, <5: ini. 50mg, then 25mg qd
Lamivudine + Zidovudine	PRC C, Lact ?
Combivir *Tab 150 + 300mg*	**HIV infx:** 1 Tab PO bid; DARF: not rec in RF
Stavudine (d4T)	EHL 0.9–1.6h, PRC C, Lact ?
Zerit *Cap 15mg, 20mg, 30mg, 40mg*	**HIV infx:** >60kg: 40mg PO bid <60kg: 30mg PO bid; **CH** <30kg: 1mg/kg PO bid, >30kg: see adults; DARF: GFR (ml/min) >50: 100% q12h, 26–50: 50% q12h, 10–25: 50% q24h
Tenofovir	EHL 17h, PRC B Lact +
Viread *Tab 300mg*	**HIV infx:** 300mg PO qd; DARF: CrCl 30–49: give q48h, 10–29: give 2x/wk, HD: give q7d after HD
Zalcitabine (ddC)	EHL 1–3h, PRC C Lact ?
Hivid *Tab 0.375mg, 0.75mg*	**HIV infx:** 0.75mg PO tid in combination with other antiretroviral drugs; **CH:** 0.015–0.04mg/kg PO qid; DARF: GFR (ml/min): 10–40: 100% q12h, <10: 100% q24h
Zidovudine (AZT, ZDV)	EHL 1h, PRC C, Lact ?
Retrovir *Cap 100mg, Syr 50mg/5ml, Inj 10mg/ml* **Generics** *Cap 100mg*	**HIV infx:** 600 mg/d PO div bid or tid; 1mg/kg IV over 1h 5–6x/d in combination with other antiretroviral drugs; **PRO of maternal-fetal HIV transmission:** mother (>14 wk of pregnancy): 100mg PO 5x/d until start of labor, during labor, 2mg/kg IV over 1h, then 1mg/kg/h until delivery; newborn: 2mg/kg PO q6h within 12h of birth for 6 wk, **CH** 3 mo–12 yr: 180mg/square meter q6h, max. 200mg q6h

7.17.8 Anti-HIV Drugs: Non-Nucleoside Reverse Transcriptase Inhibitors

MA/Ind (efavirenz, nevirapine): direct binding on the reverse transcriptase ⇒ blockage of DNA-polymerase of HIV-1;
AE (delavirdine): N/V, rash, headache, fatigue
AE (efavirenz): dizziness, drowsiness, impaired concentration, sleeplessness, exanthema, liver enzymesm
AE (nevirapine): rash, nausea, diarrhea, fever, headache, liver enzymesm, hypersensitivity to product ingredients;
CI (delavirdine): hypersensitivity to delavirdine products, concomitant use with rifampin or rifabutin
CI (efavirenz): combination with astemizole, cisapride, midazolam, triazolam, fexofenadine, ergotamine derivatives; children < 3 yr, hypersensitivity to product ingredients
CI (nevirapine): hypersensitivity to nevirapine products

Delavirdine (DLV)	EHL 2–11h, PRC C, Lact ?
Rescriptor *Tab 100mg*	**HIV infx:** 400mg PO tid combined with other antiretroviral; **CH** >16yr: see adults
Efavirenz (EFV)	EHL 52–76 h (1 dose), 40–55 h (x dose), Lact -
Sustiva *Cap 50mg, 100mg, 200mg, 600mg*	**HIV infx:** 600mg PO qd combined with other antiretroviral drugs; **CH** >3 yr: 10–15kg: 200mg PO qd, 15–20kg: 250mg PO qd, 20–25kg: 300mg PO qd, 25–32.5kg: 350mg PO qd, 33–40kg: 400mg PO qd, >40kg: 600mg qd
Nevirapine (NVP)	EHL 22–84h, PRC C, Lact ?
Viramune *Tab 200mg*	**HIV infx:** 200mg PO qd for 14d, then 200mg PO bid combined with other antiretroviral drugs; **CH** 2 mo–8 yr: 4mg/kg PO qd for 14d, then 7mg/kg bid, >8 yr: 4 mg/kg PO qd x 2 wk, then 4 mg/kg bid, max. 400mg/d; **PRO of maternal-fetal HIV transmission:** mother 200mg PO as single dose at onset of labor; neonate 2mg/kg PO within 3d of birth

7.17.9 Anti-HIV Drugs: Protease Inhibitors

MA/Ind: specific inhibition of HIV protease ⇒ protein production↓ (i.e. rev. transcriptase) fosamprenavir is a pro-drug of amprenavir;
AE (amprenavir): N/V, diarrhea, rash, paresthesia;
AE (indinavir, ritonavir): nausea, headache, diarrhea, tiredness, exanthema;
AE (nelfinavir, saquinavir): diarrhea, nausea, exanthema
CI (amprenavir): concomitant interacting drugs, hypersensitivity to amprenavir products, children < 4yr, hepatic or RF, under metronidazole Tx;
CI (indinavir): hypersensitivity to indinavir products;
CI (nelfinavir): combination w/rifampicin, fexofenadine;
CI (ritonavir): severe hepatic insufficiency;
CI (saquinavir): combination w/rifampicin

Amprenavir (APV)	EHL 7–10h, PRC C, Lact -
Agenerase *Cap 50, 150mg, Sol (oral) 15mg/ml*	**HIV-1 infx:** 1200mg PO bid in combination with ohther antiretroviral drugs; **CH** 4–16yr, <50kg: Cap: 20mg/kg PO bid, max. 2400mg/d, Sol: 22.5mg/kg bid
Atazanavir	EHL 7h, PRC B, Lact ?
Reyataz *Cap 150mg, 200mg*	**HIV-1 infx:** 300–400mg PO qd
Darunavir	EHL 15h, PRC B, Lact +
Prezista *Tab 300mg*	**HIV infx:** 600mg PO bid, give with ritonavir 100mg PO bid; DARF: not req
Fosamprenavir	PRC C, Lact ?
Telzir *Tab 700mg, Sol (oral) 50mg/ml*	**HIV infx:** 1400mg PO qd or 700mg PO bid with ritonavir 200mg PO qd or 100mg PO bid; DARF: not req
Indinavir (IDV)	EHL 1.5–2h, PRC C, Lact -
Crixivan *Cap 200mg, 400mg*	**HIV infx:** 800mg PO tid in combination with other antiretroviral drugs; DARF: not req
Nelfinavir (NFV)	EHL 3.5–5h, PRC B, Lact ?
Viracept *Tab 250mg, 625mg Susp 50mg/scoopful*	**HIV infx:** 750mg PO tid or 1250mg PO bid in combination with other antiretroviral drugs; **CH** 2–13 yr: 20–30 mg/kg tid

Ritonavir (RTV)	EHL 3–3.5h, PRC B, Lact ?
Norvir *Cap 100mg, Sol (oral) 80mg/ml*	**HIV infx:** ini. 300mg PO bid, incr. at 2–3d intervalls by 100mg bid to 600mg bid in combination with other antiretroviral drugs; **CH:** ini 250mg/m2 PO bid, incr. at 2–3d intervalls by 50mg/m2/dose to 400 mg/m^2 PO bid, max. 600mg PO bid
Ritonavir + lopinavir	
Kaletra *Cap 33.3mg + 133.3mg, 50mg + 200mg, Sol 20 + 80mg*	**HIV infx:** ini 100 + 400mg PO bid
Saquinavir (SQV)	EHL 13h, PRC B Lact?
Fortovase *Cap 200mg* **Invirase** *Cap 200mg, 500mg*	**HIV infx:** Fortovase: 1200mg PO tid; Invirase: 600mg PO tid in combination with other antiretroviral drugs
Tipranavir	EHL 6h, PRC C Lact +
Aptivus *Cap 250mg*	**HIV infx:** 500mg PO bid

7.17.10 Anti-HIV Drugs: Other

ME/EF: CCR5 antagonists, binds to human chemokine receptor CCR5 and inhibits interaction with envelope glycoprotein (gp120)
AE: cough, pyrexia, upper respiratory tract infections, rash, musculoskeletal symptoms, abdominal pain, dizziness CI: hypersensativity to drug

Maraviroc	EHL 14-18h, PRC C Lact ?
Celsentri *Tab 150mg, 300mg*	**CCR5-tropic HIV-1 infx (with multiple resistance):** 300 mg PO bid

7.18 Antifungals

7.18.1 Drugs for Subcutaneous and Systemic Mycoses

Ind (amphotericin B): Candida-species, Aspergillus, Histoplasma, Sporothrix, Blastomyces, Cryptococcus, Coccidoides; **Ind** (fluconazole): Candida-species (except C. krusei, C. glabrata), Cryptococcus, Histoplasma, Trichosporon, Dermatophytes, Blastomyces
AE (amphotericin B): fever, chills, N/V, diarrhea, generalized pains, anemia, renal dysfunction, hypokalemia, thrombocytopenia; **AE** (caspofungin): neutropenia, anemia, headache, hypokalemia, fever, phlebitis, increased liver enzymes; **AE** (fluconazole): nausea, stomachache, diarrhea, exanthema, headache, peripheral neuropathy, LFT↑, itching; **AE** (itraconazole): N/V, hypokalemia, LFT↑, rash; serious cardiovascular events, rare cases of serious hepatotoxicity; **AE** (ketoconazole): hepatitis, N/V, adrenal insuff.; **AE** (micafungin): rash, pruritus, facial swelling, vasodilatation; **AE** (posaconazole): nausea, headache; **CI** (amphotericin B): severe hepatic, kidney dysfunct., hypersensitivity to amphotericin B; **CI** (caspofungin): hypersensitivity to caspofungin; **CI** (fluconazole): severe hepatic dysfunction, great caution with children, hypersensitivity to fluconazole; **CI** (itraconazole): hypersensitivity to itraconazole, concurrent use with astemizole, fexofenadine, triazolam, cisapride, oral midazolam, pimozide, quinidine, HMG-CoA reductase inhibitors, ergot alkaloids, congestive heart failure; **CI** (ketoconazole): hypersensitivity to ketoconazole prod., concurrent use with astemizole, fexofenadine, cisapride, oral triazolam; **CI** (micafungin): hypersensitivity to micafungin; **CI** (posaconazole): hypersensitive to this drug, co-administration with ergot alkaloids, co-administration with medicinal prod. metabolized through the CYP3A4 system

Amphotericin B	EHL 15 d, PRC B Lact ?
Fungizone *Inj 50mg/vial*	**Severe fungal infx:** test dose 1mg slow IV, if tolerated start 0.25 mg/kg IV qd, incr. to 0.5–1.5 mg/kg/d, max. 1.5 mg/kg/d, administra-tion time: 2–6h DARF: GFR (ml/min) >50: 100% q24h, 10–50: 100% q24h, <10: 100% q24–36h
Amphotericin B Lipid Complex	EHL 170h, PRC B, Lact ?
Abelcet *Inj lipid complex 5mg/ml*	**Severe fungal infx:** 5 mg/kg IV qd administration time: 2.5mg/kg/h
Amphotericin B Liposome	EHL 7–153h, PRC B, Lact ?
AmBisome *Inj liposomal 50mg/vial*	**Severe fungal infx:** 3–5 mg/kg IV qd; administration time: 2h; **CH** 1mo–16 yr: 3mg/kg IV qd
Caspofungin	EHL 9–11h, PRC C, Lact ?
Cancidas *Inj 50mg/vial, 70mg/vial*	**Invasive aspergillosis**: d1 70mg IV over 1h, then 50mg IV qd; DARF: not req

Fluconazole	EHL 30 h
Diflucan *Tab 50mg,100mg, Cap 150mg, Susp 50mg/5ml, Inj 2mg/ml* **Generics** *Tab 50mg,100mg, Cap 150mg, Inj 2mg/ml*	**Oropharyngeal/esophageal candidiasis:** d1 200mg PO/IV qd, then 100 mg qd; **vaginal candidiasis:** 150mg PO as single dose; **systemic candidiasis:** 400 mg PO/IV qd; **CH oropharyngeal/esophageal candidiasis:** d1 6mg/ kg PO/IV qd, then 3mg/kg qd; **syst. candidiasis:** 6–12 mg/kg PO/IV qd; DARF: GFR (ml/min) >50: 100%, <50: 50%
Itraconazole	EHL 64h (x dose)/24h (1x), IV35h, PRC C, Lact ?
Sporanox *Cap 100mg, Inj 10mg/ml, Sol (oral) 10mg/ml*	**Aspergillosis:** 200mg IV bid x 2d, then 200mg IV qd; 200–400mg/d PO for 3 mo; **blastomycosis:** 200mg IV bid x 2d, then 200mg IV qd; 200–400mg/d PO; **oropharngeal/esophageal candidiasis:** 100–200mg PO swish and swallow; **onychomycosis, toenails:** 200mg PO qd for 12 wk; DARF: GFR (ml/min) > 30: 100%, <30: IV not rated
Ketoconazole	EHL 2–12h, PRC C, Lact ?
Generics *Tab 200mg*	**Various fungal infx:** 200–400mg PO qd; **CH** >2 yr: 3.3– 6.6mg/kg PO qd; DARF: not req
Micafungin	EHL 14-17.2, PRC C, Lact ?
Mycamine *Inj 25mg/vial, 50mg/vial*	**Esophageal candidiasis:** 150mg IV qd; **PRO in stem cell transplant:**50mg IV qd; DARF: not req
Posaconazole	EHL 14-17.2, PRC C, Lact ?
Spriafil *Susp (oral) 40mg/ml*	**PRO Aspergillus/Candida infx:** 200 mg PO tid; **Invasive aspergillosis:** 400mg PO bid; **Oropharyngeal candidiasis:** ini 100mg PO bid x 1 day, then 100 mg PO qd x 13days
Voriconazole	PRC D, Lact ?
Vfend *Tab 50mg, 200mg, Susp. (oral) 3g, Inj 200mg/vial*	**Invasive fungal infections:** ini 6 mg/kg IV q12h x 2 doses, then 4 mg/kg IV q12h; Oral: <40 kg: 100 mg PO q12h, >40 kg: 200 mg PO q12h; **Esophageal candidiasis:** <40 kg: 100 mg PO q12h, >40 kg: 200 mg PO q12h

7.18.2 Drugs for Superficial Mycoses

Ind (clotrimazole): cutaneous, oral, vaginal candidiasis, dermatomycosis
Ind (nystatin): Candida, Blastomyces, Coccidioides, Histoplasma, Aspergillus
Ind (terbinafine): dermal fungal infx, onychomycosis
AE (clotrimazole): N/V, transient elevations in LFT, contact dermatitis;
AE (nystatin): in high doses: diarrhea, vaginal irritation/pain, N/V, rash
AE (terbinafine): local irritation, N/V, LFT↑
CI (clotrimazole): hypersensitivity to clotrimazole;
CI (nystatin): hypersensitivity to nystatin products;
CI (terbinafine): hypersensitivity to terbinafine products

Clotrimazole	EHL 3.5–5h, PRC B, Lact ?
Generics *lozenge (oral) 10mg*	**Oropharyngeal candidiasis:** 1 troche dissolved slowly in the mouth 5x/d for 14d; **PRO:** 1 troche dissolved slowly in mouth tid; **CH** >3 yr: see adults
Nystatin	EHL no data, PRC C, Lact +
Candistatin *Tab vag 100,000 U* **Nilstat** *Powder (oral) 100%, Tab 500,000 U, Tab (vag) 100,000 U, Susp 100,000 U/ml* **Nyaderm** *Susp 100,000 U/ml* **Generics** *Susp 100,000 U/ml*	**Oral candidiasis:** 400,000–600,000 U PO qid **GI andidiasis:** 0.5–1 mio U PO tid; **infants:** 200,000 U PO qid; **CH** see adults
Terbinafine	EHL 22–26h, PRC B, Lact -
Lamisil *Tab 250mg* **Generics** *Tab 250mg*	**Onychomycosis, fingernails:** 250mg PO qd for 6 wk; **onychomycosis, toenails:** 250mg PO qd for 12 wk; **superficial mycoses:** 250mg PO qd for 1–4 wk; **systemic mycoses:** 250–500mg PO qd for 1–16 mo; DARF: GFR (ml/min) <50: 50%

7.19 Antiparasitics

AE (atovaquone): fever, rash, N/V, diarrhea;
AE (iodoquinol): optic neuritis/atrophy, peripheral neuropathy;
AE (mebendazole): abdominal pain, diarrhea, rash
AE (metronidazole): seizures, N/V, metallic taste;
AE (pentamidine): leukopenia, thrombocytopenia, hypotension, chest pain, rash;
AE (praziquantel): malaise, headache
AE (pyrantel): N/V, headache;
AE (pyrimethamine): Steven's-Johnson syndrome, megaloblastic anemia, leukopenia;
CI (albendazole): hypersensitivity to albendazole or benzimidazoles
CI (atovaquone, ivermectin, mebendazole, metronidazole): hypersensitivity to product
CI (iodoquinol): hepatic damage, hypersensitivity to iodine + 8-hydroxyquinolones
CI (pentamidine): hypersensitivity to pentamidine
CI (praziquantel): hypersensitivity to praziquantel, ocular cysticercosis
CI (pyrantel): liver disease, myasthenia gravis
CI (pyrimethamine): hypersensitivity to pyrimethamine products, megaloblastic anemia (folate deficiency)

Atovaquone	EHL 50–84h, PRC C, Lact ?
Mepron *Susp 750mg/5ml*	**Pneumocystis carinii Tx:** 750mg PO bid for 21d; **pneumocystis carinii PRO:** 1500mg PO qd **toxoplasmosis:** 750mg PO qid; **CH** 13–16 yr: see adults
Iodoquinol	EHL no data, PRC C, Lact ?
Diodoquin *Tab 210mg, 650 mg*	**Intestinal amebiasis:** 630–650mg PO tid for 20d; **CH:** 40 mg/kg/d PO div tid for 20d; max. 1.95g/d
Mebendazole	EHL 1.5–5.5h, PRC C, Lact ?
Vermox *Tab (chew) 100mg*	**Roundworm, whipworm, hookworm:** 100mg PO bid for 3d; **pinworm**: 100mg PO as single dose; **CH** >2 yr: see adults; DARF: not req

Metronidazole	EHL 6–11h, PRC B, Lact ?
Flagyl *Cap 500mg* **Florazole ERT** *ab ext. release 750mg* **Generics** *Tab 250mg, Inj 5mg/ml*	**Amebic dysentery:** 750mg PO tid for 5–10d **amebic liver abscess:** 500–750mg PO tid for 5–10d; **giardiasis:** 250mg PO tid for 5d; **trichomoniasis:** 250mg PO tid for 7d; **CH amebic dysentery:** 35–50mg/kg/d PO, max. 750mg/ dose, div tid for 10 d; **amebic liver** abscess: 50mg/kg/d PO div tid, max. 2.4g/d, for 7d; **giardiasis:** 15mg/kg/d PO div tid for 7–10d; **trichomoniasis:** 15mg/kg/d PO div tid for 7d; DARF: GFR(ml/min) >10:100%, <10: 50%
Pentamidine	EHL 6.4 h–9h, PRC C, Lact -
Generics *Inj 300mg/vial*	**Pneumocystis carinii Tx:** 4mg/kg IM/IV qd for 14–21d; **pneumocystis carinii PRO:** 300mg nebulized 1x q4 wk or 4mg/kg IV 1x q4 wk; **CH** >5 yr: see adults; DARF: not req
Praziquantel	EHL 0.8–3h, PRC B
Biltricide *Tab 600mg*	**Schistosomiasis:** 60mg/kg PO div tid for 1d **liver flukes:** 75mg/kg PO div tid for 1d **neurocysticercosis:** 50mg/kg/d PO div tid for 15d; **cestodiasis:** 10mg/kg PO as single dose; **CH** >4 yr: **schistosomiasis:** 60mg/kg PO div tid for 1d; DARF: not req
Pyrantel	EHL no data, PRC C, Lact ?
Combantrin *Tab 125 mg, Susp 50 mg/ml*	**Pinworm, roundworm:** 11 mg/kg PO, max. 1g as single dose
Pyrimethamine	EHL 80–96h, PRC C, Lact +
Daraprim *Tab 25mg*	**Toxoplasmosis, immunocompetent patients:** 50–75mg PO qd for 1–3 wk, then 50% of first dose for 4–5 wk; **toxoplasmosis in AIDS:** ini. 200mg PO, then 50–100mg qd; **secondary PRO of toxoplasmosis in AIDS:** 50mg PO qd, give with folinic acid (10–15 mg qd) and sulfadiazine or clindamycin; **CH toxoplasm.:** 1mg/kg/d PO div bid 2–4 d, then 50% of 1st dose for 1 mo; DARF: not req

7.20 Antimalarials

7.20.1 Antimalarials - Single Ingredient Drugs

AE (chloroquine): corneal clouding, pigmented retinopathy, methemoglobinemia, ECG changes, exanthema, muscle weakness; **AE** (doxycycline): photosensitivity, epigastric distress; **AE** (mefloquine): GI/CNS DO, psychoses, dysrhythmias, leuko-/ thrombopenia, sinus bradycardia, seizures, liver transaminases↑; **AE** (primaquine): anemia, leukocytosis, abdominal pain; **AE** (quinine): thrombocytopenia, convulsions, urticaria, hypoglycemia, hemolytic uremic syndrome; **CI** (chloroquine): retinopathy, G6PD deficiency, hypersensitivity to product, retinal/visual field changes; **CI** (doxycycline): hypersensitivity to doxycycline/ tetracycline, children < 8yr; **CI** (mefloquine): psychoses, cardiomyopathy, epilepsy; **CI** (primaquine): concomitant medications which cause bone marrow suppression, rheumatoid arthritis, lupus erythematosus; **CI** (quinine): hypersensitivity to quinine, glucose-6-phosphate dehydrogenase deficiency, myasthenia gravis

Chloroquine Phosphate	EHL 6–60 d, PRC C, Lact +
Generics *Tab 250mg*	**Malaria PRO:** 500 mg PO 1x/wk from 2 wk before exposure to 4 wk after, **malaria Tx:** d1: 1g PO, then 500mg PO after 6h, then 500mg PO qd on d2 and 3; **extraintestinal amebiasis:** 1g PO qd for 2d, then 500mg PO qd for 2–3 wk; **CH malaria PRO:** 5mg/kg PO 1x/wk from 2 wk before exposure to 6 wk after **malaria Tx:** 10mg/kg PO, max. 600mg, then 5mg/kg, max. 300mg after 6, 18 and 24h; DARF: GFR (ml/min) <10: 50%
Doxycycline	EHL 12–24h, PRC D, Lact ?
Apo-Doxy *Cap 100mg, Tab 100mg* **Doxycin** *Cap 100mg, Tab 100mg* **Doxytec** *Cap 100mg, Tab 100mg* **Novo-Doxylin** *Cap 100mg, Tab 100mg* **Vibra-Tabs** *Cap 100mg, Tab 100mg* **Generics** *Cap 100mg, Tab 100mg*	**Malaria PRO:** 100mg PO qd from 2d before exposure to 4 wk after **malaria Tx:** 200mg PO qd for 7 d with quinine; DARF: not req
Hydroxychloroquine	PRC D, Lact -
Plaquenil *Tab 200mg* **Generics** *Tab 200mg*	**RA:** ini 400–600mg PO qd, maint 200–400mg PO qd; **Malaria**: 400mg PO qwk; **SLE:** ini 400mg PO qd–bid, maint 200–400mg PO qd

Mefloquine	EHL 13–30 d, PRC C, Lact ?
Lariam *Tab 250mg*	**Malaria PRO:** 250mg PO 1x/wk from 1wk before exposure to 4 wk after **malaria Tx:** 1250mg PO single dose; **CH malaria PRO:** 1x/wk, 15–19kg: 1/4 Tab PO, 20–30kg: 1/2 Tab PO, 31–45kg: 3/4 Tab PO, >45kg: 1 Tab PO; **malaria Tx** <45 kg: 15mg/kg PO, then 10 mg/kg given 6–8h after first dose
Primaquine Phosphate	EHL 4–7h, PRC C, Lact ?
Primaquine *Tab 15mg*	**PRO of p. vivax and p. ovale relapse:** 15mg PO qd for 14d; **CH** 0.3mg/kg PO for 14d
Quinidine Gluconate	EHL no data, PRC ? Lact ?
Generics *Inj 80mg/ml, Tab ext.rel. 324mg*	**Severe p. falcip. malaria:** ini. 10 mg/kg IV over 1–2h, then 0.02 mg/kg/min for 72 h or until parasitemia <1%, or PO meds tolerated
Quinine Sulfate	EHL no data, PRC X, Lact ?
Quinine-odan *Cap 200mg, 300mg* **Generics** *Cap 200mg, 300mg*	**Malaria Tx:** 650mg PO tid for 3–7 d with doxycycline or pyrimethamine/sulfadoxine

7.20.2 Antimalarials - Combinations

AE (a. + p.): fever, headache, myalgia
CI (a. + p.): hypersensitivity to atovaquone, hypersensitivity to proguanil

Atovaquone + Proquanil	PRC C, Lact ?
Malarone *Tab 250 + 100mg*	**Malaria PRO:** 1 Tab PO qd from 2d before to 7d after exposure; **malaria Tx:** 4 Tab PO qd for 3d; **CH malaria PRO:** from 2d before to 7d after exposure, 11–20kg: 1 ped Tab PO qd, 21–30kg: 2 ped Tab PO qd, 31–40kg: 3 ped Tab PO qd, >40kg: 1 adult Tab PO qd; **malaria Tx:** for 3 d, 11–20kg: 1 adult Tab PO qd, 21–30kg: 2 adult Tab PO qd, 31–40kg; 3 adult Tab PO qd, >40kg: 4 adult Tab PO qd

8 Immunology

8.1 Vaccines

8.1.1 Combinations

AE (Diphtheria + Tetanus + Acellular Pertussis vaccine): injection site reaction, fever, irritability, drowsiness; **CI** (Diphtheria + Tetanus + Acellular Pertussis vaccine): hypersensitivity to the vaccine or thimerosal, adults and children > 7y, active infection, febrile illness, history encephalopathy secondary to DPT vaccine

Diphtheria + Tetanus + Acellular Pertussis Vaccine (DTaP)	EHL no data, PRC C, Lact -
Adacel *Inj 2 IU of diphtheria toxoid + 20 IU tetanus toxoid + 2.5 mcg pertussis toxoid/ 0.5ml single dose* **Boostrix** *Inj 2 IU of diphtheria toxoid + 20 IU tetanus toxoid + 8 mcg pertussis toxoid/ 0.5ml single dose*	**Diphtheria, tetanus, pertussis immunization:** 0.5ml IM for age 11–54 years
Diphtheria + Tetanus + Poliomyelitis Vaccine (DT Polio)	
Generics *0.5ml single dose*	**Diphtheria, tetanus, poliomyelitis immunization:** 0.5ml IM at 2, 4, 6 and 18mo of age; booster dose at 4–6y
Diphtheria + Tetanus + acellular Pertussis + Poliomyelitis Vaccine (DTaP Polio)	
Quadracel *0.5ml single dose*	**Diphtheria, tetanus, acellular pertussis, poliomyelitis:** 0.5ml IM at 2, 4, 6 and 18mo of age; booster dose at 4–6y
Diphtheria + Tetanus + acellular Pertussis + Poliomyelitis Vaccine + Haemophilus b	
Pentacel *Inj 0.5ml single dose*	**Diphtheria, tetanus, acellular pertussis, poliomyelitis, haemophilus b:** 0.5ml IM at 2, 4, 6 and 18mo of age
Diphtheria + Tetanus Toxoid (Td)	EHL no data
Generics *Inj 2LF U + 5 LF U/0.5ml*	**Tetanus, diphtheria immunization:** >7y: 0.5ml IM, rep after 4–8wk and after 6–12mo; 0.5ml booster dose q10y
Measles + Mumps + Rubella Vaccine (MMR)	
MMR II *Inj >1000 + >5000 + >1000 $CCID_{50}$/0.5ml* **Priorix** *Inj >10^3 + >$10^{3.7}$ + >10^3 $CCID_{50}$/0.5ml*	**Measles, mumps, rubella immunization:** 0.5ml IM at 12mo and 18mo or 4–6 years of age

8.1.2 Toxoids (Bacteria)

AE (tetanus toxoid): injection site pain, fever
CI (tetanus toxoid): hypersensitivity to tetanus tox. products, infx, poliomyelitis outbreak

Tetanus Toxoid	EHL no data, PRC C, Lact ?
Generics *Inj 5 LF U/0.5ml*	**Tetanus immunization:** 0.5ml IM, rep after 4–8wk and after 6–12mo; give 0.5ml booster dose q10y; **CH** <1y: 0.5ml IM, rep after 4 and 8wk and after 6–12mo; > 1y: see adults
Vi Polysaccharide Typhoid + Inactivated Hepatitis A	
ViVaxim *Inj 1ml*	**Typhoid and Hepatitis A immunization:** 1ml IM

8.1.3 Polysaccharid-Vaccines (Bacteria)

AE (pneumococcal vaccine): injection site pain, anaphylaxis;
AE (meningococcal vaccine): see Prod Info;
CI (pneumococcal vaccine): hypersensitivity to pneumococcal vaccine products, Hodgkin's disease within 10d of or during Tx;
CI (meningococcal vaccine): any acute illness, sensitivity to thimerosal or any other component of the vaccine

Haemophilus B Vaccine	PRC X
Act-HIB *Inj 10mcg purified polysaccharide/0.5ml* **PedvaxHIB** *Inj 7.5mcg purified polysaccharide/0.5ml*	**Haemophilus B:** 0.5ml IM at 2, 4, 6 and 18mo of age
Meningococcal Polysaccharide Vaccine	EHL no data, PRC C
Menactra *Inj 0.5ml conjugates from Groups A, C, Y and W-135* **Menjugate** *Inj 0.5ml Group C-CRM197 conjugate vaccine* **Menomune** *Inj 0.5ml conjugates from Groups A, C, Y and W-135* **Meningitec** *Inj 0.5ml Group C-CRM197 conjugate vaccine* **NeisVac-C** *Inj 0.5ml Group C-TT conjugate vaccine* **Generics** *Inj 50mcg of conjugate from each of Groups A, C, Y and W-135/0.5ml*	**Meningococcal infx PRO:** 0.5ml IM; **CH** 3–18mo: 0.5ml SC, rep after 3mo; > 2y: see adults

Pneumococcal Vaccine	EHL no data
Pneumo 23 *Inj 25mcg of each of the 23 polysaccharide types/0.5ml* **Pneumovax 23** *Inj 25mcg of each of the 23 polysaccharide types/0.5ml Prevnar Inj 25mcg of each of the 23 polysaccharide types/0.5ml*	**Pneumococcal infx PRO:** 0.5ml IM/SC

Salmonella TyphiVi Vaccine	PRC C, Lact ?
Typherix *Inj 25mcg polysaccharide/0.5ml* **Typhim Vi** *Inj 25mcg polysaccharide/0.5ml*	**Salmonella Typhi immunization:** 0.5ml IM

8.1.4 Inactivated Vaccines (Bacteria)

AE (cholera vaccine): fever, malaise, headache
CI (cholera vaccine): illness, hypersensitivity to cholera vaccine

Cholera Vaccine	EHL no data, PRC C, Lact ?
Mutacol Berna *Sol (oral) 2–10 X 108 CFU viable V. Cholerae + 20–100X108 CFU non-viable V. Cholerae/package*	**Cholera immunization:** 1 packet PO

8.1.5 Live Attenuated Vaccines (Bacteria)

AE: flu-like syndrome, hematuria, urinary frequency, dysuria
CI: positive tuberculin tests, burns, AIDS, immunocompromised status, fever unknown origin, UTI (intravesical BCG), hypersensitivity to BCG vaccine

BCG Vaccine	EHL no data
BCG Vaccine *Inj 50mg/vial*	**Different BCG vaccine products are available for TB immunization;** route of immunization and dose depends on product; see Prod Info; **TB immunization**: 0.2–0.3ml percutanous; **CH** >1mo: see adults, **CH** <1mo: 50%

8.1.6 Inactivated Vaccines (Viruses)

AE (hepatitis A vaccine): fever, injection site pain/soreness, headache
AE (hepatitis B vaccine): fever, injection site soreness/erythema
AE (influenza vaccine): fever, pain, redness at injection site, malaise
AE (japanese encephalitis vaccine): fever, headache, injection site pain
AE (poliovirus vaccine): fever, injection site reaction, fussiness and crying in children
AE (rabies vaccine): dizziness, malaise, injection site reaction, myalgias, nausea
CI (hepatitis A vaccine): hypersensitivity to hepatitis A vaccine
CI (hepatitis B vaccine): hypersensitivity to hepatitis B vaccine/yeast
CI (influenza vaccine): allergy to chicken feathers/dander/eggs, hypersensitivity to vaccine/thimerosol, active acute respiratory disease/infections
CI (japanese encephalitis vaccine): hypersensitivity to japanese encephalitis vaccine
CI (poliovirus vaccine): hypersensitivity to streptomycin, neomycin, polymixin B, hypersensitivity to polio vaccine products
CI (rabies vaccine): hypersensitivity to rabies vaccine products, fever

Hepatitis A Vaccine	EHL no data, PRC C, Lact ?
Avaxim *Inj 160U/0.5ml* **Avaxim-Pediatric** *Inj 80U/0.5ml* **Havrix** *Inj 720U/ml, 1,440U/ml* **Vaqta** *Inj 25U/0.5ml, 50U/ml*	**Hep. A immunization:** Avaxim, Epaxal Berna: 0.5ml IM, rep after 6–12mo Havrix: 1,440 U IM, rep after 6–12mo; Vaqta: 50 U IM, rep after 6mo; **CH** 2–17y: Havrix: 720 U IM, rep after 6–12mo; Vaqta: 25 U IM, rep after 6–18mo
Hepatitis B Vaccine	EHL no data, PRC C, Lact ?
Engerix-B *Inj 10mcg/0.5ml (pediatric), Inj 20mcg/ml, 200mcg/10ml (adult)* **Recombivax HB** *Inj 10mcg/ml, 40mcg/ml*	**Hep. B immunization:** Engerix-B: 20mcg IM, rep after 1 + 6mo **Recombivax HB:** 10mcg IM, rep after1 + 6mo; **CH Engerix-B:** 10mcg IM within 7d of birth, rep after 1 + 6mo; **Recombivax HB:** 5mcg IM within 7d of birth, rep after 1 + 6mo
Hepatitis A + B Vaccine	PRC C, Lact ?
Twinrix *Inj 360U + 10mcg/0.5ml (Junior), 720U + 20mcg/ml (adult)*	**Hep. A+B immunization:** 720 + 20mcg IM, rep after 1 + 6mo
Influenza Vaccine	EHL no data, PRC C, Lact +
Fluviral S/F *Inj 45mcg/0.5ml* **Influvac** *Inj 45mcg/0.5ml* **Vaxigrip** *Inj 45mcg/0.5ml*	**Influenza virus PRO:** 0.5ml IM once yearly; **CH** 6–35mo: 0.25ml IM, rep after 4wk; 3–8y: 0.5ml IM, rep after 4wk; 9–12y: see adults

Japanese Encephalitis Vaccine	EHL no data
JE-Vax *Inj single dose vial*	**Japanese encephalitis immunization:** 1ml SC on d 0, 7, 30; 1ml booster dose may be given after 2y; **CH** 1–3y: 0.5ml SC on d 0, 7, 30; > 3y: see adults

Papillomavirus Vaccine	EHL no data, PRC B, Lact ?
Gardasil *Inj 20 mcg HPV 6 L1 + 40 mcg HPV 11 L1 + 40 mcg HPV 16 L1 + 20 mcg HPV 18 L1 protein*	**human papillomavirus immunization:** 0.5ml IM x 3 at 0, 2, 6mo

Poliovirus Vaccine	EHL no data
IMOVAX Polio *Inj 40 D antigen U of Type1 + 8 D antigen U of Type2 + 32 D antigen U of Type 3 poliovirus/0.5ml*	**poliomyelitis immunization:** IPOL: 0.5ml SC, rep after 1 and 6–12mo

Rabies Vaccine 9	EHL no data, PRC C, Lact ?
Imovax Rabies *Inj: 1ml is equal to or greater than 2.5 U of rabies antigen*	**Rabies immunization, pre exposure:** 1ml IM on d 0, 7, 21 or 28; **post exposure:** 1ml IM on d 0, 3, 7, 14, 28, 90 with a concomittant dose of 20 U/kg rabies IG on d 0; **CH** see adults

8.1.7 Live Attenuated Vaccines (Viruses)

AE (varicella vaccine): fever, N/V, injection site pain/swelling
AE (yellow fever vaccine): fever, malaise, headache
CI (varicella vaccine): hypersensitivity to varicella vaccine products, blood dyscrasias, immunodeficiency, active TB
CI (yellow fever vaccine): hypersensitivity to yellow virus vaccine products/eggs, child younger than 4mo of age, blood transfusion or IG therapy within 8wk

Rotavirus Vaccine	EHL no data
Rotateq *Susp (oral) 2ml of 5 live reassortant viruses (G1, G2, G3, G4, P7)*	**Rotavirus immunization: CH** 6–32wk: 2ml PO q4–10wk x 3, 1st dose at 6–12wk and 3rd dose prior to 32wk old

Varicella Vaccine	EHL no data, PRC C, Lact ?
Varivax *Inj 1350 PFU (plaque forming U) of Oka/Merck varicella virus/0.5ml*	**Varicella immunization:** 0.5ml SC, rep after 4v8wk; **CH** > 12y: see adults; 1–12y: 0.5ml SC as single dose

Yellow Fever Vaccine	EHL no data, PRC C, Lact +
YF-Vax *5.04 Log 10 Plaque Forming Units (PFU)/0.5ml*	**Yellow fever immunization:** 0.5ml SC as single dose; **CH** > 9mo: see adults

8.1.8 Other Vaccines

AE (plague vaccine): see Prod Info
AE (typhoid vaccine): fever, rash, N/V, myalgia, diarrhea
CI (plague vaccine): see Prod Info
CI (typhoid vaccine): hypersensitivity to typhoid vaccine products, immunodeficiency, persistent diarrhea, GI illness

Typhoid Vaccine	EHL no data
Vivotif Berna *Cap 2–10 X 109 colony-forming U of viable S. typhi Ty21a / 5–60 X 109 bact. cells of non-viable S. typhi Ty21a*	1 Cap PO 1h ac on d 1, 3, 5, 7 **CH** >6y: see adults

8.2 Immunoglobulins

AE (hepatitis B IG): rash, pain at injection site, joint pain
AE (IG): flushing of face, hypotension, tachycardia, chest tightness, rash
AE (rabies IG human): fever, pain at injection site, hypersensitivity reaction
AE (tetanus IG): fever, redness, pain at injection site, myalgia
AE (varicella-zoster IG): injection site reaction
CI (hepatitis B IG): hypersensitivity to IG products;
CI (IG): hypersensitivity to IG, blood products, IgA deficiency
CI (rabies IG human): hypersensitivity to rabies IG/thimerosal
CI (tetanus IG): hypersensitivity to tetanus IG products, patients with IgA deficiency
CI (varicella-zoster IG): IgA deficiency, hypersensitivity to IG products/neomycin, immunodeficiency, blood dyscrasias, fever/ respiratory, illness/active TB

Anti-Thymocyte Globulin	EHL 5.7d, PRC C, Lact ?
Atgam *Inj 50mg/ml*	**Immunosupression:** 7–30mg/kg IV qd, duration is dependent on indication for immunosuppresion
Black Widow Spider Antivenin	PRC C, Lact ?
Antivenin (Latrodectus Mactans) *Inj 6,000 U/vial*	**Black widow spider bite:** 1 vial IM/IV

Botulism Antitoxin	EHL n/a,
Botulism Antitoxin *Inj 5,000 U/vial (type E)*	**Botulism toxin poisoning:** 1 vial IV (1:10 dilution) or IM
Diphtheria Antitoxin	PRC D, Lact ?
Diphtheria Antitoxin *Inj 20,000 U/vial*	**Diphtheria:** 10,000–150,000 U IV (1:10 dilution) or IM
Hepatitis B Immune Globulin	EHL 17.5d/25d, PRC C, Lact ?
Bayhep B *Inj 0.5ml syringe, 1ml vial, 5ml vial*	**Post-exposure PRO:** 0.06ml/kg IM, repeat in 1mo for persons, who are not given hepatitis B vaccine. Initiate hepatitis B vaccine series PRO of infants born to HBsAG (+) mothers: 0.5ml IM within 12h of birth. Initiate hepatitis B vaccine series
Hepatitis A Immune Globulin	EHL 3–5wk, PRC C, Lact no data
Baygam *Inj (IM form) 2ml, 5ml, 10ml single dose vials* **Gammagard S/D** *Inj 0.5g, 1g, 2.5g, 5g, 10g size vials* **Iveegam Immuno** *Inj 5g/vial*	**Hep. A post-exposure PRO (i.e. household or institutional contacts):** 0.02ml/kg IM; hep. A pre-exposure PRO: < 3mo length of stay = 0.02ml/kg IM;> 3mo length of stay = 0.06ml/kg IM and rep. q4–6mo; measles: 0.2–0.25ml/kg IM within 6d of exposure, max 15ml; **CH** pediatric HIV: 400mg/kg IV inf q28d; measles: 0.2–0.25ml/kg IM within 6d of exposure, max 15ml
Rabies Immune Globulin	EHL 21d, PRC C, Lact ?
Bayrab *Inj 300 U/vial, 1500 U/vial* **Imogam Rabies Pasteurized** *Inj 150 U/ml*	**Post-exposure PRO:** 20IU/kg (0.133ml/kg), infiltrated in the area around the wound and the rest given IM
Tetanus Immune Globulin	EHL 3–5wk, PRC B/C, Lact no data
Baytet *Inj 250U/vial, 250U/single dose syringe* **Tetanus Immune Globulin** *Inj 250U/vial*	**Tetanus PRO:** 250U IM at time of injury; higher doses in severe injuries, severely contaminated wounds, or wounds >24h old, see Prod Info **tetanus Tx:** dose adjusted to severitiy of infx/clinical situation; usually TIG 3,000–6,000 U IM; **CH** >7y: see adults; **CH** <7y: 4 U/kg IM

Varicella-Zoster Immune Globulin	EHL 3wk, PRC C, Lact ?
VariZIG *Inj 125 U/vial* **Varicella-Zoster mmune Globulin** *Inj 100 U/ml*	**Passive immunization to varicella:** **IM (gluteal):** ≤10kg: 125U at one site; 10.1–20kg: 250U at a single site, 20.1–30kg: 375U with no > 2.5ml at a single site, 30.1–40kg: 500 U with no > 2.5ml at a single site, > 40kg: 625U with no > 2.5ml at a single site; spezialized dosing for post-exposure PRO in immundeficient patients

8.3 Immunosuppressives

MA (anakinra): recombinant interleukin-1 receptor antagonist
AE (cyclosporine): renal damage, hepatic DO, cardiotoxic, tremors, hirsutism, gingival hypertrophy, edema;
AE (daclizumab): N/V, headache, dizziness, tremor;
AE (mycophenolate mofetil): myelosuppression, HTN, tremor, diarrhea, N/V;
AE (sirolimus): thrombocyto-, leukopenia, hyperlipidemia, headache, periph. edema;
AE (anakinra): neutropenia, infections, headache, injection site reactions;
AE (tacrolimus): HTN, N/V, diarrhea, headache/tremor, infx;
CI (cyclosporine): renal dysfunction, uncontrollable HTN, uncontrollable infx, tumors, severe hepatic diseases;
CI (daclizumab, sirolimus, tacrolimus): hypersens. to product;
CI (anakinra): hypersensitivity to E. coli-derived products;
CI (mycophenolate mofetil): hypersens. to mycophenolate mofetil/mycophenolic acid, hypersens. to IV formulation

Anakinra	EHL 4–6h, PRC B, Lact ?
Kineret *Inj 150mg/ml*	**Rheumatoid arthritis**: 100mg sc qd; DARF: CrCl<30 decrease by 70–75%
Basiliximab	EHL 7.2 +/- 3.2d, PRC B, Lact ?
Simulect *Inj 20mg/vial*	**Renal transplant:** 20mg IV 2h prior to transpl., rep after 4d; **CH** 2–15y: 12mg/square meter 2h prior to transpl., rep after 4d

Cyclosporine	EHL 19h, PRC C, Lact -
Neoral *Cap 10mg, 25mg, 50mg, 100mg, Sol (oral) 100mg/ml* **Sandimmune** *Inj 50mg/ml* **Generics** *Cap 100mg*	**Organ transplant:** ini 15mg/kg/d PO for 7–14d, then decrease 5%/wk, maint 5–10mg/kg/d; IV: 1/3 of PO dose; **rheum. arthritis:** ini 2.5mg/kg/d PO div bid, incr prn after 8–12wk by 0.5–0.75mg/kg/d, max 4mg/kg/d
Daclizumab	EHL 44–360h, PRC C, Lact ?
Zenapax *Inj 25mg/5ml*	**Renal transplant:** 1mg/kg IV 24h prior to transpl., rep q14d for a total of 5 doses
Muromonab-CD3	
Orthoclone OKT 3 *Inj 1mg/ml*	**Acute allograft rejection:** 5mg IV qd for 10-14d
Mycophenolate Mofetil	EHL 16–18h, PRC C, Lact ?
Cellcept *Tab 500mg, Cap 250mg, Susp 200mg/ml, Inj 500mg/vial*	**Renal transplant:** 1g IV/PO bid; **heart transplant:** 1.5g IV/ PO bid; **liver transplant:** 1.5g PO bid; 1g IV bid
Sirolimus	EHL 57–63h, PRC C, Lact ?
Rapamune *Sol (oral) 1mg/ml, Tab 1mg*	**Renal transplant:** ini 6mg for 1d, maint 2mg PO qd; DARF: not req
Tacrolimus	EHL 8.7–11.3h, PRC C, Lact -
Prograf *Cap 1mg, 5mg, Inj 5mg/ml*	**Liver/renal transplant:** ini 0.03–0.05mg/kg/d IV contin. inf, maint 0.1–0.2mg/kg PO div bid

8.4 Recommended Childhood Immunization Schedule

Vaccine	Months					Years		
	Birth	2	4	6	12	18	4–6	14–16
Diphtherie, tetanus, pertussis (acell.) [1]		DTap	DTap	DTap		DTap	DTap	
Inactivated poliovirus		IPV	IPV	IPV[5]		IPV	IPV	
Haemophilus influenza type b[2]		Hib	Hib	Hib		Hib		
Measles, mumps and rubella					MMR	MMR[5] or	MMR[6]	
Tetanus[3] **and diphteriea toxoid**[10]								Td
Hepatitis B (3 doses)[4]	**Infancy or preadolescence (9–13 years)**							
Varicella					V[7]			
Pneumococcal conjugate		PC[8]	PC	PC	PC			
Meningococcal conjugate		MC[9]	MC	MC	**or**			MC[9]
Influenza				**6–23mo, 1–2doses**				

Canadian Immunization Guide Seventh Edition-2006; National Advisory Committee on Immunization (NACI)

1. **Diphtheria, tetanus, acellular pertussis and inactivated polio virus vaccine (DTaP-IPV):** DTaP-IPV(± Hib) vaccine is the preferred vaccine for all doses in the vaccination series, including completion of the series in children who have received one or more doses of DPT (whole cell) vaccine (e.g., recent immigrants).
2. **Hib** schedule shown is for PRP-T vaccine. If PRP-OMP is used, give at 2, 4 and 12 months of age.
3. Td (tetanus and diphtheria toxoid), a combined adsorbed "adult type" preparation for use in people > 7 years of age, contains less diphtheria toxoid than preparat. given to younger childr. and is less likely to cause react. in older people.
4. **Hepatitis B vaccine** can be routinely given to infants or preadolescents, depending on the provincial/territorial policy; three doses at 0, 1 and 6 month intervals are preferred. The second dose should be administered at least 1 month after the first dose, and the third at least 2 months after the second dose. A two-dose schedule for adolescents is also possible (see Guide).
5. This dose of **MMR** is not needed routinely, but can be included for convenience.
6. A second dose of **MMR** is recommended, at least 1 month after the first dose for the purpose of better measles protection. For convenience, options include giving it with the next scheduled vaccination at 18 months of age or with school entry (4–6 years) vaccinations (depending on the provincial/territorial policy), or at any intervening age that is practicle. The need for a 2nd dose of mumps and rubella vaccine is not estab. but may benefit (given for conven. as MMR). The 2nd dose of MMR should be given at the same visit as DTaP IPV (+ Hib) to ensure high uptake rates. 7. Children aged 12 months to 12 years should receive one dose of varicella vaccine. Individuals > 13 years of age should receive two doses at least 28 days apart.
8. **Pneumococcal conjugate vaccine ñ 7-valent (Pneu-C-7):** recommended for all children under 2 years of age. The recommended schedule depends on the age of the child when vaccination is begun (see Guide)
9. **Meningococcal C conjugate vaccine (Men-C):** recommended for children < 5 years of age, adolescents, young adults. Recomm. schedule age of the child (see Guide)
10. **dTap** adult formulation with reduced diphtheria toxoid and pertussis component

9 Antirheumatics, Analgesics

9.1 Antirheumatics

9.1.1 Gold

MA: inhibition of leukocyte migration into synovial membrane; **EF:** influence on rheumatoid process; **AE:** hair loss, dermatitis, stomatitis, pancytopenia, renal damage
AE (auranofin): rash, abdominal cramps, N/V, pruritus, proteinuria, diarrhea, anemia
AE (aurothioglucose): stomatitis, proteinuria, blood dyscrasias, pruritus/dermatitis
AE (gold sodium thiomalate): pruritus/rash, mucous membrane reactions, nephrotic syndrome, hematologic toxicity; **CI:** renal insufficiency, complete blood count changes, hepatic damage; **CI** (auranofin): hypersensitivity to gold salts, severe colitis, pulmonary fibrosis, exfoliative dermatitis, bone marrow aplasia, hematological DO;
CI (aurothioglucose): SLE, untreat. CHF/DM, blood DO, severe HTN, urticaria, eczema, colitis
CI (gold sodium thiomalate): toxicity to gold/heavy metals, SLE, severe debilitation

Auranofin	EHL 15–31d, PRC C, Lact ?
Ridaura *Cap 3mg*	**Rheumatoid arthritis:** 3mg PO bid or 6mg PO qd, max 9mg/d; **CH:** 0.1–0.15mg/kg/d PO; max 0.2mg/kg/d
Gold Sodium Thiomalate	EHL 5d, PRC C, Lact ?
Myochrysine *Inj 10mg/ml, 25mg/ml, 50mg/ml*	**Rheumatoid arthritis:** 1st wk: 10mg IM, 2nd wk: 25mg, then 25–50mg/wk until cumulative dose of 0.8–1g; maint 25–50mg q other wk for 2–20wk; **CH:** test dose 10mg IM, then 1mg/kg/wk until cumulative dose of 0.8–1g; max 50mg/dose maint 1mg/kg q2–4wk; DARF: GFR (ml/min) >50: 100%, <50: not rec

9.1.2 Hydroxychloroquin

AE: agranulocytosis, ocular toxicity, skin/mucosal pigmentation, N/V; **CI:** retinal or visual field changes from prior use, hypersens. to hydroxychloroquine, long-term use in children

Hydroxychloroquine Sulfate	EHL 40d, PRC C, Lact ?
Plaquenil *Tab 200mg*	**Rheumatoid arthritis:** 400–600mg PO qd maint. 200–400mg PO qd; LE: 400mg PO qd–bid maint 200–400mg PO qd; **CH:** 3–5mg/kg/d PO, max 400mg/d or max 7mg/kg/ d

9.1.3 Sulfasalazine

MA: prostaglandin synthesis ↓ ⇒ influence on rheumatoid process
AE: headache, N/V, GI distress, reversible oligospermia
CI: hypersensitivity to sulfasalazine/sulfa drugs/salicylates

Sulfasalazine	EHL 7.6h, PRC B, Lact ?
Salazopyrin *Tab 500mg* **Salazopyrin En-Tabs** *Tab ent. coat. 500mg* **Generics** *Tab 500mg, Tab ent. coat. 500mg*	**Rheumatoid arthritis:** ini 500mg PO qd–bid; maint 1g bid; **CH:** ini 10mg/kg/d PO; maint 30–50mg/kg/d div bid, max 2g/d

9.1.4 Immunosuppressants

MA (azathioprine, mercaptopurine, methotrexate): immunosuppressive, synthesis of cytokines ↓
EF: influence on rheumatoid process
AE (azathioprine, mercaptopurine): leukopenia/thrombocytopenia, N/V, pancreatitis, GI hypersensitivity, hepatitis
AE (methotrexate): exanthema, hair loss, GI ulcers, N/V, hematopoietic DO, lung fibrosis
CI (azathioprine, mercaptopurine): hypersensitivity to azathioprine
CI (methotrexate): acute infx, severe bone marrow depression, hepatic DO, GI ulcers, RF

Azathioprine	EHL 3h, PRC D, Lact -
Imuran *Tab 50mg, Inj 100mg/20ml* **Generics** *Tab 50mg*	**Rheumatoid arthritis:** ini 1mg/kg/d PO, maint 1–2.5mg/ kg/d; **Crohn's disease, Ulcerative colitis:** ini 50mg PO qd, maint 100-250mg PO qd, max 2.5mg/kg/d; DARF: GFR (ml/min) >50: 100%, 10–50: 75%, <10: 50%
Mercaptopurine (6-MP)	PRC D, Lact ?
Purinethol *Tab 50mg*	**ALL:** 2.5-5mg/kg PO qd, maint 1.25-2.5mg/kg PO qd; **Crohn's disease, Ulcerative colitis:** ini 50mg PO qd, maint 75-125mg PO qd, max 1.5mg/kg/d
Methotrexate	EHL no data, PRC X, Lact -
Generics *Tab 2.5mg, 10mg* *Inj 10mg/ml, 25mg/ml*	**Rheumatoid arthritis:** 7.5–15mg/wk PO/IM; **Crohn's disease:** ini 25mg IM qwk x 16 wks, maint 15mg IM qweek; DARF: GFR (ml/min) >50: 100%, 10–50: 50%;

9.1.5 Disease-Modifiying Anti-Rheumatic Drugs

MA (abatacept): modulates T-cell activation; **MA** (adalimumab): human antibody, binds TNF-alpha; **MA** (anakinra): recombinant interleukin-1 receptor antagonist; **MA** (efalizumab): monoclonal antibody binds to CD11 leukocyte surface antigen, reducing T cell activation and function; **MA** (etanercept): genetically engineered fusion protein composed of TNF receptors ⇒ binds 2 molecules of TNF and prevents them from binding to cellular receptors; **MA** (infliximab): murine antibody, binds TNF-alpha; **MA** (leflunomide): inhibition of dihydroorotate dehydrogenase ⇒ inhibition of pyrimidine synthesis ⇒ lymphocyte proliferation↓; **EF:** influence on rheumatoid process; **AE** (anakinra): neutropenia, infections, headache, injection site reactions; **AE** (etanercept): injection site reaction, headache, rhinitis; **AE** (infliximab): dyspnea, urticaria, headache, infusion reaction **AE** (leflunomide): diarrhea, HTN, transaminases↑, exanthema, hair loss, bone marrow depression, susceptibility to infx↑; **CI** (abatacept): active infection; **CI** (anakinra): hypersensitivity to E. coli-derived products; **CI** (etanercept): hypersensitivity to etanercept products; **CI** (infliximab): severe infections, Class III/IV CHF, hypersensitivity to murine proteins; **CI** (leflunomide): severe immunodeficiencies, restricted hematopoiesis, severe infections, hepatic dysfunction, moderate and severe RF, children and adolescents < 18

Abatacept	EHL 13d, PRC C, Lact ?
Orencia *Inj 250mg/15ml*	**Rheumatoid arthritis:** <60kg: ini 500mg IV at week 0,2,4 then q4wk; 60–100kg: ini 750mg IV at week 0,2,4 then q4wk; >100kg: ini 1g IV at week 0,2,4 then q4wk
Adalimumab	EHL 14d, PRC B, Lact ?
Humira *Inj 40mg/0.8ml*	**Ankylosing spondylitis, psoriatic arthritis, rheumatoid arthritis:** 40mg SC q2wk
Anakinra	EHL 4–6h, PRC B, Lact ?
Kineret *Inj 150mg/vial*	**Rheumatoid arthritis**: 100mg SC qd
Efalizumab	EHL 5–8d, PRC C, Lact -
Raptiva *Inj 150mg/vial*	**Psoriasis:** ini 0.7mg/kg SC x1, then 1mg/kg SC qwk, max 200mg/dose; DARF: not req
Etanercept	EHL 90–300h, PRC B, Lact ?
Enbrel *Inj 25mg/vial*	**Rheumatoid arthritis:** 25mg SC 2x/wk; **CH** 4–17y: 0.4mg/ kg SC 2x/wk; max 25mg/dose; **Psoriasis**: ini 50mg SC 2x/wk x 3mo, maint. 25mg SC 2x/wk or 50mg SC qwk; **Psoriatic arthritis:** 25mg SC 2x/wk or 50mg SC qwk; DARF: not req

Infliximab	EHL 9.5d, PRC B, Lact ?
Remicade *Inj 100mg/vial*	**Ankylosing spondylitis:** 5mg/kg IV week 0,2,6 then q6 weeks (ank. spondylitis), q8wks (psoriasis); **Rheumatoid arthritis:** 3mg/kg IV week 0,2,6 then q 8 weeks; DARF: not req
Leflunomide	EHL 4–28d, PRC X, Lact -
Arava *Tab 10mg, 20mg, 100mg* **Generics** *Tab 10mg, 20mg*	**Rheumatoid arthritis:** 100mg PO qd for 3d; maint 10- 20mg PO qd; DARF: not req

9.2 Nonsteroidal Anti-Inflammatory Drugs

9.2.1 NSAID - Salicylates

MA/EF: inhibition of cyclooxygenase ⇒ synthesis of prostaglandins ↓ ⇒ analgesic, anti-inflammatory, antipyretic; inhibition of blood platelet aggregation (aspirin); **Note:** salicylate-containing products are not recommended for use in children or teenagers with chicken pox, influenza or flu symptoms; **AE:** allergic skin reactions, dizziness, nausea, tinnitus, GI ulcerations, bronchospasm, hematopoietic DO, renal dysfunctions, abscess formation after IM administration; **AE**(aspirin): pancytopenia, acid-base balance DO, bleeding time ↑; **AE** (diflunisal): GI distress, rash; **CI** (acid NSAIDs): GI ulcerations,hematopoietic DO; **CI** (aspirin): restricted use in children and adolescents with febrile diseases (danger of Reye's syndrome; **CI** (diflunisal): hypersensitivity to diflunisal, asthma, allergic reactions to ASA or other anti- inflammatories

Aspirin (Acetylsalicylic Acid)	EHL 4.7–9h, PRC D, Lact ?
Asaphen *Tab 80mg* **Asaphen E.C.** *Ent. coated tab 80mg* **Asatab** *Tab 80mg* **Aspirin** *Tab 80mg, 325mg, 500mg, 650mg, Coated Tab 81mg* **Entrophen** *Cap 325mg, 650mg, Tab 325mg, 500mg, 650mg* **MSD Enteric Coated ASA** *Tab 325mg, 650mg* **Novasen** *Ent. coated tab 325mg, 650mg* **Generics** *Tab 325mg*	**Pain,fever:** 325–650mg PO/PR q4h prn, max 3.9g/d; **rheumatoid arthritis:** 3.2–6g/d in div doses; **rheumatic fever:** 1g q3–6h; **CH** 2–14y: **fever:** 10–15mg/kg PO q4h, max 60–80mg/kg/d; DARF GFR < 10ml/h: not rated
Diflunisal	EHL 8–12h, PRC C, Lact ?
Generics *Tab 250mg, 500mg*	**Pain:** ini 1g PO, maint 250–500mg q8–12h; **rheumatoid arthritis, osteoarthritis:** 500mg–1g PO div bid, max 1.5g/d; DARF: GFR (ml/min) > 50: 100%, <50: 50%

9.2.2 NSAID - Propionic Acid Derivatives

MA/EF: see NSAID, Aspirin + other salicylates →197 ;
AE (flurbiprofen): headache, GI distress, ocular burning/ stinging, rash, ulcers;
AE (ibuprofen): nausea, heartburn, ulcers, rash;
AE (ketoprofen): malaise, dizziness, GI distress, rash, tinnitus;
AE (ketorolac): GI distress, ulcers, headache/dizziness;
AE (naproxen): GI upset, headache, edema, dizziness;
AE (oxaprozin): GI distress, rash
CI (ibuprofen, ketoprofen, naproxen): hypersensitivity to product ingredients, asthma, allergic reactions to ASA, other anti-inflammatories;
CI (flurbiprofen): hypersensitivity to flurbiprofen products, asthma, allergic reaction to ASA/other anti-inflammatories, ocular epithelial herpes simplex keratitis;
CI (ketorolac, oxaprozin): hypersensitivity to product ingredients, allergy to ASA or other inflammatories, syndr. of nasal polyps and angioedema

Flurbiprofen	EHL 5.7h, PRC B, Lact ?
Ansaid *Tab 50mg, 100mg* **Froben** *Tab 50mg, 100mg* **Froben SR** *Cap sust rel 200mg* **Novo-Flurprofen** *Tab 50mg, 100mg* **Generics** *Tab 50mg, 100mg*	**Rheumatoid arthritis, osteoarthritis:** 200-300mg/d PO div bid-qid
Ibuprofen	EHL 1.8-2.0h, PRC D, Lact +
Advil *Tab 200mg, Cap 200mg, Susp 100mg/5ml* **Novo-Profen** *Tab 200mg, 300mg, 400mg, 600mg* **Generics** *Tab 200mg, 300mg, 400mg, 600mg*	**Rheumatoid arthritis, osteoarthritis:** 1200-3200mg/d PO div tid-qid; **pain, dysmenorrhea:** 400mg PO q4-6h; **CH juv. rheum. arthritis:** 30-50mg/kg/d PO div tid-qid, max 2.4g/d; **CH fever, pain:** 5-10mg/kg PO q6-8h prn, max 40mg/kg/d; DARF: not req
Ketoprofen	EHL 2-4h, PRC B, Lact ?
Apo-Keto-E *Ent coat Tab 50mg, 100mg* **Apo-Keto SR** *Ent coat Tab Sust Rel 200mg* **Oruvail** *Cap ext.rel. 150mg, 200mg* **Generics** *Cap 50mg, Ent Coat Tab 50, 100mg*	**Rheumatoid arthritis, osteoarthritis:** 100-300mg/d PO div tid-qid; pain, **dysmenorrhea:** 25-50mg PO q6-8h **CH juv. rheumatoid arthritis:** 25-50mg bid; DARF: see Prod Info

Ketorolac	EHL 5.3h, PRC C, Lact ?
Toradol *Tab 10mg, Inj 10mg/ml, 30mg/ml* **Generics** *Tab 10mg, Inj 30mg/ml*	**Pain:** ini 30–60mg IM or 15–30mg IV or 15–30mg IV/IM q6h; max IV/IM, 120mg/d; 10mg PO q4–6h prn; max PO 40mg/d; DARF: see Prod Info

Naproxen	EHL 12–15h
Anaprox *Tab 275mg, 550mg* **Apo-Napro-Na** *Tab 275mg, 550mg* **Naprelan** *Tab cont. rel. 375mg, 500mg* **Naprosyn** *Supp 500mg, Susp 125mg/5ml, Tab 500mg, Ent coat tab 250mg, 375mg, 500mg, Sust rel tab 750mg* **Novo-Naprox** *Tab 125mg, 250mg, 275mg, 375mg, 500mg, 550mg,* **Novo-Naprox SR** *Sust rel tab 750mg* **Novo-Naprox-EC** *Ent. coated Tab 250mg, 375mg, 500mg* **Nu-Naprox** *Tab 125mg, 250mg, 375mg, 500mg* **Generics** *Tab 125mg, 250mg, 375mg, 500mg, Sust rel tab 750mg, Supp 500mg*	**Rheumatoid arthritis, osteoarthritis, ankylosing spondylitis:** 250–500mg PO bid; **pain, dysmenorrhea:** ini 500mg, maint 250mg q6–8h prn; **CH** (rheumatoid arthritis): 10mg/kg/d div bid; DARF: not req

Oxaprozin	EHL 24–69h, PRC C, Lact ?
Daypro *Tab 600mg* **Generics** *Tab 600mg*	**Rheumatoid arthritis, osteoarthritis:** 1200mg PO qd, max 1800mg/d; DARF: severe renal impairment: 600mg PO qd

Tiaprofenic Acid	EHL 1.7h, PRC C, Lact ?
Surgam *Tab 300mg* **Surgam SR** *Cap sust rel 300mg* **Generics** *Tab 200mg, 300mg*	**Rheumatoid arthritis, osteoarthritis:** 300–600mg PO daily in div doses, max 600mg/d

9.2.3 NSAID - Acetic Acid Derivatives

MA/EF: see NSAID, Aspirin + other salicylates →197
AE (diclofenac): nausea/diarrhea, constipation, headache, burning/stinging, ulcers;
AE (diclofenac): abdominal pain, nausea, diarrhea;
AE (etodolac): GI distress, malaise, dizziness;
AE (indomethacin): headache, GI distress;
AE (nabumetone): headache/dizziness, edema, GI distress;
AE (sulindac): headache, dizziness, rash/pruritus, GI distress, edema;
AE (tolmetin): edema, dizziness, GI distress, BP ↑
CI (diclofenac): hypersensitivity to diclofenac or misoprostol, asthma or allergic reactions with aspirin or NSAIDS
CI (diclofenac, etodolac, nabumetone, sulindac): hypersensitivity to product ingredients, allergic reactions to ASA or other anti-inflammatories, asthma
CI (indomethacin, in addition): history of recent rectal bleeding or proctitis

Diclofenac	EHL 2h, PRC B, Lact ?
Apo-Diclo *Tab 25mg, 50mg, Tab ext.rel. 75mg, 100mg* **Novo-Difenac-K** *Tab 50mg* **Nu-Diclo** *Tab 25mg, 50mg* **Nu-Diclo SR** *Tab ext.rel. 75mg, 100mg* **Voltaren** *Tab 25mg, 50mg, Supp 50mg, 100mg* **Voltaren-SR** *Tab ext.rel. 75mg, 100mg* **Generics** *Tab 25mg, 50mg, Tab ext.rel. 75mg, 100mg, Supp 50mg, 100mg*	**Osteoarthritis, rheumatoid arthritis:** 50mg PO bid-tid or 75mg bid or 100mg qd; **ankylosing spondylitis:** 25mg PO qid **pain, dysmenorrhea:** 50mg PO tid

Diclofenac + Misoprostol	
Arthrotec *Tab ext. rel. 50mg + 200mcg, 75mg + 200mcg*	**Osteoarthritis:** 50mg/200mcg PO bid-tid or 75mg/ 200mcg bid; **rheumatoid arthritis:** 50mg/200mcg PO bid-qid or 75mg/200mcg bid ; DARF: GFR < 30ml/min: contraind.

Etodolac	EHL 6-7h, PRC C, Lact ?
Ultradol *Cap 200mg, 300mg* **Generics** *Cap 200mg, 300mg*	**Pain:** 200-400mg PO q6-8h; max 1,000 mg/d; max in patients weighing < 60kg is 20mg/kg/d; **rheumatoid arthritis, osteoarthritis:** ini 400-500mg PO bid or 300mg bid-tid; maint 400-1,000mg/d

Indomethacin	EHL 4.5h, PRC D, Lact +
Indotec *Cap 25mg, 50mg, Supp 50mg, 100mg* **Novo-Methacin** *Cap 25mg, 50mg, Supp 50mg, 100mg* **Nu-Indo** *Cap 25mg, 50mg* **Generics** *Cap 25mg, 50mg*	**Rheumatoid arthritis, osteoarthritis:** 25mg PO bid-tid, max 200mg/d **bursitis, tendinitis:** 75-150mg/d PO/PR div tid-qid; DARF: not req
Ketorolac	EHL 5.3h, PRC C, Lact ?
Toradol *Tab 10mg, Inj 10mg/ml, 30mg/ml* **Generics** *Tab 10mg, Inj 30mg/ml*	**Pain:** ini 30-60mg IM or 15-30mg IV or 15-30mg IV/IM q6h; max IV/IM 120mg/d; 10mg PO q4-6h prn; max PO 40mg/d; DARF: see Prod Info
Nabumetone	EHL unknown, PRC C, Lact ?
Generics *Tab 500mg*	**Rheumatoid arthritis, osteoarthritis:** 500mg PO bid, maint 1-2g/d; DARF not req
Sulindac	EHL 7.8h, PRC D, Lact -
Apo-Sulin *Tab 150mg, 200mg* **Novo-Sundac** *Tab 150mg, 200mg* **Generics** *Tab 150mg, 200mg*	**Rheumatoid arthritis, osteoarthritis, ankylosing spondylitis:** 150mg PO bid **bursitis, tendinitis, gout:** 200mg PO bid; max 400mg/d; **CH** limited data, 4mg/kg/d PO div bid has been used; DARF: not req

9.2.4 NSAID - Cyclooxygenase-2-Inhibitors

MA/EF: high selectivity for cyclooxygenase-2; inhibition of cyclooxygenase ⇒ synthesis of prostaglandins ↓
AE: dyspepsia, abdominal pain, GI effects
CI: hypersensitivity to celecoxib products, hypersensitivity to ASA or other anti-inflammatory drugs, hypersensitivity to sulfonamides

Celecoxib	EHL 11h , PRC C, Lact ?
Celebrex *Cap 100mg, 200mg*	**Osteoarthritis:** 100mg PO bid or 200mg qd; **rheumatoid arthritis:** 100-200mg PO bid

9.2.5 Other NSAIDs

MA/EF: see NSAID, Aspirin + other salicylates →197
AE (meloxicam): dyspepsia, flatulence, abdominal pain, diarrhea
AE (piroxicam) GI distress, rash, dizziness, ulcers, edema
CI (meloxicam): hypersensitiviy to meloxicam, allergic reactions to aspirin/NSAIDS
CI (piroxicam): hypersensitivity to piroxicam products, asthma, allergic reactions to ASA or other anti-inflammatories

Floctafenine	EHL 8h, PRC C, Lact -
Generics *Tab 200mg, 400mg*	**Pain:** 200–400mg PO q6–8 h PRN, max 1 200 mg/d
Mefenamic Acid	EHL 3–4h, PRC D, Lact -
Generics *Cap 250mg*	**Muscular aches, pain, primary dysmenorrhea, headache, dental pain:** ini 500mg PO then 250mg PO q6h PRN
Meloxicam	EHL 15–20h, PRC N, Lact ?
Mobicox *Tab 7.5mg, 15mg* **Generics** *Tab 7.5mg, 15mg*	**Osteoarthritis:** 7.5mg PO qd, max 15mg/d; DARF: see Prod Info
Piroxicam	EHL 50h, PRC C, Lact +
Novo-Pirocam *Cap 10mg, 20mg* **Nu-Pirox** *Cap 10mg, 20mg* **Generics** *Cap 10mg, 20mg*	**Rheumatoid arthritis, osteoarthritis:** 20mg PO qd or div bid; DARF: not req
Tenoxicam	EHL 60–75h, PRC D, Lact ?
Generics *Tab 20mg*	**Rheumatoid arthritis, osteoarthritis, ankylosing spondylitis, acute gouty arthritis, dysmenorrhoea:** 20mg PO qd

9.3 Other Non-Opioid Analgesics

9.3.1 Aniline Derivatives

MA: inhibition of cyclooxygenase ⇒ synthesis of prostaglandins ↓; **EF:** anti-inflammatory, analgesic, only mildly antiphlogistic; **AE:** allergic skin reactions, headache, bronchospasm, renal damage (tubular and papillary necrosis, interstitial nephritis), hepatic damage
CI: restricted use in presence of hepatic DO, Meulengracht's syndrome, renal DO

Acetaminophen (Paracetamol)	EHL no data, PRC B, Lact +
Abenol *Supp 120mg, 325mg, 650mg* **Atasol** *Cap 325mg, 500mg, Drops 80mg/ml, Tab 325mg, 500mg* **Novo-Gesic** *Tab 325mg, 500mg* **Pediatrix** *Drops 80mg/ml, Sol (oral) 160mg/5ml* **Tempra** *Drops 80mg/ml, Syr 80mg/5ml, 160mg/5ml, Tab (chew) 80mg, 160mg, Tab (quick dissolve) 160mg* **Tylenol** *Cap 325mg, 500mg, 650mg, Soft chews 80mg, Elixir 160mg/5ml, Susp (oral) 160mg/5ml, Gelcaps 500mg, Drops 80mg/ml, Tab (chew) 160mg, Tab 325mg, 500mg* **Generics** *Cap 325mg, 500mg, Tab 325mg, 500mg*	**Pain, fever:** 325–1,000mg PO/PR q4–6h, max 4g/d; **CH:** 10–15mg/kg/dose PO/PR q4–6h, max 5 doses/d; DARF: GFR (ml/min) >50: q4h, 10–50: q6h, <10: q8h

9.3.2 Non-Opioid Analgesic Combinations

Acetaminophen + Methocarbamol	PRC D, Lact ?
Methoxacet Extra Strength *Tab 500+400mg*	**Acute painful musculoskeletal conditions:** 2 Tab PO qid
Aspirin + Butalbital + Caffeine	PRC D, Lact ?
Fiorinal *Tab 330 + 50 + 40mg, Cap 330 + 50 + 40mg* **ratio-Tecnal** *Tab 330 + 50 + 40mg, Cap 330 + 50 + 40mg* **Trianal** *Tab 330 + 50 + 40mg, Cap 330 + 50 + 40mg*	**Tension headache:** 1–2 Tab/Cap PO q4h
Aspirin + Methocarbamol	PRC D, Lact ?
Aspirin Night-Time *Tab 500 + 400mg* **Methoxisal** *Cap 325 + 400mg, 500 + 400mg* **Robaxisal** *Cap 325 + 400mg* **Robaxisal Extra Strength** *Cap 500 + 400mg*	**Acute painful musculoskeletal conditions:** 2 Tab PO qid

9.4 Opioids

9.4.1 Opioid Agonists

MA/EF: stimulation of central opiate receptors ⇒analgesic, sedative, respiratory depression, antitussive, emetic and antiemetic (see AE); **AE:** respiratory depression, sedation, bradycardia, hypotensive circulation DO, pruritus, bronchospasm, transpiration, spasms of pancreatic and bile ducts, constipation, seizures, miosis, tolerance development, urinary retention; **CI:** restricted use for children < 1, addiction to opiates, pancreatitis, respiratory DO; Note: all are PRC D if used for prolonged periods or in high doses at term

Codeine	EHL 2.5–3.5h, PRC C, Lact + Equivalent dose compared to morphine 10mg IM (IM/oral): 120 / 200
Linctus codeine *Liq (oral) 0.2%* **Generics** *Tab 15mg, 30mg, 50mg, 100mg, 150mg, 200mg, Inj 30mg/ml, 60mg/ml, Liq (oral) 143mg/30ml*	**Pain:** 15–60mg PO/IM//SC q4–6h; **cough:** 10–20mg PO/ SC q4–6h prn; **CH pain:** > 2y: 0.5–1mg/kg/dose PO/SC/IM q4–6h; **CH cough:** 2–6y: 1mg/kg/d PO div qid, max 30mg/ 24h; 6–12y: 5–10mg PO q4–6h prn; max 60mg/24h; DARF: GFR (ml/min) > 50: 100%, 10–50: 75%, <10: 50%
Fentanyl	EHL no data, PRC C, Lact ? Equivalence (IM/oral): 0.1–0.2 / -
Duragesic *Film (ext.rel, TD) 0.6mg/24h, 1.2mg/24h, 1.8mg/24h, 2.4mg/24h* **Generics** *Inj 0.05mg/ml, Film (ext.rel, TD) 2.5mg/patch (25mcg/h), 5mg/patch (50mcg/h), 7.5mg/patch (75mcg/h), 10mg/patch (100mcg/h); 4.125mg/patch (25 µg/h); 8.25mg/patch (50 µg/h), 12.375mg/patch (75 µg/h), 16.5mg (100 µg/h)*	**Chronic pain:** 25–100mcg/h patch q72h **breakthrough CA pain:** ini 200mcg PO (oral transmucosal), titrate dose
Hydromorphone	EHL 2.5h, PRC C, Lact ? Equivalence (IM/oral): 1.5 / 7.5
Dilaudid *Tab 1mg, 2mg, 4mg, 8mg, Liquid (oral) 1mg/ml, Supp 3mg, Inj 2mg/ml* **Dilaudid-HP** *Inj 10mg/ml, 20mg/ml, 50mg/ml, 250mg/vial* **Hydromorph Contin** *Tab cont rel 3mg, 6mg, 12mg, 24mg, 30mg* **Generics** *Supp 3mg, Syr 1mg/ml, Tab 1mg, 2mg, 4mg, 8mg, Inj 2mg/ml, 10mg/ml, 20mg/ml, 50mg/ml, 100 mg/ml*	**Pain:** 2–4mg PO q4–6h; 1–2mg IM/SC/IV q4–6h prn; 3mg PR q6–8h

Meperidine (Pethidine)	EHL 3.2–3.7h, PRC B, Lact + Equivalence (IM/oral): 75 / 300
Demerol *Tab 50mg, Inj 50mg/ml, 75mg/ml, 100mg/ml* **Generics** *Inj 10mg/ml, 25mg/ml, 50mg/ml, 75mg/ml, 100mg/ml*	**Pain:** 50–150mg IV/IM/SC/PO q3–4h prn **CH:** 1–2mg/kg q3–4h IM/SC/PO; DARF: GFR (ml/min) > 50: 100%, 10–50: 75%, <10: 50%
Methadone	EHL 23h, PRCB, Lact ? Equivalence (IM/oral): variable
Metadol *Sol (oral) 10mg/ ml*	**Pain:** 2.5–10mg PO/SC/IM q3–4h prn; **narcotic addiction:** 40–180mg PO qd, taper dose as appropriate to avoid withdrawal symptoms; **CH pain:** 0.1–0.2mg/kg PO q6h; DARF: GFR (ml/min) > 50: q6h, 10–50: q8h, <10: q8–12h
Morphine Sulfate	EHL no data, PRC C, Lact ? Equivalence (IM/oral): 10 / 20–30
Kadian *Cap ext.rel. 20mg, 50mg, 100mg* **M-Eslon** *Cap 10mg, 15mg, 30mg, 60mg, 100mg, 200mg* **M.O.S. (morphine HCl)** *Conc (oral) 20mg/ml, 50mg/ml, Supp 10mg, 20mg, 30mg, Syr 1mg/ml, 5mg/ml, 10mg/ml, Tab 10mg, 20mg, 40mg, 60mg* **M.O.S. Sulfate** *Tab 5mg, 10mg, 25mg, 50mg* **M.O.S. SR (morphine HCl)** *Tab slow rel. 30mg, 60mg* **MS Contin** *Supp sust. rel. 30mg, 60mg, 100mg, 200mg, Tab sust. rel. 15mg, 30mg, 60mg, 100mg, 200mg* **MSIR** *Supp 10mg, 20mg, 30mg, Tab 5mg, 10mg, 20mg, 30mg* **Statex** *Drops 20mg/ml, 50mg/ml, Supp 5mg, 10mg, 20mg, 30mg, Syr 1mg/ml, 5mg/ml, 10mg/ml, Tab 5mg, 10mg, 25mg, 50mg* **Generics** *Inj 0.5mg/ml, 1mg/ml, 2mg/ml, 5mg,ml, 10mg/ml, 15mg/ml, 25mg/ml, 50mg/ml, Syr 1mg/ml, 5mg/ml, 10mg/ml, 20mg/ml, Tab sust. release 15mg, 30mg, 60mg*	**Pain:** 5–30mg PO q4h; 10mg IM/SC q4h; 2–10mg IV q4h; 10–20mg PR q4h; **CH:** 0.1–0.2mg/kg IM/SC/IV q2–4h, max 15mg/dose; DARF: GFR (ml/min) > 50: 100%, 10–50: 75%, <10: 50%

Oxycodone	EHL 3.2–8h, PRC C, Lact ? Equivalence (IM/oral): - / 10–15
OxyContin *Tab ext.rel. 10mg, 20mg, 40mg, 80mg* **Oxy IR** *Tab 5mg, 10mg, 20mg* **Supeudol** *Supp 10mg, 20mg, Tab 5mg, 10mg*	**Pain:** 10–30mg PO q6h prn; ext.rel.: 10mg PO q12h

Propoxyphene	EHL 6–12h, PRC D, Lact + Equivalence (IM/oral): 50 / 100
642 Tablets *Tab 65mg* **Darvon-N** *Tab 100mg*	**Pain:** 65mg PO q4h prn, max 390mg/d; DARF: GFR (ml/min) > 50: 100%, 10–50: 100%, <10: not rec

Tramadol	EHL 6.3h, PRC C, Lact +
Ralivia *Tab ext. rel. 100, 200, 300mg* **Tridural** *Tab ext. rel. 100, 200, 300mg* **Zytram XL** *Tab cont. rel. 150, 200, 300, 400mg*	**Pain:** ini 25mg PO qam, maint. 50–100mg PO q4–6h prn; DARF: GFR (ml/min) <30: give q12h, max 200mg/d; cirrhosis: 50mg q12h, max 100mg/d

9.4.2 Opioid Agonist-Antagonists

MA/EF: (buprenorphine, butorphanol, nalbuphanol): partial agonist and antagonist activity at the mu-opioid receptor and agonist activity at the kappa-opioid receptor;
AE (butorphanol): sedation, drowsiness, N/V, diplopia;
AE (nalbuphine): sedation, sweatiness, N/V, dizziness, resp. depression;
AE (pentaz.): physical dependence, resp. depression, hallucinations, confusion, N/V;
CI (butorphanol): hypersens. to butorphanol, benzethonium;
CI (nalbuphine): hypersens. to nalbuphine, oxymorphone, naloxone;
CI (pentaz.): hypersens. to pentazocine, naloxone (PO)

Buprenorphine + Naloxone	EHL 37h, PRC C, Lact +
Suboxone *Tab 2mg + 0.5mg, 8mg + 2mg*	**Treatment in opioid drug dependence** ini 4 mg/d; max 24mg/d; DARF: not req; contraindicated in patients with severe hepatic dysfunction

Butorphanol	EHL 4–7h, PRC C, Lact + Equivalence (IM/oral): 2 / -
Generics *Spray (Nasal) 10mg/ml*	**Postop pain, pain:** 1mg intranasally q3–4h prn; DARF: GFR (ml/min) > 50: 100%, 10–50: 75%, < 10: 50%
Nalbuphine	EHL 2.2 + 2.6h, PRC B, Lact ? Equivalence (IM/oral): 10 / -
Nubain *Inj 10mg/ml, 20mg/ml*	**Pain:** 10–20mg SC/IM/IV q3–6h prn; anesth: 0.3–3mg/kg IV, then 0.25–0.5mg/kg prn
Pentazocine	EHL 2–3.6h, PRC C, Lact ? Equivalence (IM/oral): 60 / 180
Talwin *Inj 30mg/ml, Tab 50mg*	**Pain:** 30mg IV/IM/SC q3–4h prn; max 360mg/d; 50–100mg PO q3–4h; max 600mg/d; DARF: GFR (ml/min) > 50: 100%, 10–50: 75%, <10: 50%

9.4.3 Opioid Antagonists

MA: competitive blockage of opiate receptors;
AE: withdrawal syndrome in opiate addicts, allergic reactions;
AE (nalmefene): N/V, headache, dizziness, tachycardia;
AE (naloxone): opiate withdrawal symptoms;
CI: hypersensitivity to product ingredients

Naloxone	EHL 30–81min, PRC B, Lact ?
Generics *Inj 0.4mg/ml, 1mg/ml*	**Opioid overdose:** 0.4–2mg IV/IM/SC, rep. prn q2–3min; **postop respiratory depression:** 0.1–0.2mg IV rep. prn q2–3min; **CH opiod overdose:** < **20kg:** 0.1mg/kg IV, > **20kg:** 2mg IV, rep. prn q2–3min; **postop respiratory depression:** 10mcg/kg IV/IM/SC rep. prn q2–3min; DARF: not req
Naltrexone	EHL 12.9h, PRC C, Lact ?
ReVia *Tab 50mg*	**Opioid dependancy/alcoholism:** ini 50mg PO qd

9.5 Opioid Analgesic Combinations

Codeine + Acetaminophen	PRC C, Lact ?
ratio-Emtec *Tab 30mg + 300mg* **ratio-Lenoltec No. 4** *Tab 60mg + 300mg* **Triatec-30** *Tab 30mg + 300mg* **Tylenol Elixir with codeine** *Sol (oral) 8mg + 160mg/5ml* **Tylenol No. 4 with codeine** *Tab 60mg + 300mg*	**Pain:** 1–2 Cap/Tab PO q4h prn

Codeine + Acetaminophen + Caffeine	
Atasol- 8, 15, 30 *Tab 8mg + 325mg + 30mg, 15mg + 325mg + 30mg, 30mg + 325mg + 30mg* **Exdol-8, 15, 30** *Tab 8mg + 300mg + 30mg, 15mg + 300mg + 30mg, 30mg + 300mg + 30mg* **ratio-Lenoltec No. 1** *Cap 8mg + 300mg + 15mg, Tab 8mg + 300mg + 15mg* **ratio-Lenoltec No. 2** *Tab 15mg + 300mg + 15mg* **ratio-Lenoltec No. 3** *Tab 30mg + 300mg + 15mg* **Triatec 8** *Tab 8mg + 325mg + 30mg, 8mg + 500mg + 30mg* **Tylenol No. 1 with codeine** *Tab 8mg + 300mg + 15mg, 8mg + 500mg + 15mg* **Tylenol No. 2 with codeine** *Tab 15mg + 300mg + 15mg* **Tylenol No. 3 with codeine** *Tab 30mg + 300mg + 15mg*	**Pain:** 1–2 Cap/Tab PO q4h prn

Codeine + Aspirin + Caffeine	
222 tablets *Tab 8mg + 375mg + 30mg* **282 tablets** *Tab 15mg + 375mg + 30mg* **292 tablets** *Tab 30mg + 375mg + 30mg*	**Pain:** 1–2 Tab PO q4h prn
Codeine + Aspirin + Caffeine + Meprobamate	
282 MEP tablets *Tab 15mg + 375mg + 30mg + 200mg*	**Pain/muscle spasm:** 1–2 Tab PO q4h prn
Codeine + Aspirin + Butalbital + Caffeine	PRC C, Lact -
Fiorinal-C ¼, ½ *Cap 15mg + 330mg + 50mg + 40mg, 30mg + 330mg + 50mg + 40mg* **ratio-Tecnal C1/4, C1/2** *Cap 15mg + 330mg + 50mg + 40mg, 30mg + 330mg + 50mg + 40mg* **Trianal C1/4, C1/2** *Cap 15mg + 330mg + 50mg + 40mg, 30mg + 330mg + 50mg + 40mg*	**Pain:** 1–2 Cap PO q4h prn, max 6 Cap/d
Hydrocodone + Ibuprofen	PRC D, Lact +
Ibucodone *Tab 7.5mg + 200mg*	**Pain:** 1 Tab PO q4-6 hours; max 6 tab/24h
Oxycodone + Acetaminophen	PRC C, Lact -
Endocet *Tab 5 + 325mg* **ratio-Oxycocet** *Tab 5 + 325mg* **Percocet Demi** *Tab 2.5 + 325mg* **Percocet** *Tab 5 + 325mg*	**Pain:** 1 Tab PO q6h prn; max 4g acetaminophen/d
Oxycodone + Aspirin	PRC D, Lact ?
Endodan *Tab 5 + 325mg* **ratio-Oxycodan** *Tab 5 + 325mg* **Percodan-demi** *Tab 2.5 + 325mg* **Percodan** *Tab 5 + 325mg*	**Pain:** 1 Tab PO q6h prn
Tramadol + Acetaminophen	PRC C, Lact ?
Tramacet *Tab 37.5 + 325mg*	**Pain:** 2 Tab PO q4–6h prn; max 8 Tabs/d; DARF CrCl (ml/min): <30: give q12h, max 4 tabs/d

10 Anesthetics

10.1 Intravenous Anesthetics and Sedatives

10.1.1 Barbiturates

MA (thiopental): barbiturate, hypnotic, anticonvulsive, decrease of intracranial pressure
AE (thiopental): BP↓↓, resp. depression, bronchospasm, hemolytic anemia, vasodilation, intracranial pressure changes, hepatotoxicity, erythema
CI (thiopental): shock, status asthmaticus, intoxications, porphyria, severe CVS disease, hypersensitivity to thiopental products/ barbiturate

Thiopental	EHL 3–18h, PRC
Pentothal *Inj (Sol) 1g/vial, 2.5g/vial, 5g/vial, Inj (Powder) 250mg/syringe, 500mg/syringe, 500mg/vial, 1g/vial*	**Anesthesia induction:** 3–5mg/kg IV convulsive state: 75–125mg IV; **CH** 1–12y: anesthesia induction: 5–6mg/kg IV; DARF: GFR (ml/min) >10: 100%, <10: 75%

10.1.2 Benzodiazepines

MA/EF: opening of chloride channels ⇒ inhibiting function of GABA neurons↑, especially in the limbic system ⇒ sedative, sleep inducing, anxiolytic, muscle relaxing
AE (midazolam): amnesia, N/V, respiratory depression
CI (midazolam): acute narrow angle glaucoma, hypersensitivity to midazolam products

Midazolam	EHL 2–5h, PRC D, Lact ?
Versed *Inj 1mg/ml, 5mg/ml* **Generics** *Inj 1mg/ml, 5mg/ml*	**Anesthesia induction:** 0.15–0.35mg/kg IV; **sedation**: 0.05–0.1mg/kg IV, maint. 0.02–0.1mg/kg/h; **CH** 0.5–5y: **sedation:** 0.05–0.1mg/kg IV; **CH** 6–12y: **sedation:** 0.025–0.05mg/kg IV; DARF: GFR (ml/min): >10: 100%, <10: 50%

10.1.3 Opioids

MA/EF: stimulation of central opiate receptors ⇒ analgesic, sedative
AE (alfentanil): muscle rigidity, arrhythmias, dizziness, N/V, apnea
AE (fentanyl): respiratory depression, muscle rigidity, N/V, urinary retention, sedation
AE (remifentanil): hypotension, bradycardia, N/V
AE (sufentanil): respiratory depression, N/V, skeletal muscle rigidity, HTN, drowsiness, urinary retention
CI (alfentanil, fentanyl, remifentanil, sufentanil): hypersensitivity to product ingredients/ opioid agonists

Alfentanil — EHL 90–111min, PRC C, Lact ?
Equivalent dose compared to morphine 10mg IM (IM/oral): 0.4–0.8 / -

Alfenta *Inj 0.5mg/ml* **Generics** *Inj 0.5mg/2ml*	**Anesthesia:** individualized according to type and duration of surg. procedure/anesthesia; 8–75mcg/kg IV, maint 0.5–3mcg/kg/min according to duration of surgical procedure

Fentanyl — EHL 2–7h, PRC C, Lact ?
Equivalence (IM/oral): 0.1–0.2 / -

Duragesic *Film (ext.rel, TD) 0.3mg/24h (12.5mcg/h), 0.6mg/24h (25mcg/h), 1.2mg/ 24h (50mcg/h), 1.8mg/24h (75mcg/h), 2.4mg/24h (100mcg/h)* **Generics** *Inj 0.05mg/ml, Film (ext.rel, TD) 2.5mg/patch (25mcg/h), 5mg/patch (50mcg/ h), 7.5mg/patch (75mcg/h), 10mg/patch (100mcg/h); 4.125mg/patch (25 µg/h), 8.25mg/patch (50 µg/h), 12.375mg/patch (75 µg/h), 16.5mg (100 µg/h)*	**Pain:** 50–100mcg IV/IM q1–2h prn; Trans. derm. patch change q72h; **anesthesia adjunct:** 2–50mcg/kg IV

Remifentanil — EHL 3–10min, PRC C, Lact ?

Ultiva *Inj 1mg/vial, 2mg/vial, 5mg/vial*	**Anesthesia induction:** 0.5–1mcg/kg/min IV, maint 0.05–2mcg/kg/min; DARF not req

Sufentanil — EHL 158–164min, PRC C, Lact ?
Equivalence (IM/oral): 0.01–0.04 / -

Sufenta *Inj 0.05mg/ml* **Generics** *Inj 0.05mg/ml*	**Analgesic adjunct:** 1–8mcg/kg IV; **anesthesia:** 8–30mcg/ kg IV, then 10–50mcg prn; **CH** < 12y: **anesthesia:** 10–25mcg/kg IV, then 25–50mcg prn

10.1.4 Ketamine

EF: analgesic, hypnotic without considerable respiratory depression
AE: BP ↑, tachycardia, intracranial pressure ↑, hypersalivation, unpleasant/vivid dreams, muscle hyperactivity, N/V
CI: severe HTN, pre-eclampsia, intracranial pressure ↑ without adequate artificial respiration, hypersensitivity to ketamine products, conditions where HTN is hazardous

Ketamine	EHL 2-3h, PRC D, Lact -
Ketalar *Inj 10mg/ml, 50mg/ml*	**Anesthesia:** 1-2mg/kg IV; 5-10mg/kg IM; maint. 0.1-0.5mg/min IV; **sedation, analgesia:** 0.2- 0.75mg/kg IV, maint 5-20mcg/kg/min, **CH anesthesia:** 1-2mg/kg IV; 5-10mg/kg IM; maint 0.01-0.03mg/kg/min IV; **CH sedation, analgesia:** 0.2-1mg/kg IV, maint 5-20mcg/ kg/min

10.1.5 Propofol

MA/EF: hypnotic for induction and maintenance of anesthesia, no analgesia
AE: BP ↑, respiratory depression, bradycardia, seizures, adrenal suppression, apnea, injection site pain, cardiac arrest
CI: decompensated cardiac insufficiency, ch < 3y, hypersensitivity to propofol products

Propofol	EHL 40-200min, PRC B, Lact ?
Diprivan *Inj 10mg/ml* **Generics** *Inj 10mg/ml*	**Anesthesia induction:** 1-2.5mg/kg IV, maint 100-200mcg/kg/min IV; **ICU sedation:** 5-50mcg/kg/min; **CH** > 3y: **anesthesia induction:** 2.5-3.5mg/kg IV, maint 125-300mcg/kg/min; **sedation:** 1-2mg/kg IV, maint 75-100mcg/kg/min; DARF: not req

10.2 Neuromuscular Blockers

10.2.1 Depolarising Muscle Relaxants

MA/EF: permanent depolarization of the motor endplate, prevention of the immediate repolarization;
AE: allerg. skin react., fasciculations, muscle pain, coronary dysrythmias, bradycardia, hyperkalemia, malignant hyperthermia, IOP ↑;
CI: impossibility of artificial respir.n, anamnestic malign.t hyperthermia, susceptibility to hyperkalemia ↑, acute phase of major trauma/major burns, hypersensit. to succinylcholine

Succinylcholine	EHL < 1min, PRC C, Lact ?
Quelicin *Inj 20mg/ml, 100mg/ml* **Generics** *Inj 20mg/ml*	**General anesthesia:** ini 0.6mg/kg IV, maint 0.5–10mg/ min; **CH general anesthesia:** ini 1–2mg/kg IV; DARF: not req

10.2.2 Non-Depolarising Muscle Relaxants

MA/EF: competitive displacement of acetylcholine at the nicotinergic receptors of the motor endplate ⇒ prevention of depolarization
AE: bronchospasm, tachycardia, urticaria, hypotension
AE (cisatracurium): bradycardia, flushing;
AE (pancuronium): HTN, salivation;
AE (rocuronium): severe pain on injection, HTN;
AE (vecuronium): brady-/tachycardia, allergic reactions, hypotension
CI: impossibility of artificial respiration; caution with myasthenia gravis and Eaton-Lambert-Syndrome
CI (cisatracurium, mivacurium): hypersensitivity to cisatracurium/benzylisoquinoliniums
CI (pancuronium): hypersensitivity to pancuronium or bromide products
CI (rocuronium, vecuronium): hypersensitivity to product ingredients

Atracurium	EHL 20min, PRC C, Lact ?
Generics *Inj 10mg/ml*	**General anesthesia:** ini 0.4–0.5mg/kg IV bolus, maint. 0.08–0.1mg/kg IV boluses
Cisatracurium	EHL 22–31min, PRC B, Lact ?
Nimbex *Inj 2mg/ml, 10mg/ml*	**General anesthesia:** ini 0.15mg/kg IV maint. 1–2mcg/kg/min IV; **ICU long-term use:** 3mcg/kg/min IV; **CH** 2–12y: **general anesthesia:** ini 0.1mg/kg IV

Pancuronium	EHL 89–140min, PRC C, Lact ?
Pancuronium *Inj 1mg/ml, 2mg/ml* **Generics** *Inj 1mg/ml, 2mg/ml*	**General anesthesia:** 0.06–0.1mg/kg IV, maint 0.01–0.06mg/kg q80–150min; DARF: GFR (ml/min) >10: 100%, <10: not rated
Rocuronium	EHL 84–131min, PRC B, Lact ?
Zemuron *Inj 10mg/ml*	**General anesthesia:** ini 600mcg/kg IV, maint 75–225mcg/kg prn
Vecuronium	EHL 65–80min, PRC C, Lact ?
Generics *Inj 10mg/vial*	**General anesthesia:** 0.075–0.1mg/kg IV, maint 0.01–0.015mg/kg, rep q15–40min prn

10.3 Local Anesthetics

MA/EF: membrane permeability for cations , especially Na+ ⇒ excitability of nerve fibers↓;
AE: dizziness, vomiting, drowsiness, convulsions, bradycardia, dysrhythmias, shock
AE (bupivacaine): arterial hypotension, ventricular arrhythmias, CNS excitation
AE (lidocaine): seizures, drowsiness, tremors, hypotension
AE (mepivacaine): fetal bradycardia, respiratory arrest, seizures, allergic reaction, porphyria
CI (topical anesthetics): severe conduction disturbances, acute decompensated coronary insufficiency, shock, infections around injection site, known allergy
CI (bupivacaine): regional IV anesthesia, paracervical block, shock or myasthenia gravis, hypersensitivity to bupivacaine products
CI (lidocaine, mepivacaine): hypersensitivity to product ingredients/amide-type anesthetics

Articaine + Epinephrine	EHL 25min, PRC C, Lact +
Astracaine *Inj 40mg + 5mcg/ml* **Astracaine forte** *Inj 40mg + 10mcg/ml*	**Local anesthesia, nerve block:** 0.5–3.6ml; oral surgery: 1–5.4ml; max 7mg/kg
Bupivacaine	EHL no data
Marcaine (with epinephrine) *1:200 000 Inj 0.25%, 0.5%* **Marcaine** *Inj (spinal) 0.75%* **Sensorcaine** *Inj 0.25%, 0.5%* **Sensorcaine with epinephrine** *1:200 000 Inj 0.25%, 0.5%* **Sensorcaine Forte with epinephrine** *1:200 000 Inj 0.5%* **Generics** *Inj 0.25%, 0.5%, 0.75%*	**Local infiltration:** 175mg (0.25% sol.); **complete motor blockade, epidural:** 75–150mg (0.5–0.75% sol.); **dental anesthesia:** 9–18mg (0.5% sol.)

Chloroprocaine	PRC C, Lact ?
Nesacaine-CE *Inj 2%, 3%*	**Mandibular nerve block:** 2–3ml (2% sol); infraorbital: 0.5–1ml (2% sol); brachial plexus: 30–40ml (2% sol); pudendal block: 10ml (2% sol); caudal and epidural block: 15–25ml (2–3% sol)
Lidocaine	EHL 1.5–2h, PRC B, Lact +
Xylocaine CO2 *Inj 17.3mg/ml* **Xylocaine** *Inj 0.5%, 1%, 1.5%, 2.0%, 4.0%* **Xylocaine (with epinephrine)** *Inj 0.5%, 1%, 1.5%, 2.0%* **Xylocaine Spinal** *Inj 5.0%* **Generics** *Inj 1%, 2.0%, 10mg/ml, Inj (with epinephrine) 1%, 2.0%*	**Caudal anesthesia:** 200–300mg (1% sol.) **epidural anesthesia:** 250–300mg (1–2% sol.);
Mepivacaine	EHL 1.9–3.2h, PRC C, Lact ?
Carbocaine *Inj 1%, 2%* **Isocaine** *Inj 3%* **Isocaine (with levonordefrin)** *Inj 2%* **Scandonest** *Inj 3%* **Scandonest (with epinephrine)** *Inj 2%* **Polocaine** *Inj 3%* **Polocaine (with levonordefrin)** *Inj 2%*	**Brachial nerve block:** 50–400mg (1–2% sol); **epidural nerve block:** 150–300mg (1–2% sol); **local infiltration:** up to 400mg (0.5–1% sol.)
Prilocaine	EHL 1.6h, PRC C, Lact +
Citanest 4% Forte *Inj (with epinephrine) 4%* **Citanest 4% Plain** *Inj 4%*	**Dental procedures:** ini 1–2ml
Ropivacaine	EHL 4h, PRC B, Lact ?
Naropin *Inj 2mg/ml, 5mg/ml, 7.5mg/ml, 10mg/ml*	**Epidural block:** 250mg

11 Neurology

11.1 Anticonvulsants

MA (carbamazepine): repeated stimulation of afferences ⇒ stimulus answer ↓
MA (benzodiazepines; clonazepam, diazepam, lorazepam): opening of chloride channels ⇒ inhibiting function of GABA neurons ↑, especially in the limbic system
MA (fosphenytoin, phenytoin): ion permeability ↓ ⇒ membrane stabilization
MA (lamotrigine): blockage of presynaptic Na+ channels ⇒ release of excitatory amino acids ↓
MA (Levetiracetam): binds synaptic vesicle protein SV2A
MA (phenobarbital): reinforcement of inhibitory effect of GABA in the CNS
MA (oxcarbazepine, topiramate): membrane stabilization by blockage of Na- channels, antagonization of the excitatory effect of glutamate, reinforcement of the inhibitory effect caused by GABA
MA (valproic acid, vigabatrin): enzymatic breakdown of GABA ↓
EF (benzodiazepines; diazepam, phenobarbital): sedative, sleep inducing, anxiolytic, anti-aggressive, anti-convulsive, muscle relaxing
AE (carbamazepine): headache, dizziness, ataxia, dysopias, cholestatic hepatitis, disturbances of haematopoiesis, bradycardic cardiac arrhythmias, allergic reactions
AE (benzodiazepines; clonazepam, diazepam, lorazepam): tiredness, sleepiness, drowsiness, confusion, paradox reactions, anterograde amnesia, respiratory depression, psychic and physical addiction
AE (fosphenytoin, phenytoin): gingival hyperplasia, hypertrichosis, dizziness, ataxia, complete blood count changes
AE (Levetiracetam): tiredness, dizziness, headache, depression
AE (oxcarbazepine): tiredness, dizziness, headache, nausea, diplopia, hyponatremia, acne, alopecia, exanthema
AE (phenobarbital): tiredness, dizziness, anterograde amnesia, dizziness, ataxia, dysopias, porphyria, N/V, hepatic dysfunction, bradycardia, respiratory depression, skin reactions, complete blood count changes, enzyme ind., addiction
AE (divalproex, valproic acid): nausea/vomiting, fatigue/sedation, tremors, hair loss, elevated transaminases, thrombocytopenia
CI (carbamazepine): AV block, severe hepatic dysfunction, combination with MAO-inhib.
CI (benzos; clonazepam, diazepam, lorazepam): myasthenia gravis, severe hepatic damage, respiratory insufficiency, ataxia
CI (fosphenytoin, phenytoin): AV block II°–III°, sick sinus, cardiac insufficiency
CI (phenobarbital): porphyria, severe hepatic and renal dysfunction, status asthmaticus, respiratory insufficiency
CI (divalproex, valproic acid): liver disease, urea cycle disorder, hypersensitivity to drug

Carbamazepine	EHL 12-17h (mult. dose), 25-65h (1x dose), PRC D, Lact +, serum-level (mcg/ml): 4-12
Novo-Carbamaz *Tab 200mg* **Tegretol** *Tab (chew) 100mg, 200mg, Tab 200mg, Susp 100mg/5ml* **Tegretol CR** *Tab sust. rel. 200mg, 400mg* **Generics** *Tab 200mg, Tab sust. rel. 200mg, 400mg, Tab (chew) 100mg, 200mg*	**Mania:** 200mg PO qd-bid, incr by 200mg/d q2-4d, maint 600-1600mg/d, max 2,000-3,000mg/d; **epilepsy:** ini 200mg PO bid, incr by 200mg/d q wk div tid-qid or bid (ext.rel.), maint 800-1,200mg/d, max 1,200mg/d, max 1,600mg/d; **CH** >12 y: ini 200 mg PO bid, or 100mg PO qid (susp), incr by 200mg/d q wk div tid-qid or bid (ext.rel.), max 1,000 mg/d (age 12-15 y), max 1,200 mg/d (age >15 y); **CH** 6-12 y: 100mg PO bid or 50mg PO qid (susp), incr by 100mg/d q wk div tid-qid or bid (ext.rel.), 15-30 mg/kg/d PO div bid-qid, maint 400-800mg/d, max 1,000mg/d; **CH** <6 y: 10-20mg/kg/d PO div bid-qid, max 35 mg/kg/d; **trigeminal neuralgia:** ini 100mg PO bid or 200mg PO qd (ext. rel.) or 50mg PO qid (susp), incr by 200mg/d prn, maint 400-800mg/d, max 1,200mg/d; **migraine PRO:** 600 mg/d, 10-20mg/kg/d PO div bid; DARF: not req
Clobazam	EHL 18h, PRC X(1st), D(2nd, 3rd), Lact -
Frisium *Tab 10mg* **Generics** *Tab 10mg*	**Epilepsy:** ini 5-15mg/d, max 80mg/d; **CH** <2yrs: ini 0.5-1mg/kg /d; 2-16yrs ini 5mg/d, max 40mg/d; DARF required, reduced dose required for impared liver function
Clonazepam	EHL 30-40h, PRC C, Lact ?, serum-level (ng/ml): 25-30
Clonapam *Tab 0.5mg, 1mg, 2mg* **Rivotril** *Tab 0.5mg, 2mg* **Generics** *Tab 0.25mg, 0.5mg, 1mg, 2mg*	**Epilepsy:** ini 0.5mg PO tid, incr by 0.5-1mg q3d, max 20mg/d; **CH** <10 y or <30kg: ini 0.01-0.03mg/kg/d (max 0.05mg/kg/d) PO div bid-tid, incr by 0.25-0.5mg q3d up to 0.1-0.2mg/kg/d div tid, **neuralgias:** 2-4mg/d PO; **anxiety, panic DO:** →249

Diazepam	EHL 22-54h, PRC D, Lact ?
Diastat *Gel (rectal) 5mg/ml* **Diazemuls** *Conc (oral) 5mg/ml* **E Pam** *Tab 2mg, 5mg, 10mg* **Novo-Dipam** *Tab 2mg, 5mg, 10mg* **Valium** *Tab 5mg* **Generics** *Tab 2mg, 5mg, 10mg* *Inj 1mg/ml, 5mg/ml*	**Status epilepticus:** 5-10mg IV, rep in 10-15min, max 30mg; **CH** 1 mo-5 y: 0.2-0.5mg/kg IV slowly q2-5min to max 5mg, >5 y: 1mg IV slowly q2-5min to max 10mg, rep q2-4h prn; **epilepsy, adj** Tx: 2-10mg PO bid-qid; **CH** >6 mo: 1-2.5mg PO tid-qid, **CH** <5 y: max 5mg/d, >5 y: max 10mg; **seizure activity**↑: 0.2-0.5 mg/kg PR or 14-27kg: 5mg, 28-50kg: 10mg, 51-75kg: 15mg, 76-111kg: 20mg, rep prn in 4-12h, max 20 mg/d or **CH** 2-5 y: 0.5 mg/kg PR, 6-11 y: 0.3 mg/kg PR, <12 y: 0.2 mg/kg PR; **alcohol withdrawal:** ini 10mg PO tid-qid x 24h, then red to 5mg tid-qid prn; DARF: not req
Divalproex Sodium	EHL 6-17h, PRC D, Lact + serum-level(mcg/ml): 70-120
Epival *Tab 125mg, 250mg, 500mg VAE, Tab ext. rel 500mg VAE* **Generics** *Tab 125mg, 250mg, 500mg VAE (VAE=valproic acid equivalents)*	**Migraine PRO:** 250mg PO bid, titrate to max 1,000mg/d; DARF: not req
Ethosuximide	PRC C, Lact ? serum-level (mcg/ml): 40-100
Zarontin *Cap 250mg, Syr 250mg/5ml*	**Epilepsy:** 500mg PO qd or div bid, incr by 250 mg/d q4-7d, maint 20-30mg/kg/d div qd-bid, max 1.5 g/d; **CH** 3-6 y: 250mg PO qd, incr by 250mg/d q4-7d, maint 20-30mg/ kg/d, >6 y: 500mg PO qd, incr by 250mg/d q4-7d, maint 20-30mg/kg/d, max 1.5g/d
Fosphenytoin	EHL (Phenytoin): 12-29h, PRC D, Lact ? serum-level (mcg/ml): 10-20
Cerebyx *Inj 50mg mg PE/ml (PE = phenytoin equivalents)*	**Status epilepticus:** 15-20mg PE/kg IV, max IV rate100-150mg PE/min; **CH:** 15-20mg PE/kg IV at rate <2mg PE/ kg/min; **seizure PRO:** 10-20mg PE/kg IM; maint 4-6mg PE/kg/d

Gabapentin	EHL 5-7h, PRC C, Lact ?
Neurontin *Tab 600mg, 800mg, Cap 100mg, 300mg, 400mg* **Generics** *Cap 100mg, 300mg, 400mg*	**Epilepsy (adj Tx):** ini 300mg PO tid, incr by 300mg/d q3-5d, maint 300-600mg PO tid, max 3,600mg/d; **CH** >12 y: adult dose; **neuropathic pain:** 300mg PO tid, max 3,600mg/d; **restless legs syndrome:** 300-2,700mg/d PO; **mania:** ini 300mg PO hs, titrate to 900-2,400 mg/d in div doses; DARF: CrCl(ml/min) 30-60: 300mg PO bid, 15-30: 300mg PO qd, <15: 300mg PO qod
Lamotrigine	EHL 25-30h, PRC C, Lact ?
Lamictal *Tab (chew) 5mg, Tab 25mg, 100mg, 150mg*	**Epilepsy (adj Tx with valproic acid):** ini 25mg PO qod x 2wk, then 25mg PO qd x 2wk, incr by 25-50mg/d q1-2wk, maint 100-400mg/d div qd-bid, maint with valproic acid alone: 100-200mg/d div qd-bid; **epilepsy (adj Tx with enzyme-inducing antiepileptic drugs):** ini 50mg PO qd x 2wk, then 50 mg PO bid x 2wk, incr by 100 mg/d q1-2wk, maint 150-250mg PO bid; **Lennox-Gastaut (adj Tx with valproic acid)** **CH** 2-12 y: ini 0.15mg/kg/d PO div qd- bid x 2wk, then 0.3mg/kg/d PO div qd-bid x 2wk, incr q1-2wk, maint 1-5mg/kg/d, max 200mg/d; **Lennox-Gastaut (adj Tx with enzyme-inducing antiepileptic drugs)** **CH** 2-12 y: ini 0.6mg/kg/d PO div bid x 2wk, then 1.2mg/kg/d PO div bid x 2wk, incr q1-2wk, maint 5-15mg/kg/d, max 400mg/d; **bipolar depression:** ini 25-50mg PO qd, incr to 100-500mg/d div bid; DARF: reduce maint dose

Levetiracetam	EHL 6-8h, PRC C, Lact ?
Keppra *Tab 250mg, 500mg, 750mg* **Generics** *Tab 250 mg, 500 mg, 750 mg*	**Partial seizures, juvenile myoclonic epilepsy:** ini 500mg PO q12h, maint. 500-1500mg PO q12h, max 3,000mg/d DARF: CrCL (ml/min) 50-80: 500-1,000mg q12h, 30-50: 250-750mg q12h, <30: 250-500mg q12h, HD: 500-1,000mg q24h, 250-500mg as suppl.; **CH:** (4-15yo) ini 20mg/kg/d PO div bid, maint. 60mg/kg/d div bid, max 3000mg/d
Lorazepam	EHL 10-20h, PRC D, Lact ?
Ativan *Tab 0.5mg, 1mg, 2mg, Tab (subling.) 0.5mg, 1mg, 2mg, Inj 4mg/ml* **Novo-Lorazem** *Tab 0.5mg, 1mg, 2mg* **Nu-Loraz** *Tab 0.5mg, 1mg, 2mg* **Generics** *Tab 0.5mg, 1mg, 2mg, Inj 4mg/ml*	**Status epilepticus:** 0.05-0.1mg/kg IV x 2-5min or 4mg IV, rep prn 0.05mg/kg in 5-15min, max single dose 4mg/ kg, max 8mg/12h; **anxiety:** 0.05mg/kg IV, max IV dose 4mg, max 2mg (preop), ini 1-2mg PO bid-tid, maint 2-6mg/d, max 10mg/d; **insomnia:** 2-4mg PO hs; DA in mild and moderate RF: use lowest effective dose in severe RF: contraind.
Methsuximide	EHL 3h, PRC D, Lact -
Celontin *Cap 300mg*	**Absence seizures:** ini 300mg PO qd, incr by 300mg/wk, maint 1,200mg/d
Nitrazepam	EHL 30h, PRC D, Lact -
Mogadon *Tab 5mg, 10mg* **Nitrazadon** *Tab 5mg, 10mg* **Generics** *Tab 5mg, 10mg*	**Insomnia:** 2.5-10mg PO qhs; **myoclonic seizures: CH** (up to 30kg): 0.3-1mg/kg/d in 3 div doses

Oxcarbazepine	EHL 1-2.5h, metabolites 8-11h, PRC C, Lact ?
Trileptal *Tab 150mg, 300mg, 600mg, Susp (oral) 60mg/ml* **Generics** *Tab 150mg, 300mg, 600mg*	**Epilepsy, monotherapy:** ini 300mg PO bid, incr by 300mg/d q3d, maint 1,200mg/d, max 2,400mg/d; **epilepsy, adj:** ini 300mg PO bid, incr by 600mg/d q wk, maint 1,200mg/d, max 2,400mg/d;**CH** 4-16 y: ini 8-10 mg/kg/d div bid, max loading dose 600mg/d, maint 900mg/d (20-29kg), 1,200mg/d (29.1-39kg), 1,800mg/d (>39kg); DARF: CrCl (ml/min) <30: reduce ini dose by 50%, titrate carefully
Paraldehyde	
Generics *Inj 1ml/ml*	**Sedation:** 0.15 ml/kg/dose PO or PR, max 5ml; seizures: 0.2-0.4ml/kg IV over 2h, max 0.4 ml/kg/d IV; 0.3ml/kg/dose PO/PR, max 5.0ml PO/PR, diluted with equal volumes of mineral or veget. oil, may repeat q4-6 h prn
Phenobarbital	EHL 1.5-4.9d, PRC D, Lact -, serum-level (mcg/ml): 15-40
Barbilixir *Elix 4mg/ml* **Generics** *Tab 15mg, 30mg, 60mg, 100mg, Elixir 5mg/ml, Inj 30mg/ml, 120mg/ml*	**Epilepsy:** 60-250mg/d PO qd or 2-3mg/kg/d; **CH** 1-5 y: 6-8mg/kg/d PO/IV, **CH** 6-12 y: 4-6mg/kg/d PO/IV, **CH** >12 y: 1-3mg/ kg/d IV/PO; **status epilepticus:** 15-20mg/kg IV, max IV rate 60mg/min, max 20mg/kg; **sedation:** 30-120mg PO qd/bid/tid, max 400mg/d; DARF: not req in mild/moderate RF, reduce in severe RF, no long term use
Phenytoin	EHL 22h, PRC D, Lact +, serum-level (mcg/ml): 10-20
Dilantin *Cap 30mg, 100mg, Susp (oral) 30mg/5ml, 125mg/ml* **Dilantin Infatabs** *Tab (chew) 50mg* **Generics** *Inj 50mg/ml*	**Epilepsy:** ini 400mg PO, then 300mg in 2h and 4h, after 1d maint 300mg PO qd (ext.rel.)/div tid; **CH** >6 y: 5mg/kg/ d PO div bid-tid, maint 4-8mg/kg/d, max 300mg/d; **status epilepticus:** 10-15mg/kg IV, max rate 50mg/min, then 100mg IV/PO q6-8h; **CH** >6 y: 10-20mg/kg IV, max 1-3mg/kg/min; DARF: no loading dose

Primidone	EHL 3.3-7h, metabol. 29-150h, PRC D, Lact ? serum-level(mcg/ml): 5-12
Generics *Tab 125mg, 250mg*	**Epilepsy:** 125mg PO qhs, incr x 10d, maint 250mg PO tid-qid, max 2g/d; **CH** <8 y: ini 50mg PO qhs x 3d, incr to 50mg PO bid x 3d, incr to 100mg PO bid x 3d, then incr to maint 125-250mg PO tid or 10-25 mg/kg/d div tid-qid, **CH** >8 y: ini 100-125mg PO qhs x 3d, incr to 100-125mg PO bid x 3d, incr to 100-125mg PO x 3d, incr to maint 250mg tid-qid or 750-1,000mg/kg/d div tid-qid; **essential tremor:** incr to 250mg PO tid; DARF: GFR (ml/min) >50: dosing q8h, 10-50: dosing q8-12h, <10: dosing q12-24h
Topiramate	EHL 18-24h, PRC C, Lact ?
Topamax *Cap 15mg, 25mg, Tab 25mg, 100mg, 200mg* **Generics** *Tab 25mg, 50mg, 100mg, 200mg*	**Epilepsy, adj Tx:** ini 50mg PO qhs, incr by 5mg/d q wk, maint 200mg PO bid, max 1,600mg/d; **CH** 2-16 y: ini 1-3mg/kg/d (or 25mg/d) PO qhs, incr by 1-3mg/kg/d q 1-2wk up to 5-9mg/kg/d div bid; DARF: CrCl (ml/min) <70: 50%
Valproic Acid	EHL 6-17h, PRC D, Lact + serum-level (mcg/ml): 50-100 (epilepsy), 25-125 (mania)
Depakene *Cap 250mg, Syr 250mg/5ml* **Generics** *Cap 250mg, 500mg, Syr 250mg/5ml*	**Seizures:**10-15mg/kg/d PO or IV inf x 60min, max 20mg/min, incr by 5-10mg/kg/d q wk, max 60mg/kg/d, div doses >250mg/d into bid-qid; **CH** >10 y: 10-15mg/kg/d PO or IV inf x 60min, max 20mg/min, incr by 5-10mg/kg/d q wk, max 60mg/kg/d, div doses >250 mg/d into bid-qid; **absence seizures:** 10-24.9kg: 250mg/d, 25-39.9kg: 500mg/d, 40-59.9kg: 750mg/d, 60-74.9kg: 1,000mg/d, 75-89.9kg: 1,250mg/d, div doses <250mg/d into bid-qid
Vigabatrin	EHL 5-8h, PRC C, Lact ?
Sabril *Powder (oral) 0.5g/sachet, Tab 500mg*	**Epilepsy:** ini 1-2g/d PO in one to two doses, maint. 2-4g/d; **CH:** ini 40mg/kg/d PO in one to two doses, maint. 80-100mg/kg/d

11.2 Migraine Therapy

11.2.1 5-HT_1 Agonists

MA/EF: serotonin agonism (5-HT1D-Rec) ⇒ vasoconstriction; Tx of migraine attack
AE: heaviness, feeling of pressure, tiredness, dizziness, flush
CI: hypersensitivity to sumatriptane, ischemic coronary diseases, heart attack, vasospastic angina, M. Raynaud, HTN, not with (dihydro-)ergotamine

Eletriptan	EHL 4h, PRC C, Lact +
Replax *Tab 20mg, 40mg*	**Migraine Tx:** 20-40mg PO, rep prn in 2h, max 80mg/d
Frovatriptan	EHL 26h, PRC C, Lact ?
Frova *Tab 2.5mg*	**Migraine Tx acute:** 2.5mg PO, rep prn in 4h, max 5mg/d
Naratriptan	EHL 5-6h, PRC C, Lact ?
Amerge *Tab 1mg, 2.5mg*	**Migraine Tx:** 1-2.5mg PO, rep prn in 4h, max 5mg/24h; >4 Tx/mo not established; DARF: CrCl (ml/min) <15: contraind., mild RF: max 2.5mg/d, reduce ini dose
Rizatriptan	EHL 2-3h, PRC C, Lact ?
Maxalt *Tab 5mg, 10mg* **Maxalt RPD** *Tab (orally disint) 5mg, 10mg*	**Migraine Tx:** 5-10mg PO, rep prn in 2h, max 30mg/24h, >4 Tx/mo not established, under propranolol Tx max 5mg PO tid
Sumatriptan	EHL 2h, PRC C, Lact -
Imitrex *Spray (nasal) 5mg/Spray, 20mg/Spray, Inj 6mg/0.5ml* **Imitrex DF** *Tab 25mg, 50mg, 100mg* **Generics** *Tab 25mg, 50mg, 100mg*	**Migraine Tx:** 6mg SC, rep prn in 1h, max 12mg/d or 25mg PO, rep q2h 25-100mg, max 200mg (if 1st dose was SC), max 300mg/d (if 1st dose was PO) or 5-20mg intranasally, rep prn q2h, max 4mg/d, >4 Tx/mo not established; **cluster headache:** 6mg SC, rep. prn in 1h, max 12mg/d
Zolmitriptan	EHL 2.5-3h, PRC C, Lact ?
Zomig *Tab 2.5mg, Nasal spray 2.5mg/spray, 5mg/spray* **Zomig Rapimelt** *Tab (dispersable) 2.5mg*	**Migraine Tx:** 1.25-2.5 mg PO, rep prn q2h, max 10mg/ 24h; DARF: not req

11.2.2 Ergot Derivates

MA/EF (dihydroergotamine): stimulation of serotonin rec. ⇒ constriction of venous capacity vessels; interval Tx; **MA/EF** (ergotamine): mostly α receptoragonism ⇒ vasoconstr. migraine attack Tx; **AE** (dihydroergotamine): N/V, peripherally inadeq. circul.; **CI** (dihydroergotamine): hypersensitivity to seca alkaloids, severe coronary insuff., vasc. diseases, severe hepat. dysfunct.

Caffeine + Ergotamine	EHL 3-6 (C.), 1.5-2.5h (E.), PRC X, Lact -
Cafergot *Supp 100mg+2mg, Tab 100mg + 1mg*	**Migraine, cluster headache:** ini 2 tab PO, then 1 tab q30min prn, max 6 tab/attack, max 10 tab/wk or max 2 supp/attack, max 5 supp/wk; DARF: contraind.
Dihydroergotamine	EHL 7-9h, PRC X, Lact -
D.H.E. 45 *Inj 1mg/ml* **Migranal** *Spray (nasal) 4mg/ml* **Generics** *Inj 1mg/ml*	**Migraine:** 1mg IV/IM/SC, rep prn q1h, max 2mg(IV) or 3mg(IM/SC)/24h or 1 spray (0.5mg) in each nostril, rep in 15min, max 4 sprays (2mg)/24h or 8 sprays (4mg)/wk; DARF: contraind. in severe RF
Methysergide	EHL 45-62min, PRC X, Lact -
Sansert *Tab 2mg*	**Migraine/cluster headache PRO:** ini 2mg PO qd, titrate to 4-8mg/d PO div bid-qid with meals, taper dose x 2-3 wk prior to discontinuation, 3-4 wk of drug-free interval after 6-mo Tx; DARF: contraind.

11.2.3 Migraine Therapy - Other Drugs

MA/EF (divalproex, valproic acid): potassium conductance↑ ⇒ neuronal activity↓;
AE (diva-lproex, valproic acid): nausea/vomiting, fatigue/sedation, tremors, hair loss, elevated transaminases, thrombocytopenia;
CI (divalproex, valproic acid): liver disease, urea cycle disorder, hypersensitivity to drug

Divalproex Sodium	EHL 6-17h, PRC D, Lact + serum-level(mcg/ml): 70-120
Epival *Tab 125mg, 250mg, 500mg VAE, Tab ext. rel 500mg VAE* **Generics** *Tab 125mg, 250mg, 500mg VAE (VAE= valproic acid equivalents)*	**Migraine PRO:** 250mg PO bid, titrate to max 1,000mg/d; DARF: not req
Flunarizine	EHL 19d, PRC ?, Lact ?
Sibelium *Cap 5mg*	**Migraine PRO:** 10mg/d
Pizotifen	EHL 26h, PRC C, Lact ?
Sandomigran *Tab 0.5mg* **Sandomigran DS** *Tab 1mg*	**Migraine PRO:** ini 0.5mg PO qhs, incr to 0.5mg PO tid, maint 1-6mg/d

Propranolol	EHL 3-4h, PRC C, Lact ?
Inderal *Tab 10mg, 20mg, 40mg, 80mg, 120mg, Inj 1mg/ml* **Inderal LA** *Cap ext.rel 60mg, 80mg, 120mg, 160mg* **Generics** *Tab 10mg, 20mg, 40mg, 80mg, 120mg*	**Migraine:** ini 80mg/d PO, maint 160-240mg/d
Tanacetum	PRC X, Lact -
Feverfew *Cap 125mg, 400mg*	**Migraine:** 125-400mg PO daily
Valproic Acid	EHL 6-17h, PRC D, Lact + serum-level(mcg/ml): 70-120
Depakene *Cap 250mg, Syr 250mg/5ml* **Generics** *Cap 250mg, 500mg, Syr 250mg/5ml*	**Migraine PRO:** 250mg PO bid, titrate to max 1,000mg/d; DARF: not req; epilepsy; mania:

11.3 Alzheimer's - Cholinesterase Inhibitors

MA/EF: reversible and noncompetitive inhibition of centrally-active acetylcholinesterase ⇒ concentration of acetylcholine ↑ ⇒ synaptic transmission ↑⇒ cognitive function ↑
AE (donepezil, rivastigmine): N/V, diarrhea, anorexia, muscle cramps, insomnia, fatigue, urinary incontinence, psychiatric disturbances, hypotension; **CI:** hypersensitivity to one of the substances or other cholinesterase inhibitors, GI disease, concurrent use of NSAIDs, asthma, obstructive pulmonary disease, sick sinus syndrome, SV cardiac conduction conditions, history of seizures, major surgery; **CI** (rivastigmine): DM, CVS/pulmonary disease, urogenital tract obstruction, Parkinson's disease (exacerbation), renal/hepatic insufficiency

Donepezil	EHL 70h, PRC C, Lact ?
Aricept *Tab 5mg, 10mg* **Aricept RDT** *Tab (rap. diss.) 5mg, 10mg*	**Alzheimer's dementia:** ini 5mg PO qhs, incr prn to 10mg PO qhs after 4-6wk, max 10mg/d; DARF: limited data
Galantamine	EHL 7-8h, PRC B, Lact -
Reminyl *Tab 4mg, 8mg, 12mg* **Reminyl ER** *Cap ext. rel. 8mg, 16mg, 24mg*	**Alzheimer's dementia:** ini 4mg PO bid, incr prn to 4mg prn by 4mg q4wk to 8-12mg PO bid, max 32mg/d; DARF: moderate RF: max 16mg/d; severe RF: not rec
Rivastigmine	PRC B, Lact ?
Exelon *Cap 1.5mg, 3mg, 4.5mg, 6mg, Sol (oral) 2mg/ml*	**Alzheimer's dementia:** ini 1.5mg PO bid, incr to 3mg PO bid >2wk, prn incr to 4.5mg PO bid up to 6mg PO bid q2wk, max 12mg/d; DARF: not req

11.4 Parkinsonian Drugs

11.4.1 Anticholinergic Parkinsonian Drugs

MA/EF: inhibition of central cholinergic neurons ⇒ plus symptoms rigor and tremor ↓
AE: confusion to psychosis, mydriasis, accommodation disturbances, glaucoma, oral dryness, micturition disturbances, fatigue, tachycardia, thermostatic dysregulation
CI: glaucoma, micturition disturbances, tachyarrhythmia, cognitive impairment; use in patients over 65 only if strictly indicated

Benztropine Mesylate	PRC C, Lact ?
Benztropine Omega *Inj 1mg/ml* **Generics** *Tab 2mg*	**Parkinsonism:** ini 0.5–2mg/qhs PO/IM/IV, incr by 0.5mg q wk, max 6mg/d, div qd-qid; **drug-induced extrapyramidal DO:** 1–4mg PO/IM/IV qd-bid; **CH** >3 y: 1–2mg/d IM/IV div qd-bid
Biperiden	EHL 18.4–24.3h, PRC C, Lact ?
Akineton *Tab 2mg*	**Parkinsonism:** 2mg PO bid-tid, incr prn to max 16mg/d; **(drug-induced) extrapyramidal DO:** 2mg PO qd-tid or 2mg IM/IV q30min prn, max 8mg/24h; **CH** 0.04mg/kg/dose IM, rep prn q30min, max 4 doses/d
Ethoprazine	
Parsitan *Tab 50mg*	**Parkinsonism:** ini 50mg PO tid, incr 50–100mg/d q2–3d, maint 100–500mg/d; **(drug-ind.) extrapyram. DO:** 100mg PO bid
Procyclidine	PRC C, Lact ?
Generics *Tab 2.5mg, 5mg, Elixir 2.5mg/5ml*	**Parkinsonism:** ini 2.5mg PO tid, maint 5mg PO tid-qid; **(drug-ind.) extrapyram. DO**: ini 2.5mg PO tid, incr by 2.5mg/d, maint 10–20mg
Trihexyphenidyl	EHL 3.7h, PRC C, Lact ?
Apo-Trihex *Tab 2mg, 5mg*	**Parkinsonism:** ini 1mg PO qd, incr by 2mg/d q3–5d, max 6–10mg/d div tid with meals, postencephalic max 15mg/d div qid with meals; **drug-induced extrapyramidal DO:** ini 1mg PO qd, titrate prn in 4–8h to 5–15mg PO/d div qd-qid; DARF: not req

11.4.2 COMT Inhibitors

MA/EF: inhibition of catechol-O-methyltransferase (COMT) ⇒ levodopa plasma levels↑ (in combination with levodopa only) ⇒ favorable on all Parkinson symptoms, particularly akinesia and psychic disturbances

Entacapone	EHL 2.4h, PRC C, Lact ?
Comtan *Tab 200mg*	**Parkinsonism, adj:** ini 200mg PO with each levodopa/ carbidopa dose, max 1,600mg/d (div 8 times/d); DARF: not req

11.4.3 Glutamate Receptor Antagonists (Dopaminergic)

MA: blockage of striatal glutamate recept. ⇒acetylcholine release ↓;
EF: influences mainly akinesia and rigor (see also: antiviral drugs); **AE:** GI disturbances, nausea, hypersensibility, paranoid psychosis with optical hallucinations;
CI: states of confusion, epilepsy, severe hepatic dysfunction, RF

Amantadine	EHL 10-14h, PRC C, Lact -
Endantadine *Cap 100mg* **Symmetrel** *Cap 100mg, Syr 50mg/5ml* **Generics** *Cap 100mg*	**Parkinsonism:** 100mg PO bid, max 400 mg/d; **drug- incuded extrapyramidal DO:** 100mg PO bid, max 300mg/d; **PRO and Tx of influenza A infx:** 200mg PO qd or 100mg PO bid; >65y: 100 mg PO qd; **CH** 1-9y: 4.5-9.0 mg/kg/d div bid-tid, max 150 mg/day; 9-12y: 200mg PO qd or 100mg PO bid; DARF: GFR (ml/min) 60–79: alt daily doses of 100 and 200 mg; 40–59: 100 mg qd; 30–39: 200 mg twice weekly; 20–29: 100 mg thrice weekly; 10–19: alt weekly doses of 100 and 200 mg; HD: 200 mg every 7 days

11.4.4 Dopamine Receptor Agonists (Dopaminergic)

MA/EF: direct dopaminergic agonist; has a favorable effect on all Parkinson symptoms, particularly akinesia and psychic disturbances
AE: CV complications, confusion, paranoid psychosis with optical hallucinations
CI: HTN, coronary heart disease, psychic disturbances, GI ulcer or bleeding

Bromocriptine	EHL 50h, PRC C, Lact -
Parlodel *Tab 2.5mg, Cap 5mg* **Generics** *Tab 2.5mg, Cap 5mg*	**Parkinsonism:** 1.25mg PO bid, incr by 2.5mg/d q14–28d, maint 10–40mg/d; max 100mg/d; **neuroleptic malignant syndr.:** 2.5–15mg PO tid; DARF: not req

Pergolide	EHL 27h, PRC B, Lact ?
Permax *Tab 0.05mg, 0.25mg, 1mg*	**Parkinsonism:** 0.05mg PO qd x 2d, incr by 0.1–0.15mg/ d q3d x 12d, then incr by 0.25mg/d q3d, maint 3.5mg/d div tid (plus levodopa 650–1,000mg/d), max 5mg/d; **acromegaly:** ini 0.05mg/d PO qd, incr q wk by 0.1mg up to 0.1–1.5mg/d; **hyperprolactinemia:** 0.025–0.6 mg/d PO qd
Pramipexole	EHL 8–14h, PRC C, Lact ?
Mirapex *Tab 0.125 mg, 0.25mg, 0.5mg, 1mg, 1.5mg* **Generics** *Tab 0.25mg, 0.5mg, 1mg, 1.5mg*	**Parkinsonism:** ini 0.125mg PO tid, incr by 0.125mg/ dose q wk, maint 0.5–1.5mg PO tid; DARF: CrCl (ml/min) 35–59: ini 0.125mg bid, max 1.5mg bid, 15–34: ini 0.125mg qd, max 1.5mg qd, <15: not defined; **restless legs syndrome:** ini 0.125mg PO qpm, maint 0.125–0.5mg PO qpm; DARF CrCl 20–60: ini 0.125mg qpm, inc by 0.125mg/d q14d prn
Ropinirole	EHL 6h, PRC C, Lact ?
Requip *Tab 0.25mg, 1mg, 2mg, 5mg*	**Parkinsonism:** 0.25mg PO tid, incr by 0.25mg PO tid q wk up to 1mg PO tid, prn incr by 0.5mg PO tid q wk up to 3mg PO tid, prn incr by 1mg PO tid q wk, max 24mg/d (8mg tid); DARF:CrCl (ml/min) 30–50: not req

11.4.5 Levodopa (Dopaminergic)

MA/EF: Levodopa (L-Dopa) crosses blood-brain-barrier, is taken up by dopaminergic cells and decarboxylated into dopamine; has a favorable effect on all Parkinson symptoms, particularly akinesia and psychic disturbances. Decarboxylase inhibitors (carbidopa, benserazide, DDI = dopamine decarboxylase inhibitors) do not cross the blood-brain-barrier preventing L-Dopa from being decarboxylated peripherally
AE: nausea, anorexia, arrhythmias, postural hypotension, nervousness, anxiety, insomnia; in course of treatment hallucinations and paranoia
Long-term AE: biphasic dystonia ("on-off" phenomenon) with a sudden onset of akinesia ("off", painful muscular cramps) followed by a sudden rebound of drug effect ("on", possibly with so-called peak-of-dose hyperkinesia)
CI: glaucoma, severe psychosis

Levodopa + Benserazide	PRC X, Lact -
Prolopa *Cap 50mg + 12.5mg, 100mg + 25mg, 200mg + 50mg*	**Parkinsonism:** ini 1 Cap (100+25) PO qd or bid, maint 4-8 Cap (100+25) qd (div into 4-6 doses)
Levodopa + Carbidopa	EHL 15min (metabol. 15h), PRC C, Lact ? ser.-lev. (mcg/ml): 0.3-1.6 (mild), 4-7 (sev. DO)
Apo-Levocarb *Tab 100mg+10mg, 100mg+ 25mg, 250mg+25mg* **Nu-Levocarb** *Tab 100mg+10mg, 100mg+ 25mg, 250mg+25mg* **Sinemet** *Tab 100mg+10mg, 100mg+ 25mg, 250mg+25mg* **Sinemet CR** *Tab ext.rel. 100mg+25mg, 200mg+50mg* **Generics** *Tab 100mg+10mg, 100mg+ 25mg, 250mg+25mg*	**Parkinsonism:** ini 1 Tab (100+25) PO tid, incr by 1 Tab/d q1-2d prn, max 8 Tab/d (800+200mg) or ini 1 Tab (100+10) PO tid-qid, incr by 1 Tab/d q1-2d prn, max 8 Tab/d (800+80mg); higher levodopa doses: 1 Tab (250+25) PO tid-qid, incr by ½-1 Tab q1-2d, max 8 Tab/d (2g+200mg); ext.rel: ini 1 Tab (200+50) PO bid, separate doses >6h, incr prn q3d; max 2g+200mg/d; DARF: not req

11.5 Mannitol

MA: osmotic binding of water in the tubule lumen of the kidney
EF: water excretion ↑ with only a small incr in electrolyte elimination
AE: exsiccation, hypernatremia, volume load; **CI:** cardiac insufficiency, pulmonary edema

Mannitol	EHL 71-100min, PRC C, Lact ?
Osmitrol 10% in water *Inj 10g/100ml* **Osmitrol 20% in water** *Inj 20g/100ml* **Generics Mannitol 25%** *Inj 12.5g/50ml*	**Intracranial HTN:** 0.25g/kg IV x 30-60min, rep q6-8h; **ICP↑, head trauma:** 0.25-1g/kg IV x 20min, rep q4-6h prn; **ICP↑/cerebral edema:** 0.25-1 g/kg/dose IV x 20-30min, then 0.25-0.5 g/kg/dose IV q4-6h prn; **CH** >12 y: 0.25g/kg/dose IV, rep q5min prn, incr dose slowly to 1g/ kg/dose prn, max 2g/kg/dose; **acute RF (Tx):** 100g/24h IV as 15%-20% sol; **acute RF(PRO):** 50-100g; **intraoc. pressure:** 1.5-g/kg IV x 30-60min as 15%-20% sol; DARF: contraind. in severe RF

11.6 Myasthenia Gravis Drugs - Cholinergics

MA/EF: inhibition (pyridostigmine, neostigmine), binding (edrophonium) of choline esterase ⇒ acetylcholine ↑;
AE: muscle spasms, abdominal/urinary cramps, salivation, diarrhea, nausea, bradycardia, miosis
CI: bronchial asthma, iritis, mechanical intestinal/urinary/biliar obstruction, intestinal/urinary/biliar spasms, Parkinsonism, myotonia

Edrophonium	EHL 1.3–2.4h, PRC C, Lact +
Enlon *Inj 10mg/ml*	**Myasthenia gravis diagnosis:** >34kg: 2mg IV in 15–30sec (test dose), if no reaction occurs in 45sec → 8mg IV; **CH** <34 kg: 1mg IV (test dose), if no reaction occurs in 45sec → 1mg IV q30–45sec, max 5mg; **CH** >34 kg: 2mg IV (test dose), if no reaction occurs in 45sec → 1mg IV q30–45sec, max 10mg; **neuromuscular blockade antagonism:** 10mg (1ml) IV slowly x 30–45sec, rep prn, max 40mg; DARF: probably req
Neostigmine	EHL 15–90min, PRC C, Lact +
Prostigmin *Tab 15mg, Inj 0.5mg/ml, 1mg/ml, 2.5mg/ml* **Generics** *Inj 0.5mg/ml, 1mg/ml, 2.5mg/ml*	**Myasthenia gravis:** 15–375mg PO qd div tid–qid,average 150mg/d or 0.5mg IM/SC prn **neuromuscular blockade reversal:** 0.5–2mg IV single shot, rep prn; **urinary reten.:** ini 0.5mg SC/IM, after the bladder is emptied, rep 0.5mg SC/IM q3h, max 5 doses
Pyridostigmine	EHL 97min (IV)–200min (oral), PRC C, Lact +
Mestinon *Tab 60mg* **Mestinon-SR** *Tab ext.rel. 180mg*	**Myasthenia gravis:** ini 60mg PO tid, incr slowly, maint 200mg PO tid, or 180mg PO qd/bid (ext.rel.) or 2mg IM/ IV q2–3h, max 1,500mg/d; **neonates:** 5mg PO q4–6h or 0.05–0.15mg/kg IM q4–6h, reduce gradually; **neuromuscular blockade reversal:** 0.1–0.25mg/kg IV bolus; DARF: probably not req

11.7 Skeletal Muscle Relaxants

MA/EF (Baclofen): inhibits transmission at spinal level, depresses CNS ⇒ muscle spasms ↓
MA/EF (Carisoprodol, Chlorzoxazone, Cyclobenzaprine, Metaxalone, Methocarbamol): CNS depressant with sedative and skeletal muscle relaxant effect;
MA/EF (Dantrolene): acts directly on skeletal muscle;
MA/EF (Orphenadrine): atropine-like on cerebral mot. centers, medulla ⇒ muscle spasm ↓;
AE (Baclofen): sedation, drowsiness, nausea, hypotonia
AE (Dantrolene): drowsiness, dizziness, weakness, malaise, fatigue, diarrhea, anorexia, nausea, headache, rash;
AE (Carisoprolol, Diazepam): drowsiness, tiredness, sleepiness, confusion, paradox reactions, anterograde amnesia, respiratory depression, psychic and physical addiction;
AE (Cyclobenzaprine): dizziness, drowsiness, lightheadedness, dry mouth;
AE (Methocarbamol): dizziness, drowsiness, lightheadedness, blurred vision, diplopia;
AE (Orphenadrine): anticholinergic, dry mouth, urinary hesitancy, blurred vision, mydriasis, drowsiness, headache, weakness, intraocular pressure ↑, palpitation, tachycardia
AE (Tizanidine): drowsiness, dizziness, dry mouth, nausea, GI Disturbances, hypotension
CI (Baclofen): peptic ulcers;
CI (Carisoprodol): porphyria, hep./renal function impairment;
CI (Cyclobenzaprine): arrhythmias, congest. heart failure, hyperthyroidism, after MI;
CI (Dantrolene): hep. impairment, acute muscle spasm;
CI (Diazepam): myasthenia gravis, severe hep. damage, respirat. insufficiency, ataxia;
CI (Methocarbamol): renal function impairment, brain damage, epilepsy;
CI (Orphenadrine): Achalasia, bladder neck obstruct., duod./pyloric obstruct., glaucoma, myasthenia gravis, prostatic hypertr. stenos. peptic ulcer
CI (Tizanidine): severe hepatic impairment

Baclofen	EHL 3-6.8h, PRC C, Lact +
Lioresal *Tab 10mg, 20mg, Inj (intrathecal) 0.05mg/ml, 0.5mg/ml, 2mg/ml* **Nu-Baclo** *Tab 10mg, 20mg* **Generics** *Tab 10mg, 20mg*	**Muscle spasticity:** 5mg PO tid; maint 40-80mg/d div tid; 300-800mg/d intrathecal **CH** 2-7y: 10-15mg/d PO div tid; max 40mg/d
Carisoprodol	EHL 8h, PRC C, Lact -
Soma *Tab 350mg*	**Musculoskeletal DO:** 350mg PO qid; DARF: not required
Cyclobenzaprine	EHL 1-3d, PRC B, Lact ?
Novo-Cycloprine *Tab 10mg* **Generics** *Tab 10mg*	**Muscle spasm:** 10mg PO tid; max 60mg/d, not longer than 2-3wk

Dantrolene	EHL 8.7h, PRC C, Lact ?
Dantrium *Cap 25mg, 100mg* *Inj 20mg/vial*	**Spasticity:** ini 25mg PO qd; maint 100mg bid-qid; **malignant hyperthermia:** 1mg/kg IV, rep.rep. until symptoms subside or to max 10mg/kg; **CH:** ini 0.5mg/kg PO bid; maint 0.5-3mg/kg bid-qid
Diazepam	EHL 0.83-2.25d, PRC D, Lact ?
Diastat *Gel (rectal) 5mg/ml* **Diazemuls** *Conc (oral) 5mg/ml* **E Pam** *Tab 2mg, 5mg, 10mg* **Novo-Dipam** *Tab 2mg, 5mg, 10mg* **Valium** *Tab 5mg* **Generics** *Tab 2mg, 5mg, 10mg* *Inj 1mg/ml, 5mg/ml*	**Muscle spasm:** 2-10mg PO/IM/IV tid-qid; DARF: not required; **sedation** →250 **anxiety** →250 **epilepsy** →218
Meprobamate	PRC C, Lact ?
Generics *Tab 200mg, 400mg*	**Muscle spasticity:** 400mg PO tid-qid or 600mg PO bid; **CH:** 100-200mg PO bid-tid
Methocarbamol	EHL 0.9-2 h, PRC C, Lact +
Robaxin *Tab 500mg, 750mg* **Robaximol** *Inj 100mg/ml* **Generics** *Inj 100mg/ml*	**Musculoskeletal pain:** 750-1500mg PO qid or 1000mg IM/IV tid for 48-72h, maint 1000mg PO qid; DARF contraind. in RF
Orphenadrine	EHL 13.2 - 20.1 h, PRC C, Lact ?
Norflex *Tab ext.rel. 100mg, Inj 30mg/ml* **Orfenace** *Tab 100mg* **Generics** *Tab ext.rel. 100mg*	**Musculoskeletal pain:** 100mg PO bid; 60mg IV/IM bid
Tizanidine	EHL 2.5 h, PRC C, Lact ?
Zanaflex *Tab 4mg* **Generics** *Tab 4mg*	**Muscle spasticity**: ini 4mg PO tid, maint 8mg tid; max 36mg/d

11.8 Other Neurology Drugs

MA/EF (betahistine): histamine H1 receptor agonist, H3 receptor antagonist;
MA/EF (natalizumab): selective adhesion molecule (SAM) inhibitor and binds to the alpha4-subunit of human integrin, expressed on the surface of all leukocytes (except neutrophils)
MA/EF (nimodipine): calcium channel blocker, predominantly arterial vasodilation, but different to other calcium channel blockers, effect on cerebral vessels ↑;
MA/EF (riluzole): presynaptic release of glutamic acid ↓, stabilization of inactivated voltage-dependent sodium channels, anticonvulsant, neuroprotective;
MA/EF (rasagiline, selegiline): selectively inhibits MAO type B, increases dopamine;
MA/EF (sodium oxybate): sodium oxybate (gamma-hydroxybutyrate) is a neurotransmitter, CNS depressant that produces dose-dependent sedation and anesthesia;
AE (natalizumab): infections, pneumonia, acute hypersensitivity reactions, depression
AE (nimodipine): hypotension, flush, reflex tachycardia, ankle edema, headache, complete blood count changes, gingival hyperplasia;
AE (riluzole): asthenia, transaminase ↑, nausea;
AE (rasagiline, selegiline): dyskinesia, headache, N/V, dry mouth ;
CI (betahistine): pheochromocytoma, peptic ulcer disease;
AE (sodium oxybate): headache, nausea, dizziness, pain (unspecified), somnolence;
CI (natalizumab): hypersensitive to this drug, progressive multifocal leukoencephalopathy (PML), immunocompromised
CI (nimodipine): shock, hypotens., significant aortic stenosis, heart failure (NYHA III–IV);
CI (riluzole): history of or current neutropen., liver/ren. impairment, HTN, other CNS DO;
CI (rasagiline, selegiline): pheochromocytoma, sympathomimetic/serotonergic use
CI (sodium oxybate): use with sedative hypnotic agents or alcohol, in patients with succinic semialdehyde dehydrogenase deficiency

Betahistine	EHL 3–4h, PRC B, Lact ?
Serc *Tab 16mg, 24mg* **Generics** *Tab 8mg, 16mg, 24mg*	**Ménière's disease, vertigo:** ini 8–16mg PO tid, max 48mg/d
Belladonna + Ergotamine + Phenobarbital	PRC X, Lact +
Bellergal Spacetabs *Tab 0.2 + 0.6 + 40mg*	**Migraine, vascular headache PRO, menopausal symptoms:** 1 tab PO bid, max 16 tabs/wk
Glatiramer	PRC B, Lact ?
Copaxone *Inj 20mg/vial*	**Multiple sclerosis:** 20mg SC qd

Meclizine	EHL 6h, PRC B, Lact ?
Bonamine *Tab (chew) 25mg*	**Motion sickness:** 25-50mg PO 1h prior to travel, rep q24h prn; **vertigo:** 25-100mg PO qd-qid; **pregnancy-induced vomiting:** 25-50mg/d; **radiation sickness:** 25-100mg/d div qd-qid
Natalizumab	PRC B, Lact ?
Tysabri *Inj 300mg/vial*	**Relapsing-remitting form of multiple sclerosis:** 300 mg IV q 4 weeks
Nimodipine	EHL 8-9h, PRC C, Lact ?
Nimotop *Cap 30mg, Inj 0.2mg/ml*	**Subarachnoid hemorrhage (Hunt/Hess grades I-III):** ini < 96h post hemorrhage, 60mg PO q4h x 21d prn, or 0.5mcg/kg/min IV (continuous inf) x 7-10d
Riluzole	EHL 12-14h, PRC C, Lact ?
Rilutek *Tab 50mg*	**Amyotrophic lateral sclerosis:** 50mg PO bid; DARF: should be considered (Prod)
Rasagiline	EHL 3h, PRC C, Lact ?
Azilect *Tab 0.5mg, 1mg*	**Parkinsonism:** ini 0.5mg PO qd, maint 1mg PO qd; ESLD (liver impair.) mild: 0.5mg qd, severe: avoid
Selegiline	EHL 10h, PRC C, Lact ?
Generics *Tab 5mg*	**Parkinsonism:** 5mg PO bid, max 10mg/d
Sodium oxybate	PRC B, Lact ?
Xyrem *Sol (oral) 500mg/ml*	**Treatment of cataplexy in patients with narcolepsy:** ini 4.5 g/night div two equal doses (1st dose at qh and 2nd dose 2.5-4hours later; incr/decr. increments of 1.5 g/night; max 9 g/night

11.9 Glasgow Coma Scale, Dermatomes

Eye opening	spontaneous	**4**
	to verbal command	**3**
	to pain	**2**
	none	**1**
Best verbal response	oriented	**5**
	confused	**4**
	inappropriate words	**3**
	incompreh. sounds	**2**
	none	**1**
Best motor response	obeys commands	**6**
	localizes pain	**5**
	withdraws from pain	**4**
	flexion to pain	**3**
	extension to pain	**2**
	none	**1**
GCS-Score		**3–15**

GCS > 8 = Somnolent		
>12	mild	
12–9	moderate	
somnolence: sleepy, easy to awake		
stupor: hypnoid, hard to awake		
GCS < 8 = Unconscious		
8–7	coma grade **I**	light coma
6–5	coma grade **II**	
4	coma grade **III**	deep coma
3	coma grade **IV**	

coma grade I: directed defensive movements, normal tone, no impairment of pupillary and eye movements, vestibulo-ocular reflex (VOR) positive
II: undirected defensive movements, normal to increased tone, light response present, pupils variable
III: undirected movements, increased tone, pupils variable, mostly contracted, unequal, decreased response to light, generalized extension and flexion, unisocoria, path. VOR
IV: No reaction to pain, flabby tone, pupils dilated and fixed, VOR -, craniocaudal loss of brainstem reflexes

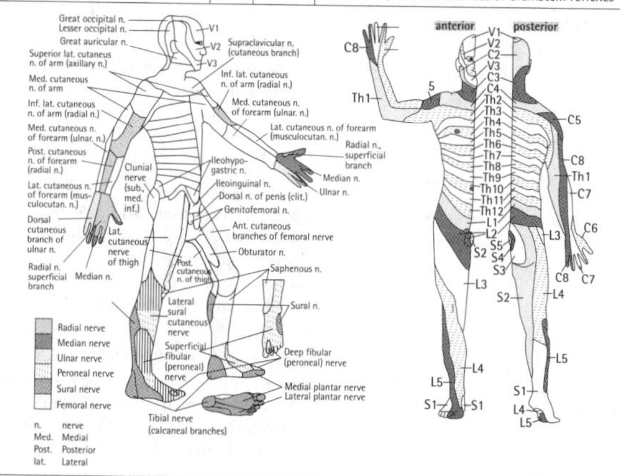

12 Psychiatry

12.1 Antidepressants

12.1.1 Serotonin-Norepinephrine Reuptake Inhibitors (SNRI) – Tricyclics, Tertiary amines

MA: inhibit reuptake of serotonin and norepinephrine into presynaptic vesicles (primarily serotonine)
AE (SNRIs): oral dryness, acute glaucoma, constipation, micturition disturbances, hypotension, arrhythmia, cardiomyopathy, dizziness, headache, restlessness, insomnia, confusion
AE (amitryptiline): drowsiness, CVS effects, seizures, hypotension, anticholinergic effects
AE (clomipramine): anticholinergic effects, somnolence, tremor, weight gain
AE (doxepin): drowsiness, CVS effects, seizures, anticholinergic effects
AE (imipramine): anticholinergic effects, seizures, weight gain, confusion, CVS effects
AE (trimipramine): sedation, weight gain, anticholinergic effects, seizures
CVS effects
CI (SNRIs): glaucoma, AV block III°, combination with MAO inhibitors or Tryptophan, hypersensitivity to product ingredients/ TCAs, recovery period after MI

Amitriptyline	EHL 15h (range 9-25h), PRC D/C, Lact ?
Elavil *Tab 50mg, 75mg* **Novo-Triptyn** *Tab 10mg, 25mg, 50mg* **Generics** *Tab 10mg, 25mg, 50mg, 75mg*	**Depression:** outpatient: ini 75mg/d PO (in div doses), gradually incr prn to max 150mg/d; **inpatient:** ini 100mg/ d PO in div doses, gradually incr prn to 200-300mg/d prn; IM: ini 80-120mg IM in 4 div doses; DARF: not req, see Prod Info
Clomipramine	EHL 19-37h (mean 32h), PRC C, Lact +
Anafranil *Tab 10mg, 25mg, 50mg* **Generics** *Tab 10mg, 25mg, 50mg*	**Obsessive compulsive DO:** ini 25mg/d PO, gradually incr over 2wk to 100mg/d, then gradually incr prn to max 250mg/d; **CH** >10 y + OCD: ini 25mg/d PO, grad.l incr over 2wk prn to max 3mg/kg/d or 100mg/d, then incr prn to max 3mg/kg/d or 200mg/d
Doxepin	EHL 16.8h (range 8-25h), PRC C, Lact -
Sinequan *Cap 10, 25, 50, 75, 100, 150mg* **Generics** *Cap 10, 25, 50, 75, 100, 150mg*	**Depression:** individualized doses, gradually incr to 75- 150mg/d (outpatients) or 150-300mg/d (inpatients); DARF: probably not req, see Prod Info

Imipramine	EHL 6-18h, PRC D, Lact ?
Tofranil *Tab 10mg, 25mg, 50mg, 75mg* **Novo-Pramine** *Tab 10mg, 25mg, 50mg* **Generics** *Tab 10mg, 25mg, 50mg, 75mg*	**Depression:** inpatients: ini 100mg/d in div doses, gradually incr to 200mg/d prn, further incr prn after 2wk up to 250-300mg/d; outpatients: ini 75mg/d (qd or in div doses) incr prn to max 150-200mg/d; DARF: not req

Trimipramine	EHL 23h, PRC C, Lact ?
Apo-Trimip *Cap 75mg, Tab 12.5mg, 25mg, 50mg, 100mg* **Generics** *Tab 12.5mg, 25mg, 50mg, 100mg*	**Depression:** outpatients: ini 75mg/d PO in div doses, maint 50-150mg/d, max 200mg/d; inpatients: ini 100mg/d in div doses, prn gradually incr to 200mg/d, max 250- 300mg/d; adolescents: ini 50mg/d, max 100mg/d

12.1.2 SNRI - Tricyclics, Secondary amines

MA: inhibit reuptake of serotonin and norepinephrine, primarily norepinephrine
Note: may cause less anticholinergic side effects than tertiary amines. Orthostatic hypotension, arrythmias. Don't use with MAOIs
AE/CI (SNRIs): see also SNRIs - tricyclics - tertiary amines →236
AE (desipramine): N/V, CVS + anticholinergic effects, sedation, seizures
AE (nortriptyline): sedation, CVS + anticholinergic effects, weight gain, seizures
CI (desipramine, nortriptyline): concomitant use of MAO inhibitors, recovery following myocardial infarction, hypersensitivity to product ingredients or TCAs

Desipramine	EHL 14.3-24.7h (average 17.1h), PRC C, Lact ?
Norpramin *Tab 25mg, 50mg* **Generics** *Tab 10mg, 25mg, 50mg, 75mg, 100mg*	**Depression:** ini 25-75mg PO qam, maint 100-200mg qd or div, max. 300mg/d; adolescents: 25-100mg/d, max 150mg/d; DARF: see Prod Info

Nortriptyline	EHL 15-39h, PRC D, Lact ?
Aventyl *Cap 10mg, 25mg* **Norventyl** *Cap 10mg, 25mg* **Generics** *Cap 10mg, 25mg*	**Depression:** ini 25-50mg PO qhs, maint 50-150mg/d (qd or div); max 150mg/d; adolescents: 30-50mg/d; DARF: not req

12.1.3 SNRI - Tricyclics/Polycyclics, 2nd Generation

MA: inhibit reuptake of serotonin and norepinephrine, primarily norepinephrine; **EF:** antidepressant, psychomotor sedation, anxiolytic; **AE/CI:** see also SNRIs - tricyclics - tertiary amines ; **AE** (maproptiline): vertigo, blurred vision, seizures, drowsiness, urinary retention; **CI** (maproptiline): hypersensitivity to product ingredients, MAO inhibitors concurrently or within 2wk of therapy, MI (during acute recovery period)

Maprotiline	EHL 27-58h (mean 43h), PRC B, Lact ?
Generics *Tab 10mg, 25mg, 50mg, 75mg*	**Depression:** ini 25-75mg PO qd x 2wk, (100-150mg PO qd in severe cases), incr prn by 25mg q2wk, maint 75- 150mg/d, max 225mg/d; DARF: not req

12.1.4 SNRI - Non-Tricyclic

MA: (atomoxetine) inhibit reuptake of norepinephrine; **MA:** (venlafaxine) inhibit reuptake of serotonin and norepinephrine; Note: Decrease dose in renal or hepatic impairment. Monitor for incr in BP; Don't use with MAOIs, caution with cimetidine and haloperidol **AE** (atomoxetine): suicidal ideation in children and adolescents, nausea, anorexia, sedation, dizziness; **AE** (venlafaxine): nausea, anorexia, sedation, dizziness; **CI** (atomoxetine): hypersensitivity to drug, concomitant use of MAOI, narrow angle glaucoma; **CI** (venlafaxine): hypersensitivity to drug, concomitant use of MAOI

Atomoxetine	EHL 5.2h, PRC C, Lact ?
Strattera *Cap 10mg, 18mg, 25mg, 40mg, 60mg, 80mg, 100mg*	**ADHD:** ini 40mg PO qam for 3 days, then incr. to 80mg PO qam, max 100mg/d **CH** <70kg: ini 0.5mg/kg PO qam for 3 days, then incr. to 1.2mg/kg PO qam, max 1.4mg/kg/day; **CH** >70kg: as per adult dose; DARF: not req.; Liver disease: CP class B decr. 50%, CP class C decr. by 75%

Venlafaxine	EHL 5h, PRC C, Lact ?
Effexor XR *Cap ext.rel. 37.5mg, 75mg, 150mg* **Generics** *Cap ext.rel. 37.5mg, 75mg, 150mg*	**Depression:** ini 75mg/d PO div bid-tid (Effexor), incr prn by 75mg/d q ≧ 4d, max 375mg/d (in div doses); ext.rel.: ini 37.5-75mg PO qd, incr by 75mg/d q ≧ 4d, max 225mg/d; **generalized anxiety DO:** ini 37.5-75mg PO qd (ext. rel.), incr prn by 75mg/d q ≧ 4d, max 225mg/d; DARF: GFR (ml/min) 10-70: 50-75%; <10, hemodialysis: 50%; see Prod Info

12.1.5 Norepinephrine-Dopamine Reuptake Inhibitors (NDRI)

MA: inhibit reuptake of norepinephrine, some dopamine
AE: N/V, seizures/tremors, agitation, insomnia, hypersensitivity reactions
CI: seizures, bulimia, anorexia, concomitant MAO inhibitors, hypersensitivity to bupropion products, concomitant use of other bupropion products

Bupropion	EHL 14h (chronic dosing: 21h), PRC B, Lact ?
Wellbutrin SR *Tab ext.rel. 100mg, 150mg* **Wellbutrin XL** *Tab ext.rel. 150mg, 300mg* **Zyban** *Tab ext.rel. 150mg* **Generics** *Tab ext.rel. 100mg, 150mg*	**Depression:** ini 100mg PO bid, after ≧ 3d incr to 300mg/d (div tid) prn; max 150mg/dose, 450mg/d; ext. rel.: ini 150mg PO qam, incr to 150mg bid as early as d4; max 400mg/d div bid; DARF: is req, see Prod Info

12.1.6 Monoamine Oxidase Inhibitors (MAOI)

MA (tranylcypromine): irreversible inhibition of MAO type A and B ⇒ oxidative break-down ↓ ⇒ synaptic conc of epinephrine, noradrenaline, serotonin ↑
EF: antidepressant, mainly psychomotor activation
AE (MAOIs): sudden changes of BP, insomnia, restlessness, dizziness, sexual dysfunction
CI (MAOIs): combination with: other antidepressants, pethidine (= meperidine), levodopa, severe hepatic dysfunction, severe HTN, acute delirium

Moclobemide	EHL 1.5h, PRC C, Lact -
Manerix *Tab 150mg, 300mg* **Generics** *Tab 100mg, 150mg, 300mg*	**Depression:** ini 150mg PO bid, incr gradually prn to max 600mg/d
Phenelzine	EHL no data, PRC C, Lact ?
Nardil *Tab 15mg*	**Depression:** ini 15mg/d PO tid, usual effective dose 45- 90mg/d in div doses; DARF: not req
Tranylcypromine	EHL 1.5-3.5h, PRC C, Lact ?
Parnate *Tab 10mg*	**Depression:** ini 10mg/d PO, incr prn by 10mg/d at 1-3wk intervals, maint 30mg/d in div doses, max 60mg/d

12.1.7 Selective Serotonin Reuptake Inhibitors (SSRI)

MA: selective inhibition of serotonin reuptake ⇒ serotonin levels in synaptic cleft ↑
EF: antidepressant, psychomotor activation
AE (SSRIs): sleeplessness, agitation, somnolence, headache, N/V, diarrhea, arrhythmias, ejaculation disturbances
AE (citalopram, escitalopram): nausea, dry mouth, sweating, somnolence, ejaculation DO
AE (fluoxetine): insomnia, asthenia, tremor, headache, GI complaints
AE (fluvoxamine): somnolence, headache, agitation, N/V, insomnia
AE (paroxetine): headache, sedation, dry mouth, insomnia, dizziness, nausea
AE (sertraline): GI complaints, tremor, headache, insomnia, male sexual dysfunction
CI (SSRIs): simultaneous treatment with MAO inhibitors, triptophan and oxitriptan; caution in children and adolescents < 18, hypersensitivity to product ingredients
CI (fluoxetine, in addition): present or recent treatment with thioridazine
CI (fluvoxamine): hypersensitivity to the drug. tizanidine or monoamine oxidase (MAO) inhibitors, thioridazine, mesoridazine, terfenadine, astemizole, or cisapride

Citalopram	EHL 33-37h, PRC C, Lact ?
Celexa *Tab 20mg, 40mg* **Generics** *Tab 20mg, 40mg*	**Depression:** ini 20mg PO qd, incr to 40mg/d at an interval of >1wk, max 60mg/d; DARF: to be used cautiously in renal impairment; see Prod Info
Escitalopram	EHL 27-32h, PRC C, Lact ?
Cipralex *Tab 10mg, 20mg*	**Depression, generalized anxiety disorder: :** ini 10mg PO qd, incr to 20mg/d at an interval of >1wk, max 20mg/d; DARF: to be used cautiously in renal impairment; see Prod Info
Fluoxetine	EHL 4-6d (chronic); 1-3d (acute), PRC C, Lact -
FXT *Cap 10mg, 40mg* **Prozac** *Cap 10mg, 20mg, Sol (oral) 20mg/5ml* **Generics** *Cap 10mg, 20mg, Sol (oral) 20mg/5ml*	**Depression/obsessive compulsive DO:** ini 20mg PO qam, incr prn q several wk, max 80mg/d; ext.rel.: 90mg PO once weekly; **bulimia:** 60mg PO qam; DARF: see Prod Info

Fluvoxamine	EHL 15.6h, PRC C, Lact ?
Luvox *Tab 50mg, 100mg* **Generics** *Tab 50mg, 100mg*	**Obsessive compulsive DO, depression:** ini 50mg PO hs, incr prn by 50mg q4-7d (doses opf > 100mg/d div bid); max 300mg/d; **CH** 8-17y + OCD: ini 25mg PO hs, incr prn by 25mg q4-7d (doses of > 50mg/d div bid), max: 200mg/d; DARF: low starting dosage + careful monitoring; see Prod Info
Paroxetine	EHL 17-22h, PRC C, Lact ?
Paxil *Tab 10mg, 20mg, 30mg* **Paxil CR** *Tab cont. rel. 12.5mg, 25mg* **Generics** *Tab 10mg, 20mg, 30mg*	**Depression:** ini 20mg PO qam, incr prn by 10mg/d q ≧ 1wk, max 50mg/d; ext.rel.: ini 25mg PO qam, incr prn by 12.5mg/d q ≧ 1wk, max 62.5mg/d; **obsessive compulsive DO:** ini 20mg PO qam, incr by 10mg/d q ≧ 1wk, rec dosage 40mg/d, max 60mg/d; **panic DO:** ini. 10mg PO qam; incr by 10mg/d, q ≧ 1wk, rec dosage 40mg/d, max 60mg/d; **social anxiety DO:** 20mg/d PO qam; DARF: ini 10mg/d, max 40mg/d; for paroxetine ext. rel. ini 12.5mg/d, max 50mg/d
Sertraline	EHL 24h, PRC C, Lact ?
Zoloft *Cap 25mg, 50mg, 100mg* **Generics** *Cap 25mg, 50mg, 100mg*	**Depression / obsessive compulsive DO:** ini 50mg/d PO, prn gradually incr at ≧ 1wk intervals, max 200mg/d; **CH** 6-12 y/OCD: 25mg/d PO, **CH** 13-17 y/OCD: 50mg/d PO; **panic/ postraumatic stress DO:** ini 25mg/d PO, incr after 1wk to 50mg/d, prn further incr q ≧1wk, max 200mg/d; DARF: not req

12.1.8 Serotonin Antagonists and Reuptake Inhibitors (SARI)

MA: serotonin antagonists and reuptake inhibitors (serotonin-5-HT2 antagonists); trazodone: selective serotonin reuptake inhibitor, at low doses, trazodone appears to act as a serotonin antagonist and at higher doses as an agonist
AE (nefazodone): dry mouth, nausea, somnolence, dizziness, blurred vision
AE (trazodone): dry mouth, dizziness, drowsiness, N/V, hypotension
CI (nefazodone): hypersensitivity to phenylpiperazine antidepressants, administration of fexofenadine/astemizole/cisapride/ MAOIs/pimozide/triazolam, caution with alprazolam, many other drug interactions; **CI** (trazodone): hypersensitivity to trazodone, carcinoid syndrome, initial recovery phase of myocardial infarction

Nefazodone	EHL 1.9-5.3h, PRC C, Lact ?
Generics *Tab 50mg, 100mg, 150mg, 200mg*	**Depression:** ini 100mg PO bid, incr prn by 100-200mg/d, div bid, at >1wk intervals, maint 300-600mg/d div bid-tid
L-Tryptophan	
Tryptan *Cap 500mg, Tab 250mg, 500mg, 750mg, 1g* **Generics** *Cap 500mg, 1,000mg*	**Depression:** ini 12g/d (div tid-qid)
Trazodone	EHL 7.1h, PRC C, Lact ?
Desyrel *Tab 50mg, 100mg* **Desyrel Dividose** *Tab 150mg* **Generics** *Tab 50mg, 75mg, 100mg, 150mg*	**Depression:** 50-150mg/d PO in div doses, incr gradually prn by 50mg q3-4d, max 400mg/d div (outpatients), 600mg/d div (inpatients); DARF: not req

12.1.9 Norepinephrine Antagonist and Serotonin Antagonists (NASA)

MA: norepinephrine antagonist and serotonin antagonist (norepinephrine, serotonin 5-HT2 and 5-HT3)
AE (Mirtazapine): drowsiness, dizziness, constipation, appetite ↑, weight gain ↑, dry mouth, agranulozytosis (0,1%)
CI (Mirtazapine): hypersensitivity to mirtazapine. Don't use with MAOIs

Mirtazapine	EHL 20-40h, PRC C, Lact ?
Remeron *Tab 30mg* **Remeron RD** *Tab (oral disint.) 15mg, 30mg, 45mg* **Generics** *Tab 30mg, Tab (oral disint.) 15mg, 30mg, 45mg*	**Depression:** ini 15mg/d PO, incr prn in intervals of >1-2wk to 15-45mg/d; DARF: see Prod Info

12.2 Antimanic (Bimodal) Drugs

MA/EF (lithium): influence on phosphatidylinositol metabolism → Tx/PRO of manic depressive states, PRO of schizoaffective psychoses
MA (valproic acid): inhibition of the enzymatic breakdown of GABA
AE (lithium): polydipsie, polyuria, GI disturbances, tremors, goiter, hypothyroidism, renal damage
AE (valproic acid): nausea/vomiting, fatigue, tremors, hair loss, elevated transaminases, thrombocytopenia
CI (lithium): severe coronary dysfunction, M. Addison, RF
CI (valproic acid): liver diseases in family, hypersensitivity to valproic acid

Lithium	EHL 14-24h, PRC D, Lact -, serum level(mEq/l): 1-1.5 (acute), 0.6-1.2 (chronic)
Carbolith *Cap 150mg, 300mg, 600mg* **Duralith** *Tab ext.rel. 300mg* **Lithane** *Cap 150mg, 300mg* **Generics** *Cap 150mg, 300mg, 600mg, Syr 300mg/5ml*	**Acute mania:** 900-1,800mg/d PO div bid-tid; long-term use: maint 300mg PO tid-qid; ext.rel. 600mg bid; DARF: GFR (ml/min): > 50: 100%, 10-50: 50-75%, < 10: 25-50%
Valproic Acid	EHL no data, PRC D, Lact + serum level: trough: 50-100mcg/ml
Depakene *Cap 250mg, Syr 250mg/5ml* **Generics** *Cap 250mg, 500mg, Syr 250mg/5ml*	**Mania:** 250mg PO tid, adjust dose rapidly to lowest therapeutic dose; DARF: see Prod Info **epilepsy** →197; **migraine** →204
see Carbamazepine →216	

12.3 Antipsychotics

12.3.1 Atypical - Serotonin Dopamine Receptor Antagonists (SDA)

AE (clozapine): agranulocytosis, sedation, salivation, CVS effects, dizziness/vertigo, seizures **AE** (olanzapine): somnolence, agitation, dizziness, constipation; **AE** (quetiapine): somnolence, dizziness, dry mouth, constipation; **AE** (risperidone): somnolence, dry mouth, constipation, blurred vision, extrapyram. effects; **CI** (clozapine): myeloproliferative DO, clozapine induced agranulocytosis, uncontrolled epilepsy, coma, hypersensitivity to clozapine products; **CI** (olanzapine, quetiapine): hypersensitivity to product ingredients; **CI** (risperidone): hyperprolactinemia, hypersensitivity to risperidone products; **CI** (paliperidone) hypersensitive to paliperidone, risperidone

Clozapine	EHL 8-12h, PRC B, Lact -
Clozaril *Tab 25mg, 100mg* **Generics** *Tab 25mg, 100mg*	**Tx-resistent schizophrenia:** ini 12.5mg PO qd-bid, incr by 25-50mg/d to 300-450mg/d (div bid-tid) by the end of 2wk, max 600-900mg/d
Olanzapine	EHL 21-54h (mean: 30h), PRC C, Lact ?
Zyprexa *Tab 2.5mg, 5mg, 7.5mg, 10mg, 15mg, 20mg, Inj 10mg/vial* **Zyprexa Zydis** *Tab (orally disint) 5mg, 10mg, 15mg, 20mg* **Generics** *Tab 2.5mg, 5mg,7.5mg,10mg,15mg*	**Psychotic DO:** ini 5-10mg PO qd, incr prn by 5mg/d qwk to usual effective dose of 10-15mg/d, max 20mg/d; DARF: see Prod Info
Quetiapine	EHL 6h, PRC C, Lact ?
Seroquel *Tab 25mg, 100mg, 200mg, 300mg* **Seroquel XR** *Tab (ext rel) 50mg, 200mg, 300mg, 400mg*	**Psychotic DO:** ini 25mg PO bid, incr by 25-50mg bid to 300-400mg/d (div bid-tid), range 150-750mg/d, max 800mg/d
Paliperidone	EHL 23h, PRC C, Lact +
Invegal *Tab (ext rel) 3mg, 6mg, 9mg*	**Schizophrenia:** ini 6mg PO qd; maint 3-12mg PO qd; DARF: CrCl 50-80 mL/min: max 6 mg qd; 10-50: max 3mg qd
Risperidone	EHL 20-30h, PRC C, Lact ?
Risperdal *Tab 0.25mg, 0.5mg, 1mg, 2mg, 3mg, 4mg, Sol (oral) 1mg/ml* **Risperdal Consta** *Inj 25mg, 37.5mg, 50mg/vial* **Risperdal M-Tab** *Tab (oral dis) 0.25mg, 0.5mg, 1mg, 2mg, 3mg, 4mg* **Generics** *Tab 0.25mg, 0.5mg, 1mg, 2mg, 3mg, 4mg, Sol (oral) 1mg/ml*	**Psychotic DO:** ini 1mg PO bid, incr prn by 1mg bid on d 2 + d 3, then at intervals >1wk, maint 4-6mg/d, max 16mg/d; Inj ini 25 mg IM q2weeks; maint. 25-50mg IM q2weeks DARF: ini 0.25-0.5mg PO qd-bid, incr prn by 0.5-1.5mg/d qwk; see Prod Info

12.3.2 Antipsychotics: D_2 Antagonists - Low Potency	
MA (D2-Antagonists): antagonism at central dopamine receptors EF (D2-Antagonists): antipsychotic and sedating (the higher the antipsychotic effect, the lower the sedating effect, and vice versa), sympathicolytic, anticholinergic, antihistaminergic, antiserotoninergic; **AE** (D2-Antagonists): early and late dyskinesias, parkinsonism, acathisia, restlessness, excitement, depression, lethargy, hyperprolactinemia, amenorrhea, mydriasis, accommodation, disturbances, micturition disturbances, constipation, glaucoma, rise in spasmophilia, hypotension, tachycardia, conduction disturbances, allergic reactions, complete blood count changes, cholestasis; **AE** (chlorprom): hypotension, akathisia, tardive dyskinesia, arrhythmias, constipation; **AE** (mesorid.): tardive dyskinesia, drowsiness, seizures, dry mouth, myelosuppression; **AE** (thioridazine): myelosuppress., arrhythmias, QT interval↑, N/V, NMS, extrapyram.effects; **CI** (D2-Antagonists): M. Parkinson, severe hepatic dysfunction, micturition DO, glaucoma, acute intoxications with sedating drugs; **CI** (chlorpromazine): hypersensitivity to chlorpromazine, myelosuppression, coma; **CI** (thioridazine): severe CNS depression, circulatory collapse, hypersensitivity to thioridazine products, HTN/hypotension/heart disease, QT interval↑, patients on drugs that prolong the QT interval, patients on drugs that inhibit cytochrome p450-2D6; **CI** (mesoridazine): hypersensitivity to mesoridazine products, coma	
Chlorpromazine	EHL 6h, PRC C, Lact ?
Generics *Inj 25mg/ml*	**Psychotic DO:** outpatients: dose range 50–400mg/d; inpatients: ini 25mg tid, incr gradually until effective dose is reached, max 800mg/d; IM: 25mg IM, can repeat with 25–50mg in 1h (severe cases: may be gradually incr over several d up to a max of 400mg q4–6h; a dose of 500mg/ d is generally sufficient); **CH** 6mo–12y: severe behavioral/psychotic DO:0.5mg/kg PO q4–6h prn or 1mg/kg PR q6–8h prn or 0.5mg/kg IM q6–8h prn
Mesoridazine	EHL no data, PRC C, Lact ? (adverse data)
Serentil *Tab 25mg*	**Alcoholism:** ini 25mg PO bid, usual dose 50–200mg/d; **Chronic brain syndrome:** ini 25mg PO tid, usual dose 75–300mg/d; **schizophrenia:** ini 50mg PO tid, usual dose 100–400mg/d
Methotrimeprazine	PRC C, Lact ?
Apo-Methoprazine *Tab 2mg, 5mg, 25mg, 50mg* **Nozinan** *Inj 25mg/ml, Liq (oral) 25mg/5ml, Oral drops 40mg/ml, Tab 2mg, 5mg, 25mg, 50mg*	**Sedation, anxiolytic:** ini 6–25mg/d PO/IM (div tid) or 10–25mg PO/IM qhs prn; **psychotic DO:**ini 50–75mg/d PO/IM (div bid–tid) **CH** PO: ini 1/4mg/kg/d PO (div bid–tid), max 40mg/d; IM: 1/16–1/8mg/kg/d IM (qd or div bid)

Pericyazine	PRC C, Lact ?
Neuleptil *Cap 5mg, 10mg, 20mg, Oral drops 10mg/ml*	**Psychotic DO:** 5-20mg PO qam and 10-40mg PO qpm, **CH** (>5 yrs): 2.5mg-10mg PO qam and 5-30mg PO qm
Pipotiazine	PRC C, Lact ?
Piportil L4 *Inj 25mg/ml, 50mg/ml*	**Schizophrenia:** ini 50-100mg IM q3-6wks, maint 75-150mg IM q4wks
Promazine	PRC C, Lact?
Generics *Inj 50mg/ml*	**Schizophrenia:** ini 50-150mg IM; repeat q30min PRN, maint 10-200mg IM q4-6h PRN; **CH** (>12yrs) 10-25mg IM q4-6 h, max 1 g/d
Thioproperazine	PRC C, Lact ?
Majeptil *Tab 10mg*	**Schizophrenia, manic syndromes:** ini 5mg PO (qd or div bid), maint 30-40mg/d PO; **CH** (>10yrs): ini 1-3mg PO qd
Thioridazine	EHL 21-24h , PRC C, Lact ?
Mellaril *Susp (oral) 10mg/5ml* **Generics** *Tab 10mg, 25mg, 50mg, 100mg*	**Psychotic DO:** ini 50-100mg PO tid, gradual incr prn, maint 200-800mg/d div bid-qid, max 800mg/d; doses > 300mg/d are only rec for patients with severe psychoses; **CH** 2-12y (if unresponsive to other agents): 0.5mg/kg/d PO divbid-tid, titrateto optimum clinical response or to max 3mg/kg/d

12.3.3 Antipsychotics: D_2 Antagonists - Mid Potency

MA, EF, AE, CI (D_2 Antagonists): see: low potency neuroleptic drugs →245;
AE (loxapine): hypotension, extrapyramidal effects, blurred vision, weight gain, sedation;
CI (loxapine): coma, hypersensitivity to loxapine products

Droperidol	PRC C, Lact -
Generic *Inj 2.5mg/ml*	**Psychosis:** 5mg IM/IV; **nausea:** 0.675mg IM/IV
Loxapine	EHL 4h (oral), 12h (IM), PRC C, Lact ?
Generics *Tab 2.5mg, 5mg, 10mg, 25mg, 50mg*	**Psychosis:** ini 10mg PO bid or up to 50mg/d in severe cases, maint 60-100mg/d div bid-qid, max 250mg/d; IM: 12.5-50mg IM q4-12h, according to response

12.3.4 Antipsychotics: D_2 Antagonists - High Potency

MA, EF, AE, CI (D_2 Antagonists): see: low potency neuroleptic drugs →245
AE (fluphenazine hydrochloride): agranulocytosis, akathisia, weight gain, hepatotoxicity, extrapyramidal effects, neuroleptic malignant syndrome
AE (haloperidol): sedation, dystonic/extrapyramidal reactions, hypotension, arrhythmias
AE (perphenazine): extrapyramidal, anticholinergic + CVS effects, seizures, sedation
AE (pimozide): extrapyramidal + CVS effects, nausea, seizures
AE (thiothixene): restlessness, blurred vision, extrapyramidal effects, N/V, myelosuppression
AE (trifluoperazine): seizures, NMS, extrapyramidal effects, blood dyscrasias
CI (fluphenazine): coma, hypersensitivity to fluphenazine products
CI (haloperidol): hypersensitivity to haloperidol products, Parkinson's disease
CI (perphenazine): blood dyscrasias, subcortical brain damage, coma, hypersensitivity to perphenazine products, severe liver disease
CI (pimozide): QT interval ↑, concomitant macrolides, hypersensitivity to pimozide, coma
CI (thiothixene): hypersensitivity to thiothixene products
CI (trifluoperazine): coma, bone marrow depression, hypersensitivity to trifluoperazine

Flupenthixol	PRC C, Lact ?
Fluonxol Depot *Inj 20mg/ml, 100mg/ml* **Fluonxol Tablets** *Tab 0.5mg, 3mg*	**Schizophrenia:** IM: ini 5mg IM test dose then 20-40mg IM, maint 20-40mg IM q2-3wks; PO: ini 1mg PO tid, maint 3-6mg/d
Fluphenazine	EHL 33h, PRC C, Lact ?
Modecate *Inj 25mg/ml, 100mg/ml* **Generics** *Tab 1mg, 2mg, 5mg Inj 25mg/ml, 100mg/ml*	**Psychosis:** 0.5-10mg/d PO div q6-8h; usual effective doses 1-20mg/d, max 40mg/d PO; IM: 1.25-10mg/d IM div q6-8h, max 10mg/d IM
Haloperidol	EHL 21h, IM: approx. 3wk;PRC C, Lact ?
Novo-Peridol *Tab 0.5mg, 1mg, 2mg, 5mg, 10mg, 20mg* **Generics** *Tab 0.5mg, 1mg, 2mg, 5mg, 10mg, Sol (oral) 2mg/ml, Inj 50mg/ml, 100mg/ml, Inj (long acting decanoate) 50mg/ml, 100mg/ml*	**IM (non depot): acutely agitated patients:** ini 2-5mg IM, may repeat q1-8h; **psychotic DO:** ini 1-6mg/d PO (moderate) and 6-15mg/d (severe symptoms) div bid-tid; usual range 1-15mg/d, max 100mg/d; decanoate (oral to depot convers.): ini: 10-20 x the previous daily oral dose, but 100mg max ini dose, at monthly intervals; **CH** 3-12 y psychotic DO: 0.05-0.15mg/kg/d PO div bid-tid, **CH** non-psychotic DO: 0.05-0.075mg/kg/d PO div bid-tid; DARF: not req

Perphenazine	EHL 8.4-12.3h, PRC C, Lact -
Trilafon *Inj 5mg/ml* **Generic** *Tab 2mg, 4mg, 8mg, 16mg*	**Psychotic symptoms:** ini 4-8mg PO tid (moderately disturbed outpatients) or 8-16mg PO bid-qid (inpatients); IM: ini 5-10mg IM, then 5mg IM q6h prn, max 15mg/d IM (out-), max 30mg/d IM (inpatients)
Pimozide	EHL 53-55h, PRC C, Lact ?
Orap *Tab 2mg, 4mg* **Generics** *Tab 2mg, 4mg*	**Tourette's syndrome:** ini 1-2mg/d PO in div doses, incr q2d prn; max 0.2mg/kg/d up to 10mg/d; **Tourette's syndrome + CH >12y:** ini 0.05mg/kg PO hs, incr prn q3d to max 0.2mg/kg up to 10mg/d; DARF: probably not req; see Prod Info
Thiothixene	EHL 34h, PRC C, Lact ?
Navane *Cap 2mg, 5mg, 10mg*	**Schizophrenia:** ini 6mg PO div tid (milder conditions) and 5mg bid (severe conditions); usual effective dose range 20-30mg/d, max 60mg/d; IM: ini 4mg bid-qid, max 30mg/d
Trifluoperazine	EHL 24h, PRC C, Lact ?
Generic *Tab 1mg, 2mg, 5mg, 10mg, 20mg*	**Non-psychotic anxiety:** 1-2mg PO bid for up to 12wk, max 6mg/d; **psychotic DO:** ini 2-5mg PO bid, usual dose is 15-20mg/d, sometimes up to 40mg/d; IM: 1-2mg q4-6h prn; **CH** 6-12y (hospitalized or under close supervision): 1mg PO qd-bid, prn gradually incr, max 15mg/d; IM: 1mg IM qd-bid
Zuclopenthixol	EHL 20h(PO), 19d(depot), PRC C, Lact -
Clopixol *Tab 10mg, 25mg, 40mg* **Clopixol-Acuphase** *Inj 50mg/ml* **Clopixol Depot** *Inj 200mg/ml*	**Schizophrenia:** Clopixol: ini 10-50mg/d PO, maint 20-60mg/d; Clopixol-Acuphase: ini 50-150mg IM, repeat q2-3d; Clopixol-Depot: 150-300mg IM q2-4wks

12.4 Anxiolytics, Hypnotics

12.4.1 Benzodiazepines

MA: opening of Cl- channels ⇒ inhibition of GABA neurons↑, especially in limbic system
EF: sedative, sleep inducing, anxiolytic, anti-aggressive, anti-convulsive, muscle relaxing
AE: tiredness, sleepiness, drowsiness, confusion, paradox reactions, anterograde amnesia, respiratory depression, psychic and physical addiction
CI: myasthenia gravis, severe hepatic damage, respiratory insufficiency, ataxia

Alprazolam	EHL 11.2h, PRC D, Lact ?
Apo-Alpraz *Tab 0.25mg, 0.5mg* **Novo-Alprazol** *Tab 0.25mg, 0.5mg* **Nu-Alpraz** *Tab 0.25mg, 0.5mg* **Xanax** *Tab 0.25mg, 0.5mg, 1mg, 2mg* **Generics** *Tab 0.25mg, 0.5mg, 1mg, 2mg*	**Anxiety:** ini 0.25-0.5mg PO tid, incr prn q3-4d to max 4mg/d, usual effective dose 0.5-4mg/d in div doses; **panic DO** ini 0.5mg PO tid, incr prn by max 1mg/d q3-4d, slower titration may be needed at doses > 4mg/d, usual effective dose 1-10mg/d (mean 5-6mg/d), max 10mg/d
Bromazepam	EHL 20h, PRC C, Lact -
Lectopam *Tab 1.5mg, 3mg, 6mg* **Generics** *Tab 1.5mg, 3mg, 6mg*	**Anxiety:** ini 6-18 mg/d in div doses, maint 6-30mg/d in div doses
Chlordiazepoxide	EHL 10-48h, PRC D, Lact ?
Generics *Cap 5mg, 10mg, 25mg*	**Anxiety:** usual oral dose range is 5-10mg PO tid-qid (mild to moderate anxiety + tension) or 20-25mg tid-qid (sev. anxiety + tension); **IV/IM: acute or severe anxiety:** 25-50mg IM/IV tid-qid; **CH** > 6y + anxiety: ini with lowest dose, incr prn, maint 5mg PO bid-qid, max 10mg bid-tid; **acute alcohol withdrawal:** 50-100mg IM/IV, repeat q2-4h prn up to 300mg/d; DARF: mild to moder.RF: not req; CrCl (ml/min)<10: 50%; see Prod Info
Clonazepam	EHL 30-40h, PRC C, Lact - serum-level (ng/ml): 25-30
Clonapam *Tab 0.5mg, 1mg, 2mg* **Rivotril** *Tab 0.5mg, 2mg* **Generics** *Tab 0.25mg, 0.5mg, 1mg, 2mg*	**Panic DO:** ini 0.25mg PO bid, gradually incr prn after 3d, max 4mg/d; (gradually decr by 0.125mg bid, q3d)

Clorazepate	EHL 2.29h, PRC D, Lact ?
Novo-Clopate *Cap 3.75mg, 7.5mg, 15mg* **Generics** *Cap 3.75mg, 7.5mg, 15mg*	**Anxiety:** ini 7.5-15mg/d PO, maint. 15-60mg/d according to patients response; DARF: not req
Diazepam	EHL 0.83-2.25d, PRC D, Lact ?
Diastat *Gel (rectal) 5mg/ml* **Diazemuls** *Conc (oral) 5mg/ml* **E Pam** *Tab 2mg, 5mg, 10mg* **Novo-Dipam** *Tab 2mg, 5mg, 10mg* **Valium** *Tab 5mg* **Generics** *Tab 2mg,5mg,10mg;Inj 1;5 mg/ml*	**Anxiety:** 2-10mg PO bid-qid; IM/IV: 2-5mg IM/IV, repeat in 3-4h prn (moderate anxiety); 5-10mg IM/IV, repeat q3-4h prn (severe DO); DARF: see Prod Info
Flurazepam	EHL 2.3h, PRC X, Lact ?
Generics *Cap 15mg, 30mg*	**Short term Tx of insomnia:** 15-30mg PO hs; DARF: see Prod Info
Lorazepam	EHL 10-20h (mean 12h) , PRC D, Lact ?
Ativan *Tab 0.5mg, 1mg, 2mg, Tab (subling.) 0.5mg, 1mg, 2mg, Inj 4mg/ml* **Novo-Lorazem** *Tab 0.5mg, 1mg, 2mg* **Nu-Loraz** *Tab 0.5mg, 1mg, 2mg* **Generics** *Tab 0.5mg, 1mg, 2mg, Inj 4mg/ml*	**Anxiety:** ini 0.5-1mg PO bid-tid, maint 2-6mg/d in div doses, max 10mg/d (div) **insomnia:** 2-4mg PO hs prn; DARF: see Prod Info
Oxazepam	EHL 2.8-8.6h, PRC D, Lact ?
Generics *Cap 10mg, 15mg, 30mg*	**Anxiety:** 10-15mg PO tid-qid (mild-to-moderate anxiety),15-30mg tid-qid (severe anxiety and agitat. with depression); **alcoholics with acute inebriation, tremulousness, or anxiety on alcohol withdrawal:** 15-30mg tid-qid; DARF: not req, see Prod Info
Temazepam	EHL 3.5-18.4h, PRC X, Lact ?
Restoril *Cap 15mg, 30mg* **Generics** *Cap 15mg, 30mg*	**Insomnia:** 7.5-30mg PO hs
Triazolam	EHL 2.3h, PRC X, Lact ?
Apo-Triazo *Tab 0.125mg, 0.25mg* **Halcion** *Tab 0.25mg* **Generics** *Tab 0.125mg, 0.25mg*	**Insomnia:** 0.125-0.25mg PO hs prn, max 0.5mg/d

12.4.2 Sedating Antihistamines

MA (diphenhydramine): antihistamine with sedative and hypnotic effect (see other antihistamines →104, →288, →289); **AE** (diphenhydramine):dizziness,headache,convulsions, cardiac arrhyt-hmia, oral dryness, micturition disturbances, paralytic ileus
CI (diphenhydramine): glaucoma, prostate hypertrophy with residual urine, acute asthma attacks, pheochromo-cytoma, epilepsy

Diphenhydramine	EHL 4–8h (prolonged with age), PRC B, Lact -
Allerdryl *Cap 25mg, 50mg* **Allernix** *Cap 25mg, 50mg, Elixir (oral) 12.5mg/5ml* **Benadryl** *Cap 25mg, 50mg, Cream 2%, Elixir (oral) 12.5mg/5ml, Liq (oral) 6.25mg/5ml, Tab (chew) 12.5mg* **Nytol** *Cap 25mg* **Nytol Extra Strength** *Cap 50mg* **Simply Sleep** *Cap 25mg* **Unisom Extra Strength/Extra Strength Sleepgels** **Generics** *Cap 25mg, 50mg, Elixir (oral) 2.5mg/ml, Inj 50mg/ml*	**Insomnia:** 50mg PO hs; **anaphylaxis , allergic rhinitis, rhinorrhea,** DARF: GFR (ml/min) >50: q6h, 10–50: q6–12h, < 10: q12–18h; see Prod Info

12.4.3 Barbiturates

MA (barbiturat.): reinforcement of the inhibitory effect caused by GABA in the CNS
EF (barbiturates): sedative, sleep inducing, anxiolytic, anti-aggressive, anti-convulsive, muscle relaxing; **AE** (barbiturates): tiredness, dizziness, anterograde amnesia, dizziness, ataxia, dysopias, porphyria, N/V, hepatic dysfunction, bradycardia, respiratory depression, skin reactions, complete blood count changes, enzyme induction, addiction; **AE** (pentobarbital): respiratory depression, tachycardia, myasthenia gravis, drowsiness; **AE** (secobarbital): vertigo, excitation, respiratory depression, CNS depression; **CI** (barbiturates): porphyria, severe hepatic and renal dysfunction, status asthmaticus, respiratory insufficiency, barbiturate sensitivity

Pentobarbital	EHL 15–48h, PRC D, Lact ?
Novo-Pentobard *Cap 100mg*	**Hypnotic:** 100mg PO hs; 120mg or 200mg PR (for patients<110 lb);150–200mg IM; **CH hypnotic:**10–20 lb. (2mo–1y): 30mg PR; 20–40 lb. (1–4y): 30mg or 60mg PR; 40–80 lb. (5–12y): 60mg PR; 80–110 lb. (12–14y): 60mg or120mg PR; IM (**CH** hypnotic): 2–6mg/kg/dose IM, not to exceed 100mg; DARF: see Prod Info

Secobarbital	EHL 19–34h, PRC D, Lact +
Novo-Secobarb *Cap 100mg* **Seconal Sodium** *Cap 100mg*	**Hypnotic:** 100mg PO hs prn; 100–200mg IM hs prn ; DARF: not req

12.4.4 Other Anxiolytics, Hypnotics

MA (chloral hydrate): hypnotic without influence on REM sleep; **MA** (zaleplon, zolpidem): benzodiazepin-like effect; **AE** (buspirone): sedation, dizziness; **AE** (chloralhydrate): arrhythmias, hallucinations, disorientation, N/V, diarrhea; **AE** (zaleplon): allergic reactions, tiredness, headache, dizziness, somnolence, nausea, development of addiction; **CI** (buspirone): hypersensitivity to buspirone products; **CI** (chloral hydrate): hypersensitivity to chloral hydrate products ; **CI** (zaleplon): Myasthenia gravis, severe liver impairment, hypersensitivity to product ingredients

Buspirone	EHL 2.4–2.7h, PRC B, Lact ?
Buspar *Tab 10mg* **Generics** *Tab 5mg, 10mg*	**Anxiety:** ini 7.5mg PO bid, incr by 5mg/d q2–3d prn, usual effective dose 20–30mg/d (in div doses), max 60mg/d DARF: see Prod Info
Chloral Hydrate	EHL no data, PRC C, Lact ?
Generics *Syr 100mg/ml*	**Alcohol withdrawal:** 0.5g–1g PO q6h prn; **Insomnia** (short-term Tx): 0.5g–1g PO/PR hs; **sedation:** 250mg PO/PR tid pc; **CH insomnia** (short-term Tx): 50mg/kg/d PO/PR, max 1g/single dose; **CH sedation:** 8mg/kg/d PO/ PR tid, max 0.5g tid; DARF: GFR (ml/min): >50: 100%, < 50: not recommend.; see Prod Info
Doxylamine	
Unisom-2 *Tab 25 mg*	**Insomnia**: 25 mg po qhs PRN
Hydroxyzine	PRC C, Lact ?
Atarax *Syr 10mg/5ml, Inj 50mg/ml* **Generics** *Cap 10mg, 25mg, 50mg, Syr 10mg/5ml, Inj 50mg/ml*	**Anxiety:** 25–100mg PO tid–qid; **CH** (<6yrs) 30–50mg/d PO in div doses, (>6yrs) 50–100mg/d PO in div doses; IM: 50–100mg IM q4–6h; **CH** 1mg/kg IM
Zaleplon	EHL 1h, PRC C, Lact -
Starnoc *Cap 5mg, 10mg*	**Short-term Tx of insomnia:** 5–10mg PO hs prn; DARF: see Prod Info
Zopiclone	EHL 5 h, PRC D, Lact +
Generics *Tab 5mg, 7.5mg*	**Insomnia**: 3.75–7.5 mg po qhs

12.4.5 Anxiolytics, Hypnotics – Combinations

AE (amitriptyline): drowsiness, anticholinergic + CVS effects, seizures, myelosuppression
AE (perphenazine): extrapyramidal, anticholinergic + CVS effects, sedation, seizures
CI (amitriptyline + chlordiazepoxide): hypersensitivity to benzodiazepines or TCAs, concomitant use with MAO inhibitors, recovery following an MI;
CI (amitriptyline + perphenazine): CVS disease, recovery period after MI, MAO Inhibitor usage, large doses of other CNS depressants, blood dyscrasias, bone marrow depression or hepatic damage, hypersensitivity to perphenazine, other piperazine phenothiazines, amitriptyline or other TCA, subcortical brain damage, coma

Perphenazine + Amitriptyline

Etrafon *Tab 2mg + 10mg, 4mg + 10mg, 2mg + 25mg, 4mg + 25mg*	**Depression/anxiety:** ini 2–4mg perphen. + 25mg amitript. tid–qid, use lowest effective level for maint; max daily dose 16mg perphenazine + 200mg amitriptyline

12.5 Drugs used in Substance Dependence

12.5.1 Smoking Cessation

MA/EF (bupropion): catecholamine reuptake in CNS↓ ⇒ local concentrations of noradrenaline + dopamine↑⇒ nicotine withdrawal symptoms↓, urge to smoke ↓
MA/EF (nicotine products): ganglionic (nicotinic) cholinergic-receptor agonists; used for nicotine replacement therapy as temporary adjunct in cessation of cigarette smoking
MA/EF (varenicline): partial agonist activity of alpha4 beta2 nicotinic acetylcholine receptor; **AE** (nicotine products): tachycardia, diarrhea, nausea/indigestion, dizziness, insomnia, headache, nasal irritation with spray, skin irritation with patch, mouth irritation (gum); **AE** (bupropion): fever, oral dryness, N/V, stomachache, constipation, insomnia, difficulty concentrating, headache, tachycardia, BP↑, depression, restlessness, fear, seizures/tremors, agitation, insomnia, hypersensitivity reactions; **AE** (varenicline): nausea, abnormal dreams, constipation, flatulence, vomiting; **CI** (nicotine products): angina, arrhythmias, active temporomandibular joint disease (gum), immediately post-MI, continued use of tobacco products, gastric ulcer, uncontrolled HTN, hypersensitivity to nicotine products; **CI** (bupropion): epilepsy, bulimia, anorexia, bipolar psychosis, severe liver cirrhosis, combination with MAO inhibitors, children and adolescents < 18, hypersensitivity to bupropion products, concomitant use of other bupropion products

Bupropion EHL 14h (chronic dosing 21h), PRC B, Lact ?

Wellbutrin SR *Tab ext.rel. 100mg, 150mg* **Wellbutrin XL** *Tab ext.rel. 150mg, 300mg* **Zyban** *Tab ext.rel. 150mg* **Generics** *Tab ext.rel. 100mg, 150mg*	**Smoking cessation:** ini 150mg PO qd x 3d, incr to 150mg PO bid x 7–12wk, max 150mg PO bid; DARF: see Prod Info

Nicotine Gum	EHL 30-120min, PRC C, Lact ?
Nicorette *Gum (chew,buccal) 2mg* **Nicorette Plus** *Gum (chew,buccal) 4mg* **Nicorette Inhaler** *Inh 4mg/inh.*	**Smoking cessation:** 1 piece (2mg) q1-2h for 6wk, then 1 piece (2mg) q2-4h for 3wk, then 1 piece (2mg) q4-8h for 3wk,max 30pieces/d of 2mg or 24 pieces/d of 4mg; 4mg pieces for high cigarette use (> 24 cigarettes/d)
Nicotine Patches	PRC (nicotine): D, Lact (nicotine): ?
Habitrol *Film (ext.rel, TD) 7mg/24h, 14mg/24h, 21mg/24h* **Nicoderm** *Film (ext.rel, TD) 7mg/24h, 14mg/24h, 21mg/24hr* **Nicotrol** *Film (ext.rel, TD) 5mg/16h, 10mg/16h, 15mg/16h*	**Smoking cessation:** see Prod Info
Varenicline	EHL 24h, PRC C, Lact ?
Champix *Tab 0.5mg, 1mg*	**Smoking cessation:** Days 1-3: 0.5mg PO qd, Days 4-7: 0.5mg PO bid, Days 8-End of treatment: 1mg PO bid

12.5.2 Alcohol Dependence

MA/EF: (acamprosate): chemical structure similar to endogenous amino acid homotaurine, modulates glutamatergic and GABAergic neurotransmission and modifies neuronal excitability
AE: diarrhoea, vomiting, adominal pain, pruritus, maculopapular rash and rare cases of bullous skin reactions have been reported
CI: hypersensitive to this drug, severe renal impairment (CrCl<30 mL/min), nursing women
see Diazepam→249, Chloral Hydrate→252, Chlordiazepoxide→249, Oxazepam→249

Acamprosate	EHL 20-33h, PRC C, Lact +
Campral *Tab del. rel 333mg*	**Maintenance of abstinence from alcohol in patients who are abstinent at treatment initiation:** 666mg PO tid (ini as soon as possible after detoxification and should be maintained if the patient relapses); DARF: CrCl 30-50 mL/min: 333 mg PO tid; <30 mL/min: not rec.; Hepatic dysf: no adj.

12.5.3 Opioid Dependence

AE (methadone): respiratory depression, dizziness, N/V, sweating, constipation
AE (naltrexone): opioid withdrawal-like syndrome, nausea, headache, dizziness, anxiety
CI (methadone): hypersensitivity to methadone;
CI (naltrexone): concomitant opioid analgesics, opioid dependency or withdrawal, hypersensitivity to naltrexone, acute hepatitis or liver failure

Methadone	EHL 23h (IV), 22h (chronic PO), PRC C, Lact ?
Metadol *Sol (oral) 10mg/ ml*	**Narcotic addiction:** 40–180mg/d PO (div), taper dose as appropr. to avoid withdrawal symptoms; DARF: see Prod Info, GFR (ml/min): > 50: q6h; 10–50: q8h, severe RF: q8–12h
Naltrexone	EHL 4h, PRC C, Lact ?
ReVia *Tab 50mg*	**Alcohol dependence:** 50mg PO qd **narcotic dependence:** ini 25mg PO qd, incr to 50mg PO qd if no signs of withdrawal

12.6 CNS Stimulants

MA/EF (caffeine): competitive inhibition of phosphodiesterase ⇒ intracellular cyclic AMP ↑ ⇒ CNS stimulation at all levels (thought flowm, wakefulness);
MA/EF (methylphenidate): amphetamine derivate → release of catecholamines ⇒ centrally stimulating;
MA/EF (modafinil): potentiation of cerebral α1-adrenergic activity ⇒ improvement of vigilance ↑, number of sudden sleep episodes ↓;
AE (caffeine): restlessness, vomiting, tachycardia;
AE (dextroamphetamine): insomnia, tachycardia, dry mouth, dependence, anorexia;
AE (methylphenidate): restlessness, behavior disturbances, slurred speech, dermatitis, skin rashes, convulsions, insomnia, states of excitability, psychoses, development of addiction;
AE (modafinil): headache, nausea, nervousness, loss of appetite, sleep DO;
CI (dextroamphetamine): hypersens. to dextroamphetamine, concomitant MAOI, CVS disease, hyperthyroidism;
CI (methylphenidate): glaucoma, marked anxiety, tension, agitation, depression, psychoses, addictions, hypersens. to methylphenidate, hyperthyroidism, prostate hypertrophy, pheochromocytoma;
CI (modafinil): combination with prazosin, addictions

Amphetamine/dextroamphetamine	EHL 9–14h, PRC C, Lact +
Adderall XR *Tab 5mg, 10mg, 15mg, 20mg, 25mg, 30mg*	**Attention deficit DO:** ini 5mg PO qd, maint 5–40mg PO qd–bid; **CH:** (3–5y) ini 2.5mg PO qam, (>6y) ini 5mg PO qam or bid, max 40mg/d; **Narcolepsy:** ini 10mg PO qam, maint 10–60 mg PO qd–bid, max 60mg/d; **CH:** (6–12y) ini 5mg PO qam, max 60mg/d, (>12y) ini 10mg PO qam, max 60mg/d; DARF: not req.

Caffeine	EHL 4–5h, PRC C, Lact +
Alert Aid *Cap 175mg, 200mg* **Destim** *Tab 200mg* **Pep-Back** *Tab 100mg* **Phenfree** *Cap 100mg* **Stay Awakes** *Tab 200mg* **Therma Pro** *Cap 100mg* **Wake Ups** *Tab 100mg* **Generics** *Tab 200mg, Liq (oral) 100mg/500ml, 200mg/500ml*	**Fatigue:** 100–200mg PO q3–4h prn

Dextroamphetamine	EHL 7–34h, PRC C, Lact -
Dexedrine *Tab 5mg, Cap ext.rel. 10mg, 15mg*	**Narcolepsy:** usual 5–60mg/d (div. qd–tid) **6–12y + narcolepsy:** ini 5mg/d PO, incr qwk by 5mg prn; >12y: ini 10mg/d PO, incr qwk by 10mg/d prn; **attention deficit hyperact. DO:** 3–5y: ini 2.5mg PO qd, incr by 2.5mg qwk prn; ≥ 6y: ini 5mg PO qd–bid, incr by 5mg qwk prn, max 40mg/d div qd–tid at 4–6h intervals

Methylphenidate	EHL PO 2–7h; IV 1–2h, PRC C, Lact ?
Biphentin *Tab 15mg, 20mg, 30mg, 40mg, 50mg, Cap cont. rel. 60mg, 80mg* **Ritalin** *Tab 10mg, 20mg* **Ritalin-SR** *Tab ext.rel. 20mg* **Generics** *Tab 5, 10, 20mg, Tab ext. rel. 20mg*	**Narcolepsy:** narcolepsy 10–60mg/d in 2–3 div doses (mean 20–30mg/d); **attention deficit DO: CH** > 6y: ini 2.5–5mg PO bid before breakfast and lunch, incr gradually by 5–10mg qwk prn to max 60mg/d

Modafinil	EHL 7.5–15h, PRC C, Lact ?
Alertec *Tab 100mg*	**Narcolepsy:** 200mg PO qam; DARF: ini 100–200mg/d, gradual incr based on safety and tolerability, see Prod Info

13 Dermatology

13.1 Acne Preparations

13.1.1 Anti-Infectives

S, R, AE, CI see Antibiotics →141

Clindamycin	PRC B, Lact -
Clindasol *Crm 1%* **Clinda-T** *Sol (top)10mg/ml* **Dalacin T Topical Solution** *Sol (top)10mg/ml*	**Acne:** apply bid; **rosacea:** apply lotion bid

Doxycycline	PRC D, Lact -
Apo-Doxy *Cap 100mg, Tab 100mg* **Doxycin** *Cap 100mg, Tab 100mg* **Doxytec** *Cap 100mg, Tab 100mg* **Novo-Doxylin** *Cap 100mg, Tab 100mg* **Vibra-Tabs** *Cap 100mg, Tab 100mg* **Generics** *Cap 100mg, Tab 100mg*	**Acne vulgaris:** 100mg PO bid; **CH** >8y: 2.2mg/kg PO qd or div bid, max 100mg PO bid; DARF: not req

Erythromycin	PRC B, Lact +
Benzamycin *Gel (top) 3%* **Erysol** *Gel(top) 2%*	**Acne:** apply bid

Sodium Sulfacetamide and Sulfur	PRC C, Lact ?
Sulfacet-R *Lot (top) 10% + 5%*	**Acne, rosacea, seborrheic dermatitis:** apply qd-tid, cleanser: qd-bid; DARF: contraind. in RF

Sulfur	EHL n/a
Sulfur Soap *Soap 10%*	**Acne:** apply qd-tid

Triclosan	EHL n/a
Adasept Skin Cleanser *Gel 0.5%, Liq (top) 0.5%* **Teraseptic** *Liq (top) 0.5%* **Trisan** *Liq (top) 0.25%*	**Acne:** apply qd-tid

13.1.2 Keratolytics

AE (benzoyl peroxide): burning/stinging, contact dermatitis, redness
CI (benzoyl peroxide): hypersensitivity to benzoyl peroxide products

Benzoyl Peroxide	PRC C, Lact ?
Acetoxyl *Gel (top) 2.5%, 5%, 10 %* **Benoxyl** *Lot (top) 5%, 10 %, 20%* **Benzac AC, Benzac W, Benzac W Wash** *Gel (top) 5%, 10 %* **Desquam-X** *Gel (top) 5%, 10%, Wash (top) 5%, 10%* **Oxyderm** *Lot (top) 5%, 10 %, 20%* **Panoxyl** *Gel (top) 5%, 10%, 15%, 20%, Bar (top) 5%, 10%* **Panoxyl Aquagel** *Gel (top) 2.5%, 5%* **Panoxyl Wash** *Cleanser (top) 5%* **Solugel** *Gel (top) 4%, 8%*	**Acne:** cleansers: wash qd/bid, cream/gel/sol: ini apply qd, prn gradually incr to bid/tid

13.1.3 Retinoids

MA/EF (acitretin): normalizes growth and differentiation of skin and mucosa cells
MA/EF (isotretinoin, tazarotene, tretinoin): mitotic rate of epidermal cells↑, keratolysis, sebaceous production↓
AE (acitretin, isotretinoin): dryness of skin and mucous membranes, lip infx, hair loss, transaminases↑, blood count changes, hyperlipidemia;
AE (isotretinoin): visual disturbances, epistaxis, conjunctivits;
AE (tazarotene): burning, itching, photosensitivity;
AE (tretinoin): leukocytosis (PO), arrhythmias (PO), headache (PO), dry skin
CI (acitretin, isotretionin): renal/hepatic insufficiency, DM,
CI (acitretin)women of childbearing age;
CI (tazarotene): hypersensitivity to tazarotene products, vitamin A/retinoids;
CI (tretinoin): hypersensitivity to tretinoin or parabens

Acitretin	PRC X, Lact ?
Soriatane *Cap 10mg, 25mg*	**Severe psoriasis:** 25–50mg PO qd; **lichen planus:** 30mg/d PO x 4wk, then titrate to 10–50 mg/d x 12wk total; **Sjogren-Larsson syndr.:** 0.47mg/kg/ d PO

Isotretinoin	PRC X, Lact -
Accutane *Cap 10mg, 40mg* **Isotrex** *Gel (top) 0.05%*	**Severe, recalcitrant cystic acne:** PO: 0.5–2 mg/kg/d PO div bid x 15–20wk, rep prn 2nd course of Tx after >2mo; Topical: apply bid; **prevention of second primary tumors in pat. treated for squamous-cell CA of head/ neck:** 50–100 mg/m^2/d PO; **neuroblastoma** (maint Tx): 100–250 mg/m^2/d PO div bid

Tazarotene	PRC X, Lact ?
Tazorac *Crm 0.05%, 0.1%; Gel (top) 0.05, 1%*	**Acne, psoriasis:** apply qhs, max x 3mo

Tretinoin	PRC X, Lact ?
Retin-A *Crm 0.01%, 0.025%, 0.05%, 0.1%, Gel 0.01%, 0.025%* **Vitamin A acid** *Crm 0.01%, 0.025%, 0.05%, 0.1%, Gel 0.01%, 0.025%, 0.05%*	**Acne:** apply qhs

13.1.4 Retinoid-Like Drugs

AE (adapalene): skin irritation
CI (adapalene): hypersensitivity to adapalene

Adapalene	PRC C, Lact ?
Differin *Sol (top) 0.1%, Gel (top) 0.1%, Crm (top) 0.1%*	**Acne:** apply qhs, therapeutic results in 8–12wk

13.2 Anti-Infectives

13.2.1 Antibacterials (topical)

AE (bacitracin): contact dermatitis;
AE (mafenide): burning sensation, rash/pruritus
AE (mupirocin): headache (nasal), rhinitis/pharyngitis (nasal), taste DO (nasal), stinging/ burning, pruritus;
AE (silver sulfadiazine): local skin irritat., skin rash, itch.;
CI (bacitracin): hypersensit. to bacitracin products;
CI (mafenide): hypersens. to mafenide prod., hypersensiti. to sulfites (metabisulfite in cream);
CI (mupirocin): hypersensit. to mupirocin products, avoid contact with the eyes, avoid prod. with polyethylene glycol on open wounds ;
CI (silver sulfadiazine): hypersens. to silver or sulfonamide prod., preterms, newborns<2mo

Bacitracin	PRC C, Lact ?
Baciquent *Oint 500 U/g*	**Minorcuts, wounds, burns, skin abras.:** apl. apply qd-tid
Gentamicin	PRC C, Lact ?
Garamycin, Generics *Crm 0.1%, Oint 0.1%*	**Skin infx:** apply tid-qid, **CH** >1y: apply tid-qid
Mafenide	PRC C, Lact ?
Sulfamylon *Crm 8.5%*	**Adj Tx of burns:** apply qd-bid
Metronidazole	PRC B/X in 1st trimester Lact -
MetroCream *Crm 0.75%* **MetroGel** *Gel (top) 0.75%* **Nidagel** *Gel (top) 0.75%* **Noritate** *Crm (top) 1%*	**Rosacea:** apply bid, therapeutical effects in 3-9wk
Mupirocin	PRC B, Lact -
Bactroban *Crm (augmented) 2%, Oint (nasal) 2%* **Generics** *Oint 2%*	**Impetigo:** apply tid x 3-5d; **wound infx:** tid x 10d; **nasal MRSA eradication:** 1g div between nostrils bid x 5 d
Neomycin + Polymyxin + Bacitracin Zinc	PRC C, Lact ?
Neosporin Ointment *Oint 5mg/g + 5,000 U/g + 400U/g*	**Minor cuts, wounds, burns or skin abrasions:** apply qd-tid
Silver Sulfadiazine	PRC B, Lact -
Dermazin, Flamazine *Crm 1%*	**Burns:** apply qd-bid; DARF: measurement of sulfadiazine levels in severe RF

13.2.2 Antifungals (topical) - Polyene Group

see systemic Antifungals →155

Nystatin	PRC C, Lact ?
Candistatin *Crm 100,000 U/g* **Mycostatin** *Powder 100,000 U/g* **Nyaderm** *Crm 100,000 U/g, Oint 100,000 U/g* **Generics** *Powder 1 billion U/bottle, Crm 100,000 U/g, Oint 100,000U/g*	**Cutaneous or mucocutaneous Candida infx:** apply bid-tid; **fungal infx of the feet, dust feet and footwear:** powder applied bid-tid; **thrush:** 4-6ml PO swish and swallow qid or suck on 1-2 troches 4-5 x/d, infants: 2ml/ dose PO with 1ml in each cheek qid

13.2.3 Antifungals (topical) - Azole Group

see systemic Antifungals →155

Clotrimazole	PRC B, Lact ?
Canesten *Crm 1%* **Clotrimaderm** *Crm 1%, Sol (top) 1%*	**Tinea pedis, cruris, corporis, versicolor/ cutaneous candidiasis:** apply bid
Econazole	PRC C, Lact ?
Ecostatin *Crm 1%, Ovule 150mg*	**Tinea pedis, cruris, corporis, versicolor:** apply qd x 2wk, tinea pedis x 4wk; **cutaneous candidiasis:** apply bid x 2wk
Ketoconazole	PRC C, Lact ?
Ketoderm *Crm 2%* **Nizoral** *Shampoo 2%*	**Tinea versicolor:** apply shampoo 2% to affected area, leave on x 5min, rinse, treat x **2wk; cutaneous candidiasis, tinea coporis, cruris, versicolor:** apply crm qd, treat x 2wk, tinea pedis x 6wk; **seborrheic dermatitis:** apply crm (2%) bid x 4wk; **3** apply shampoo (1%) 2x/wk
Miconazole	PRC, Lact ?
Micatin *Crm 2%, Spray 2%* **Monistat** *Crm 2%*	**Tinea pedis, cruris, corporis, versicolor/ cutaneous candidiasis:** apply bid x 2wk, tinea pedis x 1mo

13.2.4 Antifungals (topical) - Allylamine Group

AE (naftifine): local burning or stinging, contact dermatitis
AE (terbinafine): local irritation, N/V, LFT's ↑
CI (naftifine, terbinafine): hypersensitivity to product ingredients

Naftifine	PRC B, Lact ?
Naftin *Gel 1%, Crm 1%*	**Tinea pedis, cruris, corporis:** apply qd (cream) or bid (gel)

Terbinafine	PRC B, Lact -
Lamisil *Tab 250mg, Spray 1%, Crm 1%*	**Tinea pedis:** apply bid x 1-4wk; **tinea cruris, corporis:** apply qd-bid x 1-4wk; tinea versicolor: apply sol bid x 1-4wk; **onychomycosis** (fingernails): 250mg PO qd x 6wk; **onychomycosis** (toenails): 250mg PO qd x 12wk; **CH** <20kg: 67.5mg PO qd, 20-40kg: 125mg PO qd, >40kg: 250 mg PO qd, x 6wk for fingernails, x 12wk for toenails; **onychomycosis "pulse dosing":** 500mg PO qd for 1st wk of mo x 2mo for fingernails, 4mo for toenails; DARF: CrCl (ml/min):<50: contraind.

13.2.5 Other Topical Antifungals

AE (butenafine): burning/stinging
AE (ciclopirox): periungual erythema, burning of surrounding skin
AE (haloprogin): dermal allergic reactions
AE (tolnaftate): irritation, contact dermatitis
CI (butenafine, ciclopirox, haloprogin, tolnaftate): hypersensitivity to product ingredients

Butenafine	PRC B, Lact ?
Dr. Scholl's Athlete's Foot Cream *Crm 1%*	**Tinea pedis:** apply qd x 4wk or bid x 7d; **tinea coporis/ cruris:** apply qd x 2wk
Ciclopirox	PRC B, Lact ?
Loprox *Lot (top) 1%, Crm 1%*	**Tinea pedis, cruris, corporis, versicolor/ candidiasis:** cream, lotion: apply bid; **onchomycosis of fingernails/ toenails:** apply nail sol qd to affected nails, over previous coat, remove with alcohol q7d
Tolnaftate	PRC N, Lact ?
Pitrex *Crm 1%* **ZeaSorb AF** *Powder 1%*	**Tinea pedis, cruris, corporis, versicolor:** apply bid, **CH** >2y: apply bid; **prevention of tinea pedis:** apply powder/ aerosol prn

13.2.6 Antivirals

AE (acyclovir): N/V, headache, renal impairment, rash, phlebitis; **AE** (imiquimod): erosion, flaking, edema, erythema; **AE** (penciclovir): erythema; **AE** (podofilox): local irritation, inflammation, itching; **CI** (podophyllin): see Prod Info; **CI** (acyclovir, imiquimod, penciclovir, podofilox): hypersensitivity to product ingredients; **CI** (podophyllin): DM, patients using steroids or with poor blood circulation, not on bleeding warts, moles, birthmarks or unusual warts with hair growing from them

Acyclovir	PRC C (top)/B (oral) Lact +
Zovirax *Tab 200mg, 400mg, 800mg, Susp 200mg/5ml, Crm 5%, Oint 5%* **Generics** *Tab 200mg, 400mg, 800mg*	**Herpes genitalis** (ini episodes): apply q3h (6x/d) x 7d or 200mg PO q4h (5x/d) x 10d for 1st episode, x 5d for recurrent episodes, **CH** 80 mg/kg/d PO div tid (max 1.2g/ d) x 7-10d; **mucocutaneous herpes simplex in immunocompromised patients** (non-life threatening): apply q3h (6x/d) x 7d; **herpes PRO:** 400 mg PO bid; **herpes zoster:** 800mg PO q4h (5x/d) x 7-10d; **varicella:** 800mg PO qid x 5d, IV: 5-10mg/kg IV q8h, each dose x 1h, **CH** >2y: 20mg/kg PO qid x 5d, >40kg: adult dose; **primary gingivostomatitis:** 15mg/kg PO 5x/d x 7d; DARF: CrCl (ml/min) 10-25, 800mg: q8h, <10, 800mg: q12h, <10, 400mg: 50% q12h, <10, 200mg: q12h
Cantharidin	PRC C, Lact -
Canthacur *Liq 0.7%* **Cantharone** *Liq 0.7%*	**Warts, molluscum contagiosum:** apply to warts, allow to dry and remove necrotic tissue, repeat prn
Cantharidin + Podophyllin + Salicylic acid	PRC C, Lact -
Canthacur-PS *Liq 1% + 5% + 30%* **Cantharone Plus** *Liq 1% + 2% + 30%*	**Warts, molluscum contagiosum:** apply to warts, allow to dry and remove necrotic tissue, repeat prn
Imiquimod	PRC B, Lact ?
Aldara *Crm 5%*	**External genital and perianal warts:** apply 3 x/wk hs, wash off in 6-10h; **giant molluscum contagiosum:** apply 3x/wk x 6-10h

Penciclovir	PRC B, Lact ?
Denavir *Crm 1%*	**Herpes labialis:** apply q2h x 4d
Podofilox	PRC C, Lact ?
Condyline *Sol (top) 0.5%* **Wartec** *Sol (top) 0.5%*	**External genital warts** (gel/sol)/ **perianal warts** (gel only): apply bid x 3 consecutive d/wk, rep x max 4wk
Podophyllin	PRC N, Lact -
Podofilm *Sol (top) 25%*	**Genital wart removal:** ini apply to wart and leave on x 30–40min to determine patient's sensitivity, then use minimum contact time necessary (1–4h), then remove dried podophyllin with alcohol or soap + water

13.2.7 Antiparasitics (topical)

AE (crotamiton): dermatitis, skin irritation;
AE (lindane): dermatitis, anxiety, dizziness, insomnia, myelosuppression;
AE (permethrin): pruritus, burning, stinging, rash
CI (crotamiton): hypersens. to crotamiton;
CI (lindane): hypersens. to lindane, premature neonates, seizure DO;
CI (permethrin): hypersens. to permethrin/chrysanthemums

Crotamiton	PRC C, Lact ?
Eurax *Crm 10%*	**Scabies:** massage cream/lotion into entire body from chin down, rep in 24h, then bathe in 48h; **pruritus:** massage into affected areas prn
Isopropyl myristate	
Resultz *Sol (top) 50%*	**Head lice:** apply 30–120ml to hair/head, remain on for 10min. then rinse with water, repeat in 7 day
Lindane	PRC B, Lact ?
Hexit *Shampoo 1%* **Lindane** *Lot (top) 1%, Shampoo 1%*	**Head/crab lice:** apply lotion 30–60ml to affected area, wash off in 12h or apply shampoo 30–60ml, wash off in 4min, then comb to remove nits, prn rep in 7d; **scabies:** apply lotion to total body from neck down, wash off in 8–12h

Permethrin	PRC B, Lact ?
Kwellada-P *Crm (rinse) 1%, Lot (top) 5%* **Nix** *Crm (rinse) 1%, Crm 5%*	**Scabies:** massage 30g (cream) into entire body, wash off in 8-14h, **CH** >2mo: <30g of cream needed; **head lice:** apply liquid to clean, towel-dried hair, saturate hair and scalp, wash off in 10min, **CH** >2mo: adult application

Pyrethrins, Piperonyl Butoxide	PRC C, Lact ?
R & C *Shampoo 0.33% + 3%* **R & C II** *Spray 0.3% + 1.5%*	**Head/crab/body lice:** apply shampoo/foam on dry hair, wash after 10min, rep in 5-7d

13.2.8 Anti-Infective Combinations

Betamethasone + Clotrimazole	PRC C, Lact ?
Lotriderm *Crm 0.05% + 1%*	**Tinea pedis, cruris, corporis:** apply bid x 2wk, tinea pedis x 4wk
Clioquinol + Hydrocortisone	
Vioform Hydrocortisone *Crm 3% + 1%*	**Skin infection**: apply 2-3 times daily
Framycetin + Gramicidin	
Soframycin Skin Ointment *Oint 15 + 0.05mg/g*	**Skin infection**: apply 2-4 times daily
Nystatin + Gramicidin + Neomycin + Trimacinolone	PRC C, Lact ?
Kenacomb *Crm 100,000U/g + 250mcg/g + 2.5mg/g + 0.025%, 100,000 U/g + 250mcg/g + 2.5mg/g + 1mg/g* *Oint 100,000U/g + 250mcg/g + 2.5mg/g + 0.025%, 100,000 U/g + 250mcg/g + 2.5mg/g + 1mg/g* **ratio-Triacomb** *Crm 100,000 U/g + 250mcg/g + 2.5mg/g + 1mg/g* **Viaderm-K.C.** *Crm 100,000U/g + 250mcg/g + 2.5mg/g + 1mg/g* *Oint 100,000U/g + 250mcg/g + 2.5mg/g + 1mg/g*	**Cutaneous candidiasis:** apply bid

Polymyxin + Bacitracin	PRC C, Lact ?
Polysporin Ointment *Oint 10,000U/g + 500U/g*	**Skin infx:** apply qd–tid
Polymyxin + Bacitracin + Gramicidin	PRC C, Lact ?
Polysporin Triple *Oint 10,000U/g + 500U/g + 250mcg/g*	**Skin infx:** apply qd–tid
Polymyxin B + Bacitracin + Lidocaine	PRC C, Lact ?
Ozonol Antibiotics Plus *Oint 10,000U + 500U + 40mg/g*	**Skin infection**: apply 1–3 times/d
Polymyxin + Bacitracin Zinc + Hydrocortisone + Neomycin	PRC C, Lact ?
Cortisporin *Oint 5,000U/g + 400U/g + 10mg/g + 5mg/g*	**Skin infx:** apply bid–qid
Polymyxin + Gramicidin	PRC C, Lact ?
Polysporin Cream *Crm 10,000U/g + 250mcg/g*	**Skin infx:** apply qd–tid
Polymyxin + Gramicidin + Lidocaine	PRC C, Lact ?
Lidosporin *Crm 10,000U/g + 250mcg/g + 50mg/g* **Polysporin Plus Pain Relief** *Crm 10,000U/g + 250mcg/g + 50mg/g*	**Skin infx:** apply qd–tid
Polymyxin + Gramicidin + Neomycin	PRC C, Lact ?
Neosporin Cream *Crm 10,000U/g + 250mcg/g + 5mg/g*	**Skin infx:** apply bid–5 times/d

13.3 Antipsoriatics

MA/EF (calcipotriene): vitamin D3 derivative; **AE** (anthralin): skin inflammation, irritiation, rash; **AE** (calcipotriene): skin irritation; **AE** (coal tar): rash; **CI** (anthralin): hypersens. to anthralin, erythroderma, psoriasis pustul., type Zumbusch (full- body psoriasis), inflammatory + acute psoriasis, renal DO, flexures; **CI** (calcipotriene): vitamin D toxicity, hypercalcemia, hypersensitivity to calcipotriene; **CI** (coal tar): hypersensitivity to coal tar

Anthralin	PRC C, Lact ?
Anthraforte *Oint 1%, 2%* **Anthranol** *Crm 0.1%, 0.2%, 0.4%* **Anthrascalp** *Lot 0.4%* **Micanol** *Crm 1%, 3%*	**Quiescent/chronic psoriasis:** apply qd

Calcipotriol	PRC C, Lact ?
Dovonex *Sol (top) 0.05mg/ml, Crm 0.005%, Oint 0.005%*	**Moderate plaque psoriasis:** apply bid
Calcipotriol + Betamethasone	PRC C, Lact ?
Dovobet *Oint 50mcg + 0.5mg/g*	**Psoriasis**: apply daily
Coal Tar	PRC N, Lact ?
Balnetar *Sol 2.5%* **Liquor Carbonis Detergens** *Sol 20%*	**Dandruff, seborrheic dermatitis:** shampoo ≧ 2x/wk; **psoriasis:** apply cream qd-qid or shampoo affected areas, **CH** >2y: as adults
see **Retinoids** →258	

13.4 Corticosteroids (topical)

13.4.1 Topical Corticosteroids - Very High Potency

Augmented Betamethasone Dipropionate	PRC C, Lact ?
Diprolene Glycol *Lot (top) 0.05%, Oint 0.05%, Crm 0.05%* **Diprosone** *Lot (top) 0.05%, Oint 0.05%, Crm 0.05%* **Taro-Sone** *Lot (top) 0.05%, Oint 0.05%, Crm 0.05%* **ratio-Topilene** *Lot (top) 0.05%, Oint 0.05%, Crm 0.05%* **ratio-Topisone** *Lot (top) 0.05%, Oint 0.05%, Crm 0.05%*	**Dermatoses:** apply qd-bid, max x 2wk, max 50g/wk resp. 50ml/wk
Clobetasol Propionate	PRC C, Lact ?
Dermovate *Crm 0.05%, Oint (top) 0.05%, Lot 0.05%* **Generics** *Sol (top) 0.05%, Crm 0.05%, Oint 0.05%*	**Dermatoses:** apply bid, max x 2wk, max 50g/wk
Halobetasol Propionate	PRC C, Lact ?
Ultravate *Crm 0.05%, Oint 0.05%*	**Dermatoses:** apply qd-bid, max x 2wk, max 50g cream or oint/wk

13.4.2 Topical Corticosteroids – High Potency

Amcinonide	PRC C, Lact ?
Cyclocort *Lot (top) 0.1%, Crm 0.1%, Oint 0.1%*	**Dermatoses:** apply bid-tid
Betamethasone Dipropionate	PRC C, Lact ?
Diprolene Glycol *Lot (top) 0.05%, Oint 0.05%, Crm 0.05%* **Diprosone** *Lot (top) 0.05%, Oint 0.05%, Crm 0.05%* **Taro-Sone** *Lot (top) 0.05%, Oint 0.05%, Crm 0.05%* **Topilene** *Lot (top) 0.05%, Oint 0.05%, Crm 0.05%* **Topisone** *Lot (top) 0.05%, Oint 0.05%, Crm 0.05%*	**Dermatoses:** apply qd-bid
Desoximetasone	PRC C, Lact ?
Topicort *Crm 0.05%, 0.25%, Oint 0.25%, Gel (top) 0.05%*	**Dermatoses:** apply bid
Fluticasone	PRC C, Lact ?
Cutivate *Oint 0.005%, 0.05%*	**Dermatoses:** apply bid-qid
Fluocinonide	PRC C, Lact ?
Lidemol *Sol (top) 0.05%* **Lidex** *Crm 0.05%, Oint 0.05%* **Lyderm** *Crm 0.05%, Oint 0.05%* **Tiamol** *Crm 0.05%* **Topsyn** *Gel (top) 0.05%*	**Dermatoses:** apply bid-qid
Halcinonide	PRC C, Lact ?
Halog *Sol (top) 0.1%, Crm 0.1%, Oint 0.1%*	**Dermatoses:** apply bid-tid

13.4.3 Topical Corticosteroids - Medium Potency	
Betamethasone Valerate	PRC C, Lact ?
Betaderm *Lot (top) 0.1%, Crm 0.05%, 0.1%, Oint 0.05%, 0.1%* **Betnovate** *Lot (top) 0.1%, Oint 0.05%* **ratio-Ectosone** *Crm 0.05%, 0.1%, Lot (top) 0.05%, 0.1%* **Prevex B** *Crm 0.1%* **Valisone** *Lot (top) 0.1%*	**Dermatoses:** apply qd-bid, for skalp: foam
Desoximetasone	PRC C, Lact ?
Topicort *Crm 0.05%, 0.25%, Oint 0.25%, Gel (top) 0.05%*	**Dermatoses:** apply bid
Fluocinolone Acetonide	PRC C, Lact ?
Capex Shampoo *Shampoo 0.1mg/ml* **Derma-Smoothe/FS** *Oil (top) 0.01%* **Synalar** *Sol (top) 0.01%, Oint 0.025%*	**Dermatoses:** apply bid-qid
Hydrocortisone Valerate	PRC C, Lact ?
Hydroval *Crm 0.2%, Oint 0.2%* **Westcort** *Crm 0.2%, Oint 0.2%*	**Dermatoses:** apply bid-tid
Mometasone Furoate	PRC C, Lact ?
Elocom *Lot (top) 0.1%, Crm 0.1%, Oint 0.1%*	**Dermatoses:** apply qd, **CH** ≧ 2y: adult application
Prednicarbate	PRC C, Lact ?
Dermatop *Crm 0.1%, Oint 0.1%*	**Dermatoses:** apply bid, **CH** ≧ 1y: adult application
Triamcinolone Acetonide	PRC C, Lact ?
Aristocort *Crm 0.1% 0.5%, Oint 0.1%* **Kenalog** *Crm 0.1%, Oint 0.1%* **Triaderm** *Crm 0.025%, 0.1%, Oint 0.025%, 0.1%*	**Dermatoses:** apply tid-qid

13.4.4 Topical Corticosteroids - Low Potency	
Desonide	PRC C, Lact ?
Desocort *Lot (top) 0.05%, Crm 0.05%, Oint 0.05%*	**Dermatoses:** apply bid-tid

Hydrocortisone	PRC C (top) Lact ?
Aquacort *Lot (top) 2.5%* **Emo-Cort** *Sol (top) 2.5%, Lot (top) 1%, 2.5%, Crm 1%, 2.5%* **Prevex HC** *Crm 1%* **Sarna HC** *Lot (top) 1%, 2.5%*	**Dermatoses:** apply bid-qid
Hydrocortisone Acetate	PRC C, Lact ?
Cortef Cream *Crm 0.5%* **Hyderm** *Crm 0.5%, 1%*	**Dermatoses:** apply bid-qid

13.5 Antipruritics

13.5.1 Histamine Receptor Blockers and Combinations

AE (doxepin): burning/stinging (cream), drowsiness, CVS/anticholin. effects, seizures
CI (doxepin): hypersensitivity to doxepin products, glaucoma, urinary retention, concomitant MAO inhibitors

Calamine + Diphenhydramine	PRC N, Lact ?
Caladryl *Crm 8% + 1%, Lot 8% + 1%*	**Itching due to poison ivy/oak/sumac, insect bites, minor irritation:** apply prn, max tid-qid
Diphenhydramine	Lact ?
Benadryl *Crm 2% w/w*	**Pruritus associated with atopic dermatitis, contact dermatitis, allergies:** apply locally tid to qid daily
Diphenhydramine + Zinc acetate	Lact ?
Benadryl Spray *2% + 0.1% w/v* **Benadryl Stick** *2% + 0.1% w/v*	**Pruritus associated with atopic dermatitis, contact dermatitis, allergies:** apply locally tid to qid daily
Doxepin	PRC B (top) Lact -
Zonalon *Crm 5% v*	**Pruritus associated with atopic dermatitis, lichen simplex chronicus, eczematous dermatitis:** qid x max 8d

13.5.2 Other Antipruritics

Oatmeal	PRC N, Lact +
Equate, Nutra Soothe *Bath Packets 100% colloidal oatmeal*	**Pruritus from poison ivy/oak, varicella:** add packet to bath qd prn

13.6 Hemorrhoid Care

MA/EF: (benzocaine, cinchocaine/dibucaine, pramozine): topical anesthetic
MA/EF: (framycetin) aminoglycoside antibiotic
AE (dibucaine): contact dermatitis, photosensitivity reactions;
AE (witch hazel): mild itching or burning;
CI (dibucaine): hypersensitivity to dibucaine
CI (witch hazel): hypersensitivity to Witch Hazel, internal consumption is not rec

Benzocaine + Zinc Sulfate	
Rectogel *Gel 10% + 0.5%*	**Anorectal pain/discomfort/pruritis:** apply PR bid and after bowel movements
Dibucaine	PRC N, Lact ?
Nupercainal *Oint 1%*	**Anorectal pain/discomfort/pruritis:** apply PR bid and after bowel movements
Hydrocortisone + Benzocaine + Zinc Sulfate	
Rectogel HC *Gel 1% + 10% + 0.5%*	**Anorectal pain/discomfort/pruritis:** apply PR bid and after bowel movements
Hydrocortisone + Framycetin + Cinchocaine + Esculin	
Proctol, Proctosedyl, ratio-Proctosone, Sandoz Proctomyxin HC, *Oint 5mg + 10mg + 5mg + 10mg/g, Supp 5mg + 10mg + 5mg + 10mg*	**Anorectal pain/discomfort/pruritis:** apply PR bid and after bowel movements
Hydrocortisone + Zinc Sulfate	PRC C, Lact ?
Anodan-HC, Anusol-HC, ratio-Hemcort-HC, PMS-Egozinc-HC, Sandoz Anuzinc HC *Oint 0.5% + 0.5%, Supp 10mg + 10mg* **Rivasol HC** *Oint 0.5% + 0.5%*	**Anorectal pain/discomfort/pruritis:** apply PR bid and after bowel movements
Pramoxine + Hydrocortisone	PRC C, Lact ?
Pramox HC *Crm 1% + 1%, Lot 1% + 1%* **Proctofoam-HC** *Foam 1% + 1%*	**Anorectal pain/discomfort/pruritis:** apply PR bid and after bowel movements
Pramoxine + Hydrocortisone + Zinc Sulfate	
Anugesic-HC *Oint 1% + 0.5% + 0.5%, Supp 20mg + 10mg + 10mg* **Sandoz Anuzinc HC Plus***Supp* **Proctodan-HC** *Oint 1% + 0.5% + 0.5%, Supp 20mg + 10mg + 10mg*	**Anorectal pain/discomfort/pruritis:** apply PR bid and after bowel movements

Pramoxine + Zinc Sulfate	PRC N, Lact ?
Anusol Plus *Oint 1% + 0.5%, Supp 20mg + 10mg*	**Anorectal pain/discomfort/pruritis:** apply PR bid and after bowel movements
Starch	PRC N, Lact +
Bum-Butt-R *Crm 50%*	**Anorectal pain/discomfort/pruritis:** apply PR bid and after bowel movements
Witch Hazel	PRC N, Lact +
Generics *Liq (top) 85%, 100%*	**Anorectal pain/discomfort/pruritis:** apply PR bid and after bowel movements
Zinc Sulfate	PRC C, Lact ?
Anusol, Sandoz Anuzinc *Oint 0.5%, Supp 10mg* **Rivasol** *Oint 0.5%*	**Anorectal pain/discomfort/pruritis:** apply PR bid and after bowel movements

13.7 Hair Restorers

MA/EF (finasteride): inhibition of 5-α-reductase ⇒ testosterone cannot be transformed to dihydro-testosterone ⇒ hair loss ↓, prostatic hyperplasia ↓
AE (finasteride): libido and erection disturbances, gynecomastia, lip swelling, skin rash; pregnant women may not touch tablet brittle!;
AE (minoxidil): hypertrichosis, pleural/pericard.effusion, reflex tachycardia, fluid retention;
CI (finasteride): women or children, hypersensitivity to finasteride products;
CI (minoxidil): hypersensitivity to minoxidil

Finasteride	EHL 6h, PRC X, Lact -
Propecia *Tab 1mg* **Proscar** *Tab 5mg*	**Androgenetic alopecia in men:** 1mg PO qd; **androgenetic alopecia in postmenopausal women:** 1mg PO
Minoxidil	EHL 2.3-28.9h, PRC C, Lact +
Apo-Gain *Sol (top) 2%* **Minox** *Sol (top) 2%* **Rogaine** *Sol (top) 2%*	**Androgenetic alopecia in men or women:** apply 1ml bid (to dry scalp)

13.8 Anesthetics

Lidocaine HCl	EHL 1.5–2h, PRC B, Lact +
Xylocaine *Jelly (top) 2%, Sol (top) 4%, 5%, Sol (viscous) 2%* **Generics** *Sol (viscous) 2%, Oint 5%*	**Topical anesthesia for minor dermal procedures** (eg, IV cannulation, venipuncture): apply 2.5g over 20–25cm^2 area or 1 disc ≧ 1h prior to procedure; **topical anesthesia for major dermal procedures** (ie, skin grafting harvesting): apply 2g per 10cm^2 area ≧ 2h prior to procedure; **topical anesthesia in CH** 1–3mo or <5kg: apply max 1g over max 10cm^2, 4–12mo and >5kg: apply max 2g over max 20cm^2, 1–6y and >10kg: apply max 10g over max 100cm^2, 7–12y and >20kg: apply max 20g over max 200cm^2; **prior to circumcision in infants >37wk gestation:** apply ma 1g over max 10cm^2;
Lidocaine + Prilocaine	PRC C, Lact +
EMLA *Crm 5% + 5%, Disc (top) 2.5% + 2.5%*	**Topical anesthesia for minor dermal procedures:** apply 2.5g/20–25cm^2 area or 1 disc ≧ 1h prior to procedure; **topical anesthesia for major dermal procedures :** apply 2g/10cm^2 area ≧ 2h prior to procedure; **topical anesthesia in CH** 1–3mo or <5kg: apply max 1g over max 10cm^2, 4–12mo and >5kg: apply max 2g over max 20cm^2, 1–6y and >10kg: apply max 10g over max 100cm^2, 7–12y and >20kg: apply max 20g over max 200cm^2; **prior to circumcision in infants > 37 wk gestation:** apply max 1g over max 10cm^2

see Local Anesthetics, →214

13.9 Other Dermatologic Agents

AE (alitretinoin): rash, pain (application site), exfoliative dermatitis, pruritus, edema;
AE (becaplermin): rash;
AE (capsaicin): cough with inhalation, local irritation;
AE (hydroquinone): urine discoloration, ochronosis, fingernail staining, local irritation;
AE (selenium sulfide): skin irritation, hair loss or disoloration, oily or dry scalp
CI (alitretinoin): hypersensitivity to retinoids or alitretinoin products; CI (becaplermin): hypersensitivity to bacaplermin or parabens, known neoplasm at application site;
CI (capsaicin, hydroquinone, selenium sulfide): hypersensitivity to product

Alitretinoin	PRC D, Lact -
Panretin *Gel (top) 0.1%*	**Cutaneous lesions of AIDS-related Kaposi's sarcoma:** apply bid–qid
Becaplermin	PRC C, Lact ?
Regranex *Gel 0.01%*	**Diabetic neuropathic ulcers:** apply qd (length x width x 0.6=amount of gel in inches), cover with saline- moistened gauze x 12h, then rinse and cover with saline gauze without medication
Botulinum Toxin Type A	PRC C, Lact ?
Botox *Inj 100U/vial* **Botox Cosmetic** *Inj 100U/vial*	**Cervical distonia**: **CH** >16y and adults: 198–300U IM; **blepharospasm**: ini 1.25–2.5U IM, max 5U/site; **strabismus**: 1.25–5U IM, max 25U/muscle; **reduction of glabellar line**: dose determined by gross evaluation
Capsaicin	PRC N, Lact ?
Zostrix Crm 0.025%, 0.075% **Generics** *Crm 0.025%, 0.075%*	**Pain due to rheumatoid arthritis, osteoarthritis, neuralgias (zoster):** apply prn, max tid–qid, **CH** >2y: adult application
Fluorouracil	PRC X, Lact -
Efudex *Crm 5%*	**Actinic/solar keratoses:** apply bid to lesions x 2–6wk; **superficial basal cell CA:** cover lesions with 5% bid x 3– 6wk, max 12wk

Hydroquinone	PRC C, Lact ?
Eldopaque, Eldoquin, Solaquin *Crm 2%, 4%* **Lustra** *Crm 4%* **Ultraquin** *Crm 4%, Gel (top) 4%*	**Temporary bleaching of hyperpigmented skin conditions** (i.e. chloasma, discoloration from oral contraceptives, pregnancy): apply bid to affected area
Hydroquinone + Octyl Methoxycinnamate + Avobenzone	PRC C, Lact ?
Lustra-AF *Crm 4% + 7.5%*	**Ultraviolet induced dyschromia and discoloration**: apply bid
Ammonium Lactate	PRC B, Lact ?
Dermalac *Crm 12%, Lot (top) 12%*	**Ichthyosis vulgaris, xerosis (dry, scaly skin)**: apply bid to affected area
Lactic Acid + Glycerin	PRC C, Lact ?
Epi-Lyt AHA Medicated Lotion *Lot (top) 5% + 25%*	**Ichthyosis vulgaris, xerosis** (dry, scaly skin): apply bid to affected area
Salicylic acid + Urea	
Kerasal *Crm 5% + 10%*	**Foot xerosis**: apply 1-2 times daily
Mequinol + Tretinoin	PRC C, Lact ?
Solage *Sol (top) 2% + 0.01%*	**Solar lentigines:** apply bid separated >8h
Pimecrolimus	PRC C, Lact ?
Elidel *Crm 1%*	**Atopic dermatitis:** apply to lesions bid
Selenium Sulfide	PRC C, Lact ?
Head & Shoulders Shampoo *Shampoo 1%* **Selegel** *Lot (top) 1%* **Selsun** *Liq (top) 2.5%* **Selsun Blue** *Shampoo 1%* **Versel** *Lot (top) 2.5%*	**Dandruff, seborrheic dermatitis:** massage 5-10ml of shampoo into wet scalp, allow to remain 2-3min, rinse, apply 2x/wk x 2wk, maint 1x/wk; **tinea versicolor:** apply 2.5% shampoo/lotion to affected area, allow to remain on skin 10min, rinse, rep qd x 7d

14 Ophthalmology

14.1 Anti-Infectives

14.1.1 Antibacterials - Single Ingredient Drugs

S, R, AE, CI see Antibiotics →141

Bacitracin	PRC C, Lact ?
Generics *Oint 500 U/g*	**Ocular infx:** apply ½ inch ribbon of oint q3-4h or bid-qid
Ciprofloxacin	PRC C, Lact ?
Apo-Ciproflox *Sol/Gtt (oph) 0.3%* **Ciloxan** *Sol/Gtt (oph) 0.3%, Oint (oph) 0.3%*	**Corneal ulcers/keratitis:** 2 Gtt q15min x 6h, then 2 Gtt q30min x 1d, then 2 Gtt q1h x 1d and 2 Gtt q4h x 3-14d; **CH:** adult dose, if ≧ 1 y use sol, ≧ 2 y use oint; **conjunctivitis:** 1-2 Gtt q2h while awake x 2d, then 1-2 Gtt q4h while awakefferve x 5d, or ½ inch ribbon of oint tid x 2d, then ½ inch ribbon bid x 5d; **CH:** adult dose, if ≧ 1 y use sol, if ≧ 2 y use oint
Erythromycin	PRC B, Lact +
Diomycin *Oint 0.5%* **Generics** *Oint 0.5%*	**Ocular infx:** ½ inch ribbon of oint to affected eye(s) q3-4h; **chlamydial infx:** ½ inch ribbon of oint bid x 2mo or bid x 5d/mo x 6mo; **ophthalmia neonatorum PRO:** ½ inch ribbon of oint to both eyes within 1h of birth
Framycetin	EHL n/a,
Soframycin Sterile Eye *Oint (oph) 5mg/ml, Sol/Gtt (oph) 5mg/ml*	**Ocular infx**: 1-2 gtts q 1-2 h in acute conditions (for 2-3 d), reducing to 1-2gtts, tid-qid
Fusidic acid	PRC C, Lact +
Fucithalmic *Sol 10mg/1g*	**Ocular infx**: 1 gtts bid
Gentamicin	PRC C, Lact ?
Diogent *Sol/Gtt (oph) 0.3%, Oint (oph) 0.3%* **Garamycin** *Sol/Gtt (oph) 0.3%, Sol/Gtt (otic) 0.3%, Oint (oph) 0.3%* **Generics** *Sol/Gtt (oph) 0.3%*	**Ocular infx:** 1-2 Gtt q4h or ½ inch ribbon of oint bid-tid, for severe infx max 2 Gtt qh

Ofloxacin	PRC C, Lact -
Ocuflox *Sol/Gtt (oph) 0.3%*	**Corneal ulcers/keratitis:** 1-2 Gtt q30min while awake and 1-2 Gtt 4h and 6h after retiring x 2d, then 1-2 Gtt q1h while awake x 5d, then 1-2 Gtt qid x 3d; **conjunctivitis:** 1-2 Gtt q2-4h x 2d, then 1-2 Gtt qid x 5d; **CH** ≧ 1 y: adult dose
Sulfacetamide	PRC C, Lact -
Diosulf *Sol/Gtt (oph) 10%*	**Ocular infx:** ini 1-2 Gtt q2-3h, then taper x 7-10d, or ini ½ inch ribbon of oint q3-4h, then taper x 7-10d; **CH** ≧ 2 mo: adult dose; **trachoma:** 2 Gtt q2h with systemic sulfonamide; **CH** ≧ 2 mo: adult dose
Tobramycin	PRC B, Lact -
Tobrex *Oint (oph) 0.3%, Sol/Gtt (oph) 0.3%* **Generics** *Sol/Gtt (oph) 0.3%*	**Ocular infx:** 1-2 Gtt q2h x 1-2d, then 1-2 Gtt q4-6h or ½ inch ribbon of oint bid-qid

14.1.2 Antibacterials - Combinations

Bacitracin + Polymyxin B	PRC C, Lact ?
LID-Pack *Oint (oph) 500 U/g + 10,000 U/g* **Optimyxin** *Oint (oph) 500 U/g + 10,000 U/g* **Polysporin** *Oint (oph) 500 U/g + 10,000 U/g*	**Ocular infx:** ½ inch ribbon of oint qd or q3-4h x 7-10d
Gentamicin + Betamethasone	PRC C, Lact ?
SAB-Pentasone *Sol (oph) 3 + 1mg/ml*	**Ocular infx:** 1-2 Gtt q4h
Polymyxin B + Bacitracin + Neomycin	PRC C, Lact ?
Neosporin *Oint (oph)* *10,000 U/g + 400 U/g + 5mg/g*	**Ocular infx:** ½ inch ribbon of oint q3-4 h x 7-10d
Polymyxin B + Bacitracin + Neomycin + Hydrocortisone	PRC C, Lact ?
Cortisporin *Oint (oph)* *10,000 U/g + 400 U/g + 5mg/g + 10mg/g*	**Ocular infx:** ½ inch ribbon of oint q3-4 h x 7-10d
Polymyxin + Gramicidin	PRC C, Lact ?
Optimyxin *Sol/Gtt (oph/otic)* *10,000U/ml + 0.025mg/ml*	**Ocular infx:** 1-2 Gtt q3-4h; **otic infx:** 4 Gtt 3-4x/d

Polymyxin + Gramicidin + Neomycin	PRC C, Lact ?
Neosporin *Sol/Gtt (oph) 10,000 U/ml + 0.025mg/ml + 2.5mg/ml* **Optimyxin Plus** *Sol/Gtt (oph) 10,000 U/ml + 0.025mg/ml + 2.5mg/ml*	**Ocular infx:** 1-2 Gtt q1-6h x 7-10d, for severe infx max 1-2 Gtt q1h
Polymyxin + Bacitracin + Gramicidin	PRC C, Lact ?
Polysporin Triple Antibiotic *Oint (oph) 10,000 U/g + 500 U/g + 0.25mg/g*	**Ocular infx:** ½ inch ribbon of oint q3-4 h x 7-10d
Polymyxin B + Trimethoprim	PRC C, Lact ?
Polytrim, Generics *Sol/Gtt (oph) 10,000 U/ml + 1mg/ml*	**Ocular infx:** 1Gtt q3-6h x7-10d,max 6 Gtt/d **CH** ≧ 2 mo: adult dose

14.1.3 Antivirals

Trifluridine	EHL 12min, PRC C, Lact ?
Viroptic *Sol/Gtt (oph) 1%*	**HSV keratitis/keratoconjunctivitis:** 1Gtt q2h, max 9 Gtt/d, after reepithelialization, decr to 1 Gtt q4h (min 5 Gtt/d) while awake x 7-14d, max contin use: 21d; **CH** ≧ 6 y: adult dose

14.2 Ophthalmic Anti-Inflammatory Agents

14.2.1 Corticosteroids - Single Ingredient Drugs

AE (corticosteroids): glaucoma, cataracts, corneal ulcers, secondary infections
CI (corticosteroids): bacterial, viral and fungal diseases of the eyes, injuries, corneal ulcers

Fluorometholone	PRC C, Lact ?
Flarex *Susp/Gtt (oph) 0.1%* **Fml** *Susp/Gtt (oph) 0.1%* **Fml Forte** *Susp/Gtt (oph) 0.25%* **Generics** *Susp/Gtt (oph) 0.1%*	**Anti-inflammatory:** prn ini 1 Gtt q4h or ½ inch of oint q4h x 1-2d, then 1 Gtt bid-qid or ½ inch of oint qd-tid; **CH** ≧ 2 y: adult dose
Prednisolone	EHL 2.6-3h, PRC C, Lact -
Diopred *Susp/Gtt (oph) 1%* **Pred Forte** *Susp/Gtt (oph) 1%* **Pred Mild** *Susp/Gtt (oph) 0.12%* **Generics** *Susp/Gtt (oph) 0.5%, 1%*	**Anti-inflammatory:** ini 1-2 Gtt q1h during the day and q2h during the night, then 1-2 Gtt q3-12h
Rimexolone	EHL 1-2h, PRC C, Lact ?
Vexol *Susp/Gtt (oph) 1%*	**Postop inflamm:** 1-2Gtt qidx2wk,ini 24h after surgery;**uveitis:** 1-2Gtt q1h while awake x1wk then 1Gtt q2h while awake x1wk,then taper

14.2.2 Corticosteroids - Combinations

Dexamethasone, Tobramycin	PRC C, Lact ?
Tobradex *Oint (oph) 0.1% + 0.3%, Susp/Gtt (oph) 0.1% + 0.3%*	**Anti-inflammatory:** 1-2 Gtt q2h x 1-2d, then 1-2 Gtt q4-6h or ½ inch ribbon of oint bid-qid, gradually taper when discontinuing
Neomycin, Polymyxin, Hydrocortisone, (Bacitracin Zinc)	PRC C, Lact ?
Cortisporin *Sol/Gtt (oph/otic) 10,000 U/ml + 3.5mg/ml + 10mg/ml*	**Anti-inflammatory:** 1-2 Gtt or ½ inch ribbon of oint q3-4h, prn more frequently, gradually taper when discontinuing
Polymyxin, Dexamethasone, Neomycin	PRC C, Lact ?
Dioptrol *Susp/Gtt (oph) 10,000 U/ml + 0.1% + 3.5mg/ml* **Maxitrol** *Oint (oph) 6,000 U/g + 0.1% + 3.5mg/g, Susp/Gtt (oph) 6,000 U/ml + 0.1% + 3.5mg/ml*	**Anti-inflammatory:** ini 1-2 Gtt q1h during the day and q2h during the night, then 1 Gtt q4-8h or ini ½ -1 inch ribbon (oint) tid-qid, then qd-bid, gradually taper when discontinuing
Prednisolone Acetate + Sulfacetamide Sodium	PRC C, Lact -
Blephamide *Susp (oph) 0.2% + 10%* **Dioptimyd** *Susp (oph) 0.5% + 10%*	**Anti-inflammatory:** 2 Gtt q4h while awake and hs or ½ inch ribbon of oint tid-qid (during the day) and 1-2x during the night, gradually taper when discontinuing

14.2.3 Nonsteroidal Anti-Inflammatory Agents

Diclofenac	EHL 2h, PRC B, Lact ?
Voltaren Ophtha *Sol/Gtt (oph) 0.1%*	**Postop inflammation following cataract removal:** 1 Gtt qid x 2wk, ini 24h postop; **photophobia associated with incisional refractive surgery:** 1 Gtt to operative eye(s) 1h prior to surgery and 1 Gtt 15min postop, then 1 Gtt qid prn x max 3 d
Ketorolac	EHL 5.3h, PRC C, Lact ?
Acular *Sol/Gtt (oph) 0.4%, 0.5%*	**Allergic conjunctivitis:** 1 Gtt (0.25 mg) qid; **inflammation after cataract removal:** 1 Gtt (0.25 mg) to affected eye(s) qid, ini 24h postop x 2wk **CH** ≥ 12 y: adult dose

14.3 Glaucoma Agents

14.3.1 Glaucoma Agents - Adrenergic Agonists

AE (dipivefrin): burning, mydriasis, blurred vision, follicular conjunctivitis
CI (dipivefrin): narrow angle glaucoma, hypersensitivity to dipivefrin

Dipivefrin	PRC B, Lact ?
Propine *Sol/Gtt (oph) 0.1%* **Generics** *Sol/Gtt (oph) 0.1%*	**Glaucoma:** 1 Gtt q12h

14.3.2 Glaucoma Agents - Alpha$_2$ Agonists

AE (apraclonidine): upper lid elevation, conjunctival blanching, mydriasis, irreg. heart beat
AE (brimonidine): lid retraction, headache, drowsiness ,conjunctival blanching;
CI (apraclonidine): hypersensitivity to apraclonidine or clonidine
CI (brimonidine): hypersensitivity to brimonidine, concomitant MAOI therapy

Apraclonidine	EHL 8h, PRC C, Lact ?
Iopidine *Sol/Gtt (oph) 0.5%, 1%*	**Glaucoma:** 1-2 Gtt (0.5%) tid; **perioperative IOP ↑:** 1 Gtt (1%) 1h prior to surgery, then 1 Gtt immediately after surgery
Brimonidine	EHL 3h, PRC B, Lact -
Alphagan *Sol/Gtt (oph) 0.2%*	**Glaucoma:** 1 Gtt tid

14.3.3 Glaucoma Agents - Beta Blockers

AE (beta blockers): eye: conjunctival irritation, dry eyes, decline of papillary blood supply; systemic: bronchospasm, bradycardia, hypotension, cardiac failure ↑
CI (beta blockers): cardiac insufficiency (NYHA III and IV), bradycardia, asthma

Betaxolol	EHL 12-22h, PRC C, Lact ?
Betoptic S *Susp/Gtt (oph) 0.25%* **Generics** *Sol/Gtt (oph) 0.5%*	**Glaucoma:** 1-2 Gtt bid
Levobunolol	EHL 6.1h, PRC C, Lact -
Betagan, Generics *Sol/Gtt (oph) 0.25%, 0.5%*	**Glaucoma:** 1-2 Gtt (0.5%) qd-bid or 1-2 Gtt (0.25%) bid
Timolol	EHL 4h, PRC C, Lact -
Apo-Timop *Sol/Gtt (oph) 0.25%, 0.5%* **Tim-AK** *Sol/Gtt (oph) 0.5%* **Timoptic** *Sol/Gtt (oph) 0.25%, 0.5%* **Timoptic-XE** *Sol (gel forming)/Gtt (oph) 0.25%, 0.5%* **Generics** *Sol/Gtt (oph) 0.25%, 0.5%*	**Glaucoma:** 1 Gtt (0.25 or 0.5%) bid or 1 Gtt of gel (0.25 or 0.5% Timoptic XE) qd

14.3.4 Glaucoma Agents - Carbonic Anhydrase Inhibitors	
AE (acetazolamide): taste DO, paresthesia, metabolic acidosis, tinnitus; **AE** (brinzolamide): blurred vision, bitter taste; **AE** (dorzolamide): bitter taste, superficial punctate keratitis, blurred vision, ocular burning, photophobia, conjunctivitis; **CI** (acetazolamide): hyponatremia, hypokalemia, severe hepatic disease, hyperchloremic acidosis, hypersens. to acetazolamide; **CI** (brinzolamide, dorzolamide): hypersens. to product ingredients	
Acetazolamide	EHL 4–8h, PRC C, Lact -
Generics *Tab 250mg*	**Glaucoma:** 250 mg PO qd-qid(immediate release) or 500 mg PO qd-bid (ext.rel); **acute glaucoma:** ini 250 mg IV q4h, then PO, or ini 500mg PO, then 125–250mg PO q4h; DARF: GFR (ml/ min) >50: q6h, 10–50: q12h, <10: contraind.
Brinzolamide	EHL 111d, PRC C, Lact -
Azopt *Susp/Gtt (oph) 1%*	**Glaucoma:** 1 Gtt tid; DARF: CrCl (ml/min) <30: contraind., caution in moderate RF
Dorzolamide	EHL 4mo, PRC C, Lact -
Trusopt *Sol/Gtt (oph) 2%*	**Glaucoma:** 1 Gtt tid; DARF: CrCl (ml/min) <30: contraind., caution in moderate RF
Dorzolamide + Timolol	PRC C, Lact -
Cosopt *Sol/Gtt (oph) 2% + 0.5%* **Cosopt Preservative Free** *Sol/Gtt (oph) 2% + 0.5%*	**Glaucoma:** 1 Gtt bid; DARF: CrCl (ml/min) <30: contraind., caution in moderate RF

14.3.5 Glaucoma Agents - Cholinergic Agonists	
AE (cholinergics): conjunctival reddening, accommodation disturbances, transient myopia, spasms of ciliary muscle, (headache, aching eyes), iridocysts, retinal detachment, cataracts **AE** (pilocarpine): blurred vision, difficulty in night vision, burning or itching of eyes **CI** (cholinergics): malignant glaucoma, secondary glaucoma, iritis, corneal damage **CI** (pilocarpine): hypersensitivity to pilocarpine products, acute iritis or glaucoma after cataract extraction, uncontrolled asthma	
Pilocarpine	EHL 0.76–1.35h, PRC C, Lact ?
Diocarpine *Sol (oph) 1%, 2%, 4%* **Isopto Carpine** *Sol (oph) 0.5%, 1%, 2%, 4%, 6%* **Pilopine HS** *Gel (oph) 4%* **Generics** *Sol (oph) 2%*	**Glaucoma:** 1–2 Gtt up to tid-qid or ½ inch ribbon (4% gel) hs; for drug delivery system see Prod Info

14.3.6 Glaucoma Agents - Prostaglandin F_2 (Alpha) Analogues

AE (prostaglandin analogues): conjunctival hyperemia, growth of eyelashes, ocular pruritus, iris pigmentation, ocular irritation
CI (prostaglandin analogues): known hypersensitivity

Bimatoprost	EHL 45min, PRC C, Lact ?
Lumigan *Sol/Gtt (oph) 0.03%*	**Glaucoma:** 1 Gtt hs
Latanoprost	EHL 17min, PRC C, Lact ?
Xalatan *Sol/Gtt (oph) 0.005%*	**Glaucoma:** 1 Gtt hs
Travoprost	EHL no data, PRC C, Lact ?
Travatan *Sol/Gtt (oph) 0.004%*	**Glaucoma:** 1 Gtt hs

14.4 Mydriatics, Cycloplegics

14.4.1 Anticholinergics

AE (cyclopentolate): IOP↑, burning, photophobia, blurred vision, conjunctivitis;
AE (homatropine): stinging/burning, keratitis, IOP↑, eye pain;
AE (tropicamide): ocular irritation, blurred vision;
CI (cyclopentolate): glaucoma, hypersensitivity to cyclopentolate products;
CI (homatropine): hypersensitivity to homatropine products, primary glaucoma
CI (tropicamide): narrow angle glaucoma, sensitivity to tropicamide

Atropine	PRC C, Lact ?
Isopto Atropine *Sol/Gtt (oph) 1%* **Generics** *Sol/Gtt 1%, Oint (oph) 1%*	**Anterior uveitis/postop mydriasis:** 1 Gtt (1–2% sol) up to tid or 1/4 inch ribbon (1% oint) up to tid; mydriasis lasts 7–14d; **preoperative mydriasis/refraction:** 1 Gtt (1% sol) with 1 Gtt phenylephrine (2.5% or 10%) prior to surgery; **ciliary block glaucoma:** ini 1 Gtt (1–2% sol) with 1Gtt phenylephrine 10% tid–qid, red to maint 1Gtt 1–2% sol qd–qod; **posterior synechiae:** 1 Gtt 2% alternately with phenylephrine 10% q5–10min x 5 applications each
Cyclopentolate	PRC C, Lact ?
Cyclogyl *Sol/Gtt (oph) 1%* **Diopentolate** *Sol/Gtt (oph) 1%* **Generics** *Sol/Gtt (oph) 0.5%*	**Refraction:** 1–2 Gtt (1–2%), rep prn in 5–10min, apply 45min prior to procedure; mydriasis lasts 6–24h

Homatropine	PRC C, Lact ?
Isopto Homatropine *Sol/Gtt (oph) 2%, 5%* **Generics** *Sol/Gtt (oph) 2%*	**Refraction:** 1-2 Gtt (sol 2%) or 1 Gtt (sol 5%) in eye(s) prior to procedure, rep prn q5-10min; **uveitis:** 1-2 Gtt (2-5%), rep up to max q3-4h; mydriasis lasts 1-3d
Tropicamide	PRC N, Lact ?
Diotrope *Sol/Gtt (oph) 0.5%, 1%* **Mydriacyl** *Sol/Gtt (oph) 0.5%, 1%* **Generics** *Sol/Gtt (oph) 1%*	**Fundus exam:** 1-2 Gtt (0.5%) in eye(s) 15-20min prior to exam, rep prn q30min; mydriasis lasts 6h

14.4.2 Sympathomimetics

AE (phenylephrine): tachycardia, HTN, MI, SAH;
CI (phenylephrine): hypersensitivity to phenylephrine products, narrow angle glaucoma, HTN, CAD, BPH

Phenylephrine	PRC C, Lact ?
Dionephrine *Sol/Gtt (oph) 2.5%* **Mydfrin** *Sol/Gtt (oph) 2.5%* **Generics** *Sol/Gtt (oph) 2.5%, 10%*	**Ophthalmologic exams:** 1-2 Gtt (2.5 or 10%) prior to procedure; **ocular surgery:** 1-2 Gtt (2.5 or 10%) prior to surgery; **glaucoma:** 1 Gtt (10%) qid with atropine; **uveitis:** 1-2 Gtt (2.5 or 10%) tid with atropine; **minor eye irritat.:**1-2 Gtt (0.12%) qid prn; **refraction:** 1 Gtt (2.5%) after atropine; mydriasis lasts 5h

14.4.3 Combination

Phenylephrine + Tropicamide	PRC C, Lact ?
Diophenyl-T *Sol/Gtt (oph) 5% + 0.8%*	**Ophthalmologic exams:** 1-2 Gtt prior to procedure
Timolol + Travoprost	PRC C, Lact ?
DuoTrav *Sol/Gtt (oph)* *6.8mg + 0.04mg/2.5ml*	**Glaucoma:** 1 Gtt to eye qd

14.5 Ocular Decongestants, Anti-Allergics

14.5.1 H_1-Receptor Antagonists

AE (levocabastine): ocular irritation, headache, drowsiness
AE (olopatadine): headache, ocular burning, dryness, cold syndrome, rhinopharyngitis, dysgeusia
CI (levocabastine): hypersensitivity to levocabastine products, soft contact lenses
CI (olopatadine): hyper-sensitivity to olopatadine

Levocabastine	EHL 33–40h, PRC C, Lact ?
Livostin *Susp/Gtt (oph) 0.05%*	**Seasonal allergic conjunctivitis:** 1 Gtt in each eye bid-qid x up to 2wk; **CH** ≧ 12 y: adult dose
Olopatadine	EHL 3h, PRC C, Lact ?
Patanol *Sol/Gtt (oph) 0.1%*	**Allergic conjunctivitis:** 1–2 Gtt bid in each eye within 6–8h; **CH** >3 y: adult dose

14.5.2 H_1-Antagonist, Mast Cell Stabilizer

CI (ketotifen fumarate): hypersensitivity to ketotifen products or benzoate compounds

Ketotifen Fumarate	EHL 21h, PRC C, Lact ?
Zaditor *Sol/Gtt (oph) 0.025%*	**Allergic conjunctivitis:** 1 Gtt q8–12h in each eye; **CH** > 3 y: adult dose

14.5.3 Mast Cell Stabilizers

Cromolyn Sodium	EHL 80–90min, PRC B, Lact ?
Opticrom, Generics *Sol/Gtt (oph) 2%*	**Allergic ocular DO:** 1–2 Gtt in each eye 4–6 x/d; **CH** ≧ 4 y: adult dose
Lodoxamide Tromethamine	EHL 8.5h, PRC B, Lact ?
Alomide *Sol/Gtt (oph) 0.1%*	**Allergic ocular DO:** 1–2 Gtt qid x up to 3mo; **CH** ≧ 2 y: adult dose
Nedocromil	EHL 1.5–3.3h, PRC B, Lact ?
Alocril *Sol/Gtt (oph) 2%*	**Allergic conjunctivitis:** 1–2 Gtt bid; **CH** ≧ 3 y: adult dose

14.5.4 Sympathomimetics

AE (naphazoline): local mucosal irritation, HTN, CNS effects, tremor, eye irritation and redness; **CI** (naphazoline): hypersensitivity to naphazoline products, narrow angle glaucoma, hyperthyroidism, CAD, BPH, HTN

Naphazoline	PRC C, Lact ?
Naphcon Forte *Sol/Gtt (oph) 0.1%*	**Ocular vasoconstrictor/decongestant:** 1 Gtt q3-4h prn up to qid

14.5.5 Sympathomimetics + H_1-Receptor Antagonists

Naphazoline + Pheniramine	PRC C, Lact ?
Naphcon-A *Sol/Gtt (oph) 0.025% + 0.3%*	**Ocular decongestant:** 1-2 Gtt bid-qid prn; **CH** ≧ 6 y: adult dose

14.6 Local Anesthetics

AE: allergic reactions, corneal damage after long-term use

Proparacaine	PRC C, Lact ?
Alcaine, Diocaine *Sol/Gtt (oph) 0.5%*	**Local anesthetic:** 1-2 Gtt prior to procedure, rep q 5-10min x 1-3 doses (suture or foreign body removal) or x 5-7 doses (cataract or glaucoma surgery)
Tetracaine	PRC C, Lact ?
Pontocaine, Generics *Sol/Gtt (oph) 0.5%*	**Local anesthetic:** 1-2 Gtt prior to procedure

14.7 Other Ophthalmologic Drugs

MA/EF(pegaptanib): selective Vascular Endothelial Growth Factor (VEGF) antagonist;
MA/EF (ranibizumab): humanised recombinant monoclonal antibody fragment targeted against human vascular endothelial growth factor-A (VEGF-A);
AE (ranibizumab): intraocular inflammation, increased intraocular pressure;
CI (pegaptanib, ranibizumab): hypersensitive to drug, active or suspected ocular or periocular infections, active intraocular inflammation.

Artifical Tears	PRC N, Lact ?
Genteal *Gel (oph) Hydroxypropyl-methylcellulose* **Isopto Tears** *Sol/Gtt(oph) Hypromellose 1%* **Thera Tears** *Sol/Gtt (oph) Sodium Carboxymethyl Cellulose 0.25%* **Visine Advance True Tears** *Sol/Gtt (oph) Hypromellose 0.2% + Glycerine 0.2%* **Refresh Liquigel** *Sol/Gtt (oph) Sodium Carboxymethyl Cellulose 1%* **Refresh Utra** *Sol/Gtt (oph) Boric acid + Castor oil + Glycerin* **Tears Plus** *Polyvinyl alcohol 1.4%* **Tears Naturale Forte** *Sol/Gtt (oph) Hydroxypropylmethylcellulose 0.3% + Dextran 70 0.1% + Glycerine 0.2%* **Tears Naturale P.M.** *Lub White petrolatum, mineral oil, lanolin* **Visine Advance True Tears** *Sol/Gtt (oph) Hydroxypropyl methylcellulose + Glycerine* **Visine Contact Lens Eye Drops** *Sol/Gtt (oph) Hydroxypropylmethylcellulose + Glycerine* **Visine True Tears Eye Drops** *Sol/Gtt (oph) Polyethylene Glycol*	**Ophthalmic lubricant:** 1–2 Gtt tid–qid prn
Oxymetazoline	PRC C
Visine Workplace Eye Drops *Sol/Gtt (oph)0.025%*	**Minor eye irritation**: **CH** >6 and adults: 1–2 gtts q6h PRN

Pegaptanib	PRC C, Lact ?
Macugen *Inj 0.3mg/syringe*	**Age-related macular degeneration:** 0.3 mg intravitreous injection every six weeks
Ranibizumab	PRC C, Lact ?
Lucentis *Inj 10mg/ml*	**Neovascular age-related macular degeneration:** 0.5mg intravitreal injection qmonth
Tetrahydrozoline	PRC C
Visine Original Eye Drops *Sol/Gtt (oph) 0.05%*	**Conjunctival congestion**: 1-2 gtts 2-4 times/d PRN
Tetrahydrozoline + Polyethylene Glycol	PRC C
Visine Cool Eye Drops *Sol/Gtt (oph) 0.05% + 1%*	**Minor eye irritation: CH** >6 and adults: 1-2 gtts q6h PR
Tetrahydrozoline + Zinc Sulfate	PRC C
Visine Allergy Eye Drops *Sol/Gtt (oph) 0.05% + 0.25%*	**Minor eye irritation**: 1-2 gtts q6h PRN

15 ENT

15.1 Antihistamines

15.1.1 Sedating Antihistamines

MA: competitive blockage of H1-receptors (see antihistamines →251, →288, →289)
AE (antihistamines): sedation, excitatory appearances (small children), dry mouth, glaucoma, micturition DO; **AE** (azatadine): drowsiness, epigastric distress, urinary retention or frequency; **AE** (cetirizine): drowsiness, fatigue (mild sedation), dry mouth, headache; **AE** (clemastine): sedation, shortness of breath; **AE** (chlorpheniramine): drowsiness, N/V; **AE** (diphenhydramine): dyskinesias, anaphylaxis, sedation; **AE** (hydroxyzine): xerostomia, drowsiness, headache; **CI** (antihistamines): urinary retention, glaucoma;
CI (azatadine): hypersens. to azatadine/related antihistamines, use of MAOI, narrow-angle glaucoma or urinary retention; **CI** (cetirizine): hypersens. to cetirizine or hydroxyzine;
CI (clemastine): hypersens. to clemastine, MAOI therapy, lower resp tract symptoms;
CI (chlorpheniramine, dexchlorpheniramine): hypersens. to product ingredients;
CI (diphenhydramine): hypersens. to diphenhydramine, MAOI Tx, chicken pox, measles, blisters (topical use), topical use on eyes; **CI** (hydroxyzine): hypersens. to hydroxyzine

Azatadine	EHL 9h, PRC B, Lact ?
Optimine *Tab 1mg*	**Allergic rhinitis, urticaria:** 1-2mg PO bid; **CH** >12y: 1-2mg PO bid; DARF not req
Cetirizine	EHL 7.4-9h, PRC B, Lact ?
Reactine *Tab 5mg, 10mg, 20 mg, Syr 5mg/5ml* **Generics** *Tab 5mg, 10mg*	**Allergic rhinitis, urticaria:** 5-10mg PO qd, max 20mg/d; **CH** 2-6y: 2.5mg PO qd, max 5mg/d, >6y: 5-10mg PO qd, max 10mg/d; DARF: GFR (ml/min): <30: max 5mg/d
Chlorpheniramine	EHL 20h, PRC B, Lact -
Novo-Pheniram *Syr 2.5g/5ml, Tab 4mg* **Generics** *Tab 4mg, Tab (ext rel) 12mg*	**Allergic rhinitis**: 4mg PO q4-6h; ext.rel 8mg PO q8-12h or 12mg PO q12h, max 24mg/d; **CH** 6-11y: 2mg PO q4-6h, max 12mg/d, >12y: adult dose; DARF: not req
Clemastine	EHL 21h, PRC B, Lact -
Tavist *Tab 1mg*	**Allergic rhinitis, urticaria:** 1.34-2.68mg PO bid-tid, max 8.04mg/d; **CH** 6-12y: 0.5mg PO bid, max 6mg/d

Diphenhydramine	EHL 4-8h, PRC B, Lact -
Allerdryl *Cap 25mg, 50mg* **Allernix** *Cap 25mg, 50mg, Elixir (oral) 12.5mg/5ml* **Benadryl** *Cap 25mg, 50mg, Cream 2%, Elixir (oral) 12.5mg/5ml, Liq (oral) 6.25mg/5ml, Tab (chew) 12.5mg* **Nytol** *Cap 25mg* **Nytol Extra Strength** *Cap 50mg* **Simply Sleep** *Cap 25mg* **Unisom Extra Strength/Extra Strength Sleepgels** **Generics** *Cap 25mg, 50mg, Elixir (oral) 2.5mg/ml, Inj 50mg/ml*	**Allergic rhinitis, rhinorrhea:** 25-50mg PO/IV/IM q4-6h, max 0.4g/d; **motion sickness:** 25-50mg PO 30min before exposure, then prn q4-6h; **CH:** 1.25mg PO qid, max 0.3g/d; **anaphylaxis** →31 ,**Insomnia** →251 , DARF: GFR (ml/min) >50: q6h, 10-50: q6-12h, < 10: q12-18h; see Prod Info
Hydroxyzine	EHL 3-20h, PRC C, Lact -
Atarax *Syr 10mg/5ml, Inj 50mg/ml* **Generics** *Cap 10mg, 25mg, 50mg, Syr 10mg/5ml, Inj 50mg/ml*	**Allergic reactions, pruritus:** 25-100mg PO/IM tid-qid; **CH** <6y: 50mg/d PO div tid-qid, >6y: 50-100mg/d PO div tid-qid

15.1.2 Nonsedating Antihistamines

MA, AE, CI (antihistamines): see antihistamines →251, →288, →289; **AE** (fexofenadine): nausea, dyspepsia, fatigue; **AE** (loratadine): sedation, dizziness, dry mouth, headache, nausea; **CI** (fexofenadine): hypersensitivity to fexofenadine; **CI** (loratadine): hypersens. to loratadine

Desloratadine	EHL 27h, PRC C, Lact ?
Aerius *Tab 5mg*	**Allergic rhinitis, urticaria:** 5mg PO qd; DARF: 5mg PO qod
Fexofenadine	EHL 14-18h, PRC C, Lact -
Allegra *Tab 60mg*	**Allergic rhinitis, urticaria:** 60mg PO bid or 180mg qd; **CH** 6-11y: 30mg PO bid, >12y: adult dose; DARF: 60mg PO qd
Loratadine	EHL 12-15h, PRC B, Lact ?
Claritin *Tab 10mg, Tab (orally disint) 10mg, Syr 1mg/ml* **Generics** *Tab 10mg*	**Allergic rhinitis, urticaria:** 10mg PO qd; **CH** 6-11y: adult dose; DARF: GFR (ml/min) <30: 10mg PO qod
Loratadine + Pseudoephedrine	PRC C, Lact +
Claritin Allergy + Sinus Extra Strength *Cap ext. release 10mg + 240mg*	**Allergic rhinitis**: 1 cap PO qd

15.2 Nasal Preparations

15.2.1 Anticholinergics

AE: dry mouth, bitter taste, epistaxis, nasal dryness, nasal congestion
CI: hypersensitivity to ipratropium products

Ipratropium Bromide	EHL 1.6h (IV), PRC B, Lact ?
Apo-Ipravent *Spray (metered, nasal) 0.03%, 0.06%* **Atrovent** *Spray (metered, nasal) 0.03% (0.021mg/spray), 0.06% (0.042mg/spray)* **Generics** *Spray (metered, nasal) 0.03% (0.021mg/spray)*	**Rhinorrhea associated with allergic rhinitis:** 2 sprays (0.03%) in each nostril bid-tid; **CH** ≧ 6y: adult dose; **rhinorrhea associated with common cold/vasomotor rhinitis:** 2 sprays (0.06%) in each nostril tid-qid; **CH** ≧ 12y: adult dose

15.2.2 Antihistamines, Mast Cell Stabilizers

MA/EF: see antihistamines →251, →288, →289

Cromolyn	EHL 22-25h, PRC C, Lact -
Generics *Spray (nasal) 1%, 2%*	**Allergic rhinitis:** 1 spray in each nostril q4-6h ; **CH** ≧ 6y: adult dose

15.2.3 Corticosteroids

AE (beclomethasone): adrenal suppression, candidiasis, nasopharyngeal irritation
AE (budesonide): nasal stinging, throat irritation, nasal dryness, epistaxis, headache
AE (flunisolide): nasal irritation, dysphonia, headache; **AE** (fluticasone): hoarseness, nasal burning/epistaxis, nasal congestion, pruritus/burning, eosinophilia; **AE** (mometasone): burning, atrophy, pruritus, headache; **AE** (triamcinolone): GI distress, fluid and electrolyte disturbances, HPA axis suppression, mild euphoria/depression
CI (beclomethasone, budesonide, flunisolide, fluticasone): hypersensitivity to product ingredients/corticosteroids, status asthmaticus or other acute episodes of asthma
CI (mometasone): hypersensitivity to mometasone or other corticosteroids
CI (triamcinolone): systemic fungal infections

Beclomethasone	EHL 3h, PRC C, Lact ?
Gen-Beclo AQ *Spray (metered, nasal) 0.05mg/spray* **Rivanase AQ** *Spray (metered, nasal) 0.05mg/spray* **Generics** *Spray (metered, nasal) 0.05mg/spray*	**Allergic rhinitis/nasal polyp PRO:** 1-2 spray(s) (0.042-0.084mg) in each nostril bid; **CH** >12y: adult dose, 6-12y: 1 spray (0.042mg) in each nostril bid, max 0.084mg bid

Budesonide	EHL 2-3hPRC C, Lact ?
Rhinocort Aqua *Spray (metered, nasal) 0.064mg/spray*	**Allergic rhinitis:** 2 sprays in each nostril bid or 4 sprays qd; **CH** ≧ 6y: adult dose, max 4 sprays/d (0.032mg/spray) or 2 sprays/d (0.064mg/spray)
Flunisolide	EHL 1-2h, PRC C, Lact ?
Rhinalar, Generics *Spray (metered, nasal) 0.025mg/spray*	**Allergic rhinitis:** 2 sprays in each nostril bid, prn incr to 2 sprays in each nostril tid, max 8 sprays/nostril/d; **CH** 6-14y: 1 spray in each nostril tid or 2 sprays in each nostril bid, max 4 sprays/nostril/d
Fluticasone	EHL 7.8h, PRC C, Lact ?
Avamys *Spray (metered, nasal) 27.5 mcg/spray* **Flonase** *Spray (metered, nasal) 0.05mg/spray* **Generics** *Spray (metered, nasal) 0.05mg/spray*	**Allergic rhinitis:** 2 sprays in each nostril qd or 1 spray in each nostril bid, decr to 1 spray in each nostril qd when appropriate; **CH** >4y: 1-2 sprays in each nostril qd, max 2 sprays/nostril/d
Mometasone	EHL 5.8h, PRC C, Lact ?
Nasonex *Spray (metered, nasal) 0.05mg/spray*	**Allergic rhinitis, nasal polyps:** 2 sprays in each nostril qd; **CH** ≧ 12y: adult dose, 3-11y: 1 spray in each nostril qd
Triamcinolone	EHL 2-3hPRC C, Lact ?
Nasacort AQ *Spray (met.nas.) 0.055mg/spray*	**Allergic rhinitis:** ini 2 sprays in each nostril bid, prn decr to 2 sprays/nostril qd, max 8 sprays/d; **CH** ≧ 12y: adult dose, 6-12y: 1-2 sprays in each nostril qd

15.2.4 Nasal (Topical) Decongestants

AE (sympathomimetic decongestants): reactive hyperemia, mucus membrane burning, dryness, tachycardia, BP↑. Long use: epithelial damage, chronic stuffy nose; **AE** (oxymetazoline): rebound congestion, mucosal irritation, CNS effects, tremors; **AE** (pseudoephedrine): restlessness, HTN, arrhythmias; **CI** (sympathomimetic decongestants): rhinitis sicca, severe coronary diseases; **CI** (oxymetazoline, phenylephrine): hypersensitivity to product ingredients, narrow angle glaucoma, hyperthyroidism, CAD, BPH, HTN; **CI** (pseudoephedrine): hypersensitivity to product ingredients or sympathomimetics, MAOI Tx, severe HTN/CAD

Oxymetazoline	EHL 5–8h, PRC C, Lact ?
Claritan Allergic Congestion Relief *Spray (nasal) 0.05%* **Claritan Eye Allergy Relief** *Sol (nasal) 0.25mg/ml* **Dristan Long Lasting** *Mist (nasal) 0.05%, Spray (nasal) 0.05%* **Drixoral** *Spray (nasal) 0.05%*	**Nasal congestion:** 2–3 sprays/Gtt (0.05%) in each nostril bid x 3d; **CH** ≧ 6y: adult dose, 2–5y: 2–3 Gtt (0.025%) in each nostril bid x 3d

Pseudoephedrine	EHL 9–16hPRC C, Lact ?
Balminil Decongestant *Syr 30mg/ml* **Contac Cold 12 Hour Relief Non Drowsy** *Cap (sust rel) 120mg* **Eltor 120** *Cap (sust rel) 120mg* **Pseudofrin** *Tab 60mg* **Sudafed Decongestant** *Tab 30mg* **Sudafed Decongestant Children's Chewable** *Tab (chew) 15mg* **Sudafed Decongestant Extra Strenght** *Tab 60mg* **Sudafed Decongestant 12 Hour** *Cap 120mg*	**Nasal congestion:** 60mg PO q4–6h or 120mg PO q12h (ext.rel) or 240mg PO qd (ext.rel), max 240mg/d; **CH** >12y: adult dose, 6–11y: 30mg PO q4–6h, max 120mg/d, 2–5y: 15mg PO q4–6h, max 60mg/d, 2–3y: 1.6ml; **pediatric Gtt** PO q4–6h: 12–23 mo: 1.2ml, 4–11 mo: 0.8ml, 0–3 mo: 0.4ml, max 4 doses/d

Xylometazoline	PRC C, Lact ?
Balminil Nasal Decongestant *Sol 0.1%* **Generics** *Sol 0.1%*	**Nasal congestion:** 1–3 Gtt/spray in each nostril q8–10h prn

15.2.5 Other Nasal Preparations

Framycetin + Phenylephrine + Gramicidin	
Soframycin Nasal Spray *Spray (nasal) 12.5 + 2.5 + 0.05mg/ml*	**Nasal infx/congestion**: 2 sprays in each nostril every 4 hours. Max 6 times per day

Saline Nasal Spray	EHLPRC A, Lact +
Generics *Spray (nasal) 0.7%*	**Nasal dryness:**1–3 sprays/Gtt in q nostril prn

15.3 Ear Preparations

15.3.1 Antibacterial/Antifungal Combinations

AE (acetic acid): local stinging or burning; **CI** (acetic acid): hypersensitivity to acetic acid products, perforated tympanic membranes, vaccinia and varicella (steroid-containing ear drops)

Acetic Acid + Aluminium Acetate	PRC C, Lact ?
Generics *Sol/Gtt (otic) 2% + 0.79%*	**Otitis externa:** 4-6 Gtt in affected ear(s) q2-3h, keep moist (cotton plug) x 24h

15.3.2 Agents for Otitis Externa Prophylaxis

Aluminium Acetate + Benzethonium	PRC N, Lact ?
Buro-Sol *Sol/Gtt (otic) 0.5% + 0.03%*	**Otitis externa** (PRO): 4-5 Gtt in ears after swimming, bathing; **CH** adult dose

15.3.3 Antibacterial/Corticosteroid Combinations

Ciprofloxacin + Hydrocortisone	PRC C, Lact -
Cipro HC *Susp/Gtt (otic) 0.2% + 1%*	**Otitis externa:** 3 Gtt into affected ear(s) bid x 7d; **CH** ≧ 1y: adult dose
Hydrocortisone + Polymyxin + Neomycin	PRC C, Lact ?
Cortisporin *Sol/Gtt (oph/otic) 10,000 U/ml + 3.5mg/ml + 10mg/ml*	**Otitis externa:** 4 Gtt in affected ear(s) tid-qid; **CH** 3 Gtt in affected ear(s) tid-qid

15.3.4 Decongestant/Analgesic Combinations

Benzocaine + Antipyrine	PRC C, Lact ?
Auralgan *Sol (otic) 14mg/ml + 54mg/ml*	**Otitis media** (adjunct): 2-4 Gtt tid-qid or q 1-2h prn;**cerumen removal:** 2-4Gtt tidx2-3d to detach cerumen, then prn for discomfort, insert moistened cotton plug (with sol)

15.3.5 Surfactants, Ceruminolytics

AE (cerumenex eardrops): localized dermatitis reactions, allergic contact dermatitis, skin ulcerations, burning and pain at the application site and skin rash; **CI** (carbamide peroxide): hypersensitivity to carbamide peroxide products, ear drainage or discharge, perforated tympanic membrane; **CI** (cerumenex eardrops): perforated tympanic membrane, otitis media, history of hypersensitivity to cerumenex eardrops or to any of its components

Triethanolamine	PRC C, Lact ?
Cerumenex *Sol/Gtt (otic) 10%*	**Cerumen removal:** fill ear canal with sol, insert cotton plug x 15-30min, then flush, max x 4d

15.4 Mouth and Lip Preparations

15.4.1 Antifungals

AE (clotrimazole):N/V, LFT's↑ (transient), contact dermatitis;**AE** (nystatin): diarrhea, vaginal irritation/pain, N/V, rash; **CI** (clotrimazole, nystatin): hypersensitivity to product ingrediens

Clotrimazole	EHL 3.5–5h, PRC C, Lact ?
Generics *lozenge (oral) 10mg*	**Oral candidiasis:**1troche dissolved slowly in mouth 5x/ d x 14d; **CH** ≧ 3y: adult dose; **prevention of oropharyngeal candidiasis in immunocompromised patients:** 1 troche dissolved slowly in mouth tid until end of chemotherapy/high-dose corticosteroids
Nystatin	PRC C, Lact +
Nilstat *Powder (oral) 100%, Tab 500,000 U, Susp 100,000 U/ml* **Nyaderm** *Susp 100,000 U/ml* **Generics** *Susp 100,000 U/ml*	**Thrush:** 5ml PO swish and swallow qid with ½ of dose in each cheek or 1–2 lozenges 4–5x/d, max 14d; **CH:** 2ml PO swish and swallow qid with 1ml in each cheek or use a cotton sqab, premature and low birth weight infants: 0.5ml PO in each cheek qid or use a cotton squab

15.4.2 Other Mouth and Lip Preparations

AE (chlorhexidine gluconate): skin irritation, tooth staining, altered taste
CI (chlorhexidine gluconate): hypersensitivity to chlorhexidine products

Anetholtrithion	PRC C, Lact ?
Sialor *Tab 25mg*	**Xerostomia:** 25mg PO tid before meals
Benzocaine	PRC C, Lact ?
Anbesol *Gel 6.4%, 7.5%, 20%, Liq 6.5%, 20%* **Zilactin Baby, Zilactin-B** *Gel 10%*	**Mouth or lip pain:** apply q4–6h
Benzydamine	PRC C, Lact ?
Sun-Benz *Sol (oral) 0.15%* **Tantum** *Sol (oral) 0.15%* **Generics** *Sol (oral) 0.15%*	**Mouth or throat pain:** 15 mL PO gargled/rinsed for 30sec. and spit q30min–6h

Chlorhexidine Gluconate	PRC B, Lact ?
Oro-Clense, Peridex, Generics *Sol (dental) 0.12%*	**Gingivitis:** apply 15ml x 30sec bid as oral rinse (qam and qpm after brushing teeth), expectorate after rinsing
Dequalinium	EHL n/a
Dequadin *Lozenges 0.25mg, Paint 0.5%*	**Mouth and throat infections:** 1 lozange PO q2-3h; **oral pain:** apply paint to area q2-3h
Hexetidine	EHL n/a
Steri/Sol *Liq 0.1%*	**Tonsillitis, pharyngitis, laryngitis, gingivitis, stomatitis, oral thrush, Vincent's angina:** swish and gargle 15ml for 30 sec. PO bid
Lidocaine	PRC C, Lact +
Zilactin-L *Liq 2.5%*	**Lip pain:** apply q1-2h
Lidocaine Viscous	PRC B, Lact +
Lidodan Viscous *Sol (top) 2%* **Xylocaine** *Sol (top) 2%*	**Mouth or lip pain:** 15ml topically or swish and spit q3h, max 8 doses/24h or 4.5mg/kg or max 300mg, use lowest effective dose, prn apply to small sore places with cotton-tipped applicator; **CH** >3y: 3.75-5ml topically or swish and spit up to q3h
Octyl Methoxycinnamate + Homosalate + Oxybenzone + Dimethicone + Menthol	
Zilactin-Lip *Balm 7% + 4% + 3% + 1.5% + 0.5%*	**Chapped lips:** apply tid-qid
Pilocarpine	PRC C, Lact ?
Salagen *Tab 5mg*	**Xerostomia:** ini 5mg PO tid-qid, max 30mg/d
Povidone-iodine	PRC D, Lact ?
Betadine *Mouth wash 1%*	**Mouth wash**
Triamcinolone Acetonide	PRC C, Lact ?
Kenalog in Orabase, Oracort *Paste 0.1%*	Apply bid-tid with finger, apply about 0.5cm of paste to the oral lesion

16 Urology

16.1 Bladder Agents

16.1.1 Antispasmodics (Parasympatholytics)

MA/EF (parasympatholytics): blockage of muscarine receptors, mainly direct action on smooth muscles (papaverine-like) ⇒ tonicity of smooth muscleso in GI + urinary tract
AE: sweat secretion↓, dry mouth, tachycardia, accommodation DO, glaucoma
AE (hyoscyamine): dry mouth, urinary hesitancy, blurred vision, tachycardia, headache
AE (oxybutynin): tachycardia, anticholinergic EF, insomnia, somnolence, sexual dysfunction
AE (tolterodine): dry mouth, headache, dyspepsia, constipation, xerophthalmia
CI: glaucoma, urinary retention, tachyarrhythmia, GI stenosis, toxic megacolon, myasthenia gravis
CI (hyoscyamine): hypersensitivity to hyoscyamine products, glaucoma, intestinal obstruction, severe liver/renal disease
CI (oxybutynin): glaucoma, GI obstruction, obstructive uropathy, myasthenia gravis, colitis
CI (tolterodine): urinary/gastric retention, glaucoma, hypersensitivity to tolterodine

Darifenacin	EHL 13–19h, PRC C, Lact ?
Enablex *Tab (ext. rel.) 7.5mg, 15mg*	**Bladder spasm:** ini 7.5mg PO qd, maint. 7.5–15mg PO qd; ESLD Child-Pugh class B: max 7.5mg qd, class C: avoid
Hyoscyamine	EHL 3.5h, PRC C, Lact -
Levsin *Tab 0.125mg, Tab ext.rel. 0.125mg, Gtt 0.125mg/ml, Inj 0.5mg/ml*	**Bladder spasm:** 0.125–0.3mg PO qid; ext.rel.: 0.375–0.75mg bid; max 1.5 g/d; **CH** 2–12y: 0.0625–0.125mg PO qid; ext.rel.: 0.375mg PO bid, >12y: 0.125–0.25mg PO qid; ext.rel.: see adults; **GI** →108
Oxybutynin	EHL 1.1–2.3h, PRC B, Lact ?
Ditropan *Syr 5mg/5ml, Tab 5mg* **Ditropan XL** *Tab ext.rel. 5mg, 10mg* **Oxybutyn** *Tab 5mg* **Oxytrol** *Patch 3.9mg/d* **Uromax** *Tab ext.rel. 10mg, 15mg* **Generics** *Syr 5mg/5ml, Tab 2.5mg, 5mg*	**Bladder spasm:** 5mg PO bid–tid, max 5mg PO qid; ext.rel.: 5–15mg PO qd, max 30mg PO qd; **CH** >5y: 5mg PO bid, max 5mg PO tid
Propantheline	EHL (biphasic) 57.9min, 2.93h, PRC C, Lact ?
Pro-Banthine *Tab 7.5mg, 15mg*	**Urinary incontinence, neurogenic bladder:** 15mg q4–6h, max 90mg PO qid;

Solifenacin	EHL 45–68h, PRC C, Lact -
Vesicare *Tab 5mg, 10mg*	**Overactive bladder:** ini 5mg PO qd, max 10mg/d; DARF CrCl <30: 5mg qhs; DAHF Child-Pugh class B: 5mg qd, class C: avoid
Tolterodine	EHL 1.9–3.7h, PRC C, Lact -
Detrol *Tab 1mg, 2mg* **Unidet** *Cap ext. release 2mg, 4mg*	**Overactive bladder:** 2mg PO bid; 1mg PO if reduced hepatic function
Trospium	EHL 20h, PRC C, Lact ?
Trosec *Tab 20mg*	**Overactive bladder:** 20mg PO bid; >75y: 20mg qhs; DARF CrCl <30: 20mg qhs

16.1.2 Bladder Spasm

AE (flavoxate): nervousness, headache, blurred vision, drowsiness, N/V
CI (flavoxate): intestinal obstruction, obstructive uropathy

Flavoxate	EHL no data, PRC B, Lact ?
Urispas *Tab 200mg*	**Incontinence, bladder spasm:** 100–200mg PO tid–qid; **CH** >12y: see adults

16.1.3 Other Bladder Agents

AE (pentosan polysulfate): peripheral edema, headache, dizziness, nausea
AE (phenazopyridine): GI DO, headache, rash, hemolytic anemia, nephrotoxicity, hepatitis
CI (pentosan polysulfate): hypersensitivity to pentosan polysulfate sodium
CI (phenazopyridine): hypersensitivity to phenazopyridine, hepatitis, renal insufficiency

Pentosan Polysulfate	EHL 4.8h, PRC B, Lact ?
Elmiron *Cap 100mg*	**Interstitial cystitis:** 100mg PO tid
Phenazopyridine	EHL no data, PRC B, Lact ?
Phenazo *Tab 100mg, 200mg*	**Dysuria:** 200mg PO tid for 2d; **CH** 6–12y: 12mg/kg/d PO div tid for 2d

16.2 Erectile Dysfunction

MA/E (alprostadil): identical to prostaglandin E1 d vasodilation
MA/EF (sildenafil): specific phosphodiesterase inhibitor ⇒ relaxation of corpus cavernosal smooth muscle cells ⇒ blood flow into cavernosal spaces ↑
MA/EF (yohimbine): alpha2-adrenergic blocker → erectogenic
AE (alprostadil): penile pain, neonatal apnea, bradycardia, fever
AE (sildenafil): headache, flushing, dyspepsia, abnormal vision, nasal congestion
AE (yohimbine): anxiety, nervousness, tremor, irritability, agitation, manic reactions, bronchospasm, cough, antidiuresis, dizziness, headache, HTN, tachycardia, N/V, flushes
CI (alprostadil): priapism, hypersensitivity to alprostadil, neonatal respir. distress syndrome
CI (sildenafil): hypersensitivity to sildenafil, concurrent use of nitrates
CI (yohimbine): chronic inflammation of sexual organs, prostatitis, antidepressants, tyramine-containing food, gastric/duodenal ulcers, hypersensitivity to yohimbine, children, psychiatric patients, renal or liver disease

Alprostadil	EHL 5–10min, PRC X, Lact -
Caverject *Inj 20mcg/vial, Inj 10mcg/ml, 20mcg/ml* **Prostin VR** *Inj 500mcg/ml* **Generics** *Inj 0.5mg/ml*	**Erectile dysfunction:** 2.5mcg intracavernosal injection, incr prn stepwise by 2.5, 5, 10mcg to max 40mcg; 125–250mcg intraurethral, incr decrease dose prn; max 1000mcg; max 2 uses in 24h
Sildenafil	EHL 4h, PRC B , Lact -
Viagra *Tab 25mg, 50mg, 100mg*	**Erectile dysfunction:** 50mg PO 0.5–4h before intercourse, incr prn to max 100mg PO; max 1dose/d; >65y: reduce dose
Tadalafil	EHL 17.5h, PRC B, Lact -
Cialis *Tab 2.5mg, 5mg, 10mg, 20mg*	**Erectile dysfunction:** 20mg PO prior to intercourse
Vardenafil	EHL 4–5h, PRC B, Lact -
Levitra *Tab 10mg, 20mg*	**Erectile dysfunction:** 5–20mg PO prior to intercourse
Yohimbine	EHL 0.6h, PRC N, Lact -
Yocon *Tab 5.4mg* **Generics** *Tab 2mg, 5.4mg, 6mg*	**Erectile dysfunction:** 5.4mg PO tid up to 10wk

16.3 Benign Prostatic Hyperplasia

16.3.1 Alpha-Reductase Inhibitors

MA/EF (finasteride): inhibition of the 5-α-reductase ⇒ inhibition of transformation of testosterone into dihydrotestosterone ⇒ prostatic hyperplasia ↓
AE (finasteride): sexual dysfunction, breast tenderness/enlargement
CI (finasteride): severe hepatic insufficiency, hypersensitivity to finasteride products

Dutasteride	EHL 5wk, PRC X, Lact +
Avodart *Cap 0.5mg*	**Benign prostatic hypertrophy:** 0.5mg PO qd
Finasteride	EHL 6h, PRC X, Lact -
Propecia *Tab 1mg* **Proscar** *Tab 5mg*	**Benign prostatic hypertrophy:** 5mg PO qd; DARF: not req

16.3.2 Peripheral Antiadrenergic Agents

MA/EF (tamsulosin, terazosin): selective blockage of α1-receptors in the smooth musculature of the prostate and the bladder neck ⇒ urine flowm
AE (doxazosin): hypotension, dizziness, vertigo, headache; **AE** (tamsulosin, terazosin): dizziness, postural hypotension, headache, palpitations, retrograde ejaculation
CI (doxazosin): hypersensitivity to doxazosin products or other quinazolines
CI (tamsulosin, terazosin): postural dysregulation, severe hepatic insufficiency

Alfuzosin	
Xatral *Tab sust. release 10mg*	**Benign prostatic hypertrophy**: 10mg PO qd
Doxazosin	EHL 8.8–22hPRC C, Lact ?
Cardura *Tab 1mg, 2mg, 4mg* **Generics** *Tab 1mg, 2mg, 4mg*	**Benign prostatic hypertrophy:** ini 1mg PO qd, incr prn to max 8mg PO qd
Tamsulosin	EHL 9–13h, PRC B, Lact -
Flomax *Cap 0.4mg* **Flomax CR** *Cap (cont. rel.) 0.4mg* **Generics** *Cap (cont. rel.) 0.4mg*	**Benign prostatic hypertrophy:** 0.4mg PO qd, incr prn after 2–4wk to 0.8mg PO qd; DARF: not req
Terazosin	EHL 9–12h, PRC C, Lact ?
Hytrin *Tab 1mg, 2mg, 5mg, 10mg* **Generics** *Tab 1mg, 2mg, 5mg, 10mg*	**Benign prostatic hypertrophy:** ini 1mg PO qd, incr prn to 2–10mg PO qd, max 20mg/d; DARF: not req

16.4 Prostate Cancer

MA/EF (bicalutamide, flutamide, nilutamide): competitive blocker of nuclear androgen receptors ⇒ action of androgens ↓; pure antiandrogen without gestagen-like effects
MA/EF (leuprolide, goserelin, triptorelin): GnRH agonist ⇒ gonadotropin secretion ↓, ovarian/testicular steroidogenesis ↓; **AE** (bicalutamide): hot flashes, diarrhea, pain
AE (flutamide): diarrhea, cystitis, rectal bleeding, hot flashes, liver injury;
AE (goserelin): bone pain, hot flashes, gynecomastia, impotence, breakthrough bleeding;
AE (leuprolide): amenorrhea, hot flashes, vaginal spotting, bone pain, N/V, edema
AE (nilutamide): hot flashes, gynecomastia, N/V, LFT ↑, blurred vision
CI (bicalutamide): hypersensitivity to bicalutamide products; **CI** (flutamide): hypersensitivity to flutamide products, severe hepatic impairment; **CI** (goserelin): hypersensitivity to goserelin products; **CI** (leuprolide): hypersensitivity to leuprolide products/GnRH agonists
CI (nilutamide): hypersensitivity to nilutamide, severe hepatic impairment, severe respiratory insufficiency

Bicalutamide	EHL 5.8d, PRC X, Lact ?
Casodex *Tab 50mg* **Generics** *Tab 50mg*	**Prostate CA:** 50mg PO qd
Flutamide	EHL 9.6h, PRC D, Lact ?
Euflex *Tab 250mg* **Generics** *Tab 250mg*	**Prostate CA:** 250mg PO tid
Goserelin	EHL 2.3–4.2h, PRC X, Lact -
Zoladex *Implants 3.6mg, 10.8mg*	**Prostate CA:** 3.6mg implant SC q4wk or 10.8mg implant SC q12wk
Leuprolide	EHL 3h, PRC X, Lact -
Eligard *Inj 10.2mg/syr, 28.2mg/syr* **Lupron** *Inj 5mg/ml* **Lupron Depot** *Inj 3.75mg/vial, 7.5mg/vial, 11.25mg/vial, 22.5mg/vial, 30mg/vial*	**Prostate CA:** 1mg SC qd or 7.5mg IM qmo or 22.5mg IM q3mo or 30mg IM q4mo; **implant:** 65mg SC q12mo
Nilutamide	EHL 38–59.1h, PRC C, Lact ?
Anandron *Tab 50mg*	**Prostate CA:** 300mg PO qd for 30d, then 150mg PO qd
Triptorelin	EHL 5.37 h, PRC X, Lact ?
Trelstar (Prostate) *Inj 3.75mg/vial* **Trelstar LA (Prostate)** *Inj 11.25mg/vial*	**Advanced carcinoma of the prostate (stage D2):** 3.75 mg IM qmonthly or 11.25mg IM q 3 months

16.5 Nephrolithiasis

MA/EF (allopurinol): inhibition of xanthine oxidase ⇒ uric acid formation ↓ ⇒ uricostatic
AE (acetoh. acid): N/V, headache; **AE** (allopurinol): pruritus, rash, allergic reactions, N/V, myelosuppression, leukopenia, hepatotoxicity, xanthic calculus; **AE** (K+ citrate): metabolic alkalosis, hyperkalemia, N/V, diarrhea; **CI** (acetoh. acid): serum creatinine > 2.5mg/dL, urine infected by non-urease-producing organism, patients amenable to surgery/antimicrobials; **CI** (allopurinol): allergy to allopurinol; **CI** (potassium citrate): severe renal impairment

Allopurinol	EHL 1–2h, PRC C, Lact ?
Zyloprim *Tab 100mg, 200mg, 300mg* **Novo-Purol** *Tab 100mg, 200mg, 300mg* **Generics** *Tab 100mg, 200mg, 300mg*	**Recurrent calcium oxalate stones:** 200–300mg PO qd; DARF: GFR (ml/min): 10–20: 200mg/ d; <10: 100mg/d
Potassium Citrate	EHL no data, PRC C, Lact ?
K-Lyte *Tab (efferv) 25mEq* **Polycitra-K** *Crystals 30mEq/pkt, Sol (oral) 10mEq/5ml*	**Nephrolithiasis:** 10–20mEq PO tid–qid, max 100mEq/d

16.6 Other Urologic Drugs

AE (bethan.): diarrhea, miosis, excessive lacrimation, flushing of skin; **AE** (desm.): nausea, flushing, headache; **CI** (bethan.): hyperthyroidism, peptic ulcer, asthma, bradycardia, hypotension, vasomotor instability, CAD, epilepsy, Parkinsonism, GI inflamm./spasms, peritonitis, vagotonia; **CI** (desm.): hypersens. to desmopressin, **CH** < 3mo, Type IIB von Willebrand's

Bethanechol	EHL no data, PRC C, Lact ?
Duvoid *Tab 10mg, 25mg, 50mg* **Myotonachol** *Tab 10mg, 25mg* **Generics, pms** *Tab 10mg, 25mg, 50mg*	**Urinary retention:** 10–50mg PO tid–qid; 2.5–5mg SC tid– qid
Desmopressin	EHL IV 75.5min, PO 90–150min, PRC B, Lact ?
DDAVP *Tab 0.1, 0.2mg, Tab (dis) 60mcg, 120mcg, Spray (nasal) 0.01mg/Spray, Inj 0.004mg/ml* **DDAVP Rhinyle Nasal Solution** *Spray 0.25mg/bot* **Minirin** *Tab 0.1mg* **Octostim** *Spray (nasal) 0.15mg/Spray, Inj 0.015mg/ml* **Generics** *Spray (nasal) 0.01mg/Spray, Tab 0.1mg, 0.2mg*	**Enuresis:** >6y: ini 20mcg, intranasally hs, maint 10–40mcg; **hemophilia A** →81 **central diabetes insipidus** →140

17 Gynecology, Obstetrics

17.1 Sex Hormones, Hormone Drugs

17.1.1 Estrogens

MA/EF: sec. female sexual characteristics ↑, proliferation of endometrium, liquefying of cervical mucus, protein anabolism, mineralocorticoid EF, Ca^{2+} resorption ↑, Ca^{2+} uptake in bone ↑
AE: thrombosis, skin reactions, edema, glucose tolerance ↓;
CI: hepatic DO, hormone dependent breast/uterus CA, previous thromboembolism, pancreatitis, severe HTN

Esterified Estrogens	EHL no data, PRC X, Lact -
Neo Estrone *Tab 0.3mg, 0.625mg, 1.25mg*	**Menopausal vasomotor symptoms:** 1.25mg PO qd, cyclically 3wk on/1wk off or contin. + progestin qd; **atrophic vaginitis:** 0.3–1.25mg PO qd, cyclically, if no response, >1.25mg/d; **female hypogonadism:** 2.5–7.5mg PO qd div x 20d followed by a 10d rest period; rep until bleeding; **female castration, primary ovarian failure:** 1.25mg PO qd, cyclically; **breast CA palliation in certain patients:** 10mg PO tid ≧ 3mo; **PRO of postmenopausal osteoporosis:** 0.3–1.25mg PO qd, estrogen qd + progestin for last 10–12d of cycle
Estradiol	EHL 1h, PRC X, Lact -
Estrace *Tab 0.5mg, 1mg, 2mg*	**Menopausal vasomotor symptoms and atrophic vaginitis, female hypogonadism, female castration and primary ovarian failure:** 1–2mg PO qd, cyclically 3wk on/1wk off or continuous + progestin qd; **breast CA palliation in certain patients:** 10mg PO tid ≧ 3mo; **PRO of postmenopausal osteoporosis:** 0.5mg PO qd, cyclically 3 wk on/1 wk off or contin. with progestin qd, estrogen qd + progestin for last 10–12d of cycle; **atrophic vaginitis:** local application

Estradiol Transdermal System	EHL no data, PRC X, Lact -
Climara *Film (ext.rel, TD) 0.05, 0.1mg/d* **Estraderm** *Film (ext.rel, TD) 0.025, 0.05, 0.1mg/d* **Estradot** *Film (ext.rel, TD) 0.0375, 0.05, 0.075, 0.1mg/d* **Oesclim** *Film (ext.rel, TD) 0.025, 0.05mg/d* **Vivelle** *Film (ext.rel, TD) 0.05mg/d*	**Menopausal vasomotor symptoms and atrophic vaginitis, female hypogonadism, female castration and primary ovarian failure:** ini 0.025-0.05mg/d patch 1-2/wk, depending on the product, typical regimen: 3wk on and 1wk off or continuously + progestin qd, **postmenopausal osteoporosis (PRO):** 0.025 mg/d- 0.1mg/d patch
Estradiol Valerate	EHL no data, PRC X, Lact -
Generics *Inj 10mg/ml*	**Menopausal vasomotor symptoms and atrophic vaginitis, female hypogonadism, female castration and primary ovarian failure:** 10-20mg IM q4wk
Estrogens, Conjugated	EHL 4-18.5h, PRC X, Lact -
Premarin *Tab 0.3mg, 0.625mg, 0.9mg, 1.25mg, Crm (vag) 0.625mg/g, Inj 25mg/vial* **Generics** *Tab 0.3mg, 0.625mg, 0.9mg, 1.25mg*	**Abnormal uterine bleeding:**25mg IV/IM q6-12h,**normalizing bleeding time in AV malformations and underlying renal impairment:** 30-70mg IV/PO qd until normal, estrogen qd + progestin for last 10-12d of cycle
Estrogens, Synthetic, Conjugated	EHL 4-18.5h, PRC X, Lact -
C.E.S. *Tab 0.3mg, 0.625mg, 0.9mg, 1.25mg* **Premarin** *Tab 0.3mg, 0.625mg, 0.9mg, 1.25mg, Crm (vag) 0.625mg/g, Inj 25mg/vial* **Generics** *Tab 0.3mg, 0.625mg, 0.9mg,1.25mg*	**Menopausal vasomotor symptoms:** 0.625-1.25mg PO qd, cyclically 3wk on/1wk off or contin. + progestin qd; estrogen qd + progestin for last 10-12d of cycle
Estropipate	EHL no data, PRC X, Lact -
Ogen *Tab 0.625mg, 1.25mg, 2.5mg*	**Menopausal vasomotor symptoms, vulvar and vaginal atrophy:** 0.625-5mg PO qd cyclically 3wk on/ 1wk off or contin. + progestin qd; **female hypogonadism, female castration, primary ovarian failure:** 1.25-7.5mg PO qd cyclically 3wk on and 8-10d off; **PRO of osteoporosis:** 0.625mg PO qd x 25d/31d cycle; estrogen qd + progestin for the last 10-12d of the cycle

17.1.2 Selective Estrogen Receptor Modulators

MA/EF: bind on estrogen receptors ⇒ selective expression of estrogen regulating genes ⇒ bone density ↑, total + LDL cholesterol ↓;
AE: hot flashes, leg cramps, higher risk of thromboembolic illnesses;
CI: women of childbearing age, history of thromboembolism, hypersensitivity to raloxifene, severe hepatic/renal insufficiency, endometrial or breast CA

Raloxifene	EHL 27.7h, PRC X, Lact ?
Evista *Tab 60mg*	**Osteoporosis PRO/Tx:** 60mg PO qd; **breast CA PRO:** 60–120mg PO qd

17.1.3 Antiestrogens

MA/EF: (anastrozole, exemestane, letrozole): aromatase inhibition
MA/EF (tamoxifen): blockage of peripheral estrogen receptors;
AE (aromatase inhibitors): hot flashes, nausea, fatigue, sweating, increased appetite,
AE (tamoxifen): alopecia, bone pain, hot flashes, vaginal bleeding, cycle DO, hyperplasia of endometrium, N/V, hypercalcemia;
CI (aromatase inhibitors): premenopausal, pregnancy, lactation
CI (tamoxifen): severe leuko- and thrombopenia, severe hypercalcemia

Anastrozole	EHL 50h, PRC D, Lact ?
Arimidex *Tab 1mg*	**Breast CA; adjuvant Tx (postmenopause):** 1mg PO qd
Exemestane	EHL 24h, PRC D, Lact ?
Aromasin *Tab 25mg*	**Breast CA; adjuvant Tx (postmenopause):** 25mg PO qd
Letrozole	
Femara *Tab 2.5mg*	**Advanced or metastatic breast CA (postmenopause):** 2.5mg PO qd
Tamoxifen	EHL 5–7d, PRC D, Lact ?
Apo-Tamox *Tab 10mg, 20mg* **Nolvadex** *Tab 10mg, 20mg* **Tamofen** *Tab 10mg, 20mg* **Generics** *Tab 10mg, 20mg*	**Breast CA, adjuvant Tx/PRO in high-risk women:** 20mg PO qd x 5 y

17.1.4 Progestins

MA/EF: secretive transformation of endometrium, pregnancy maintenance, inhibition of ovulation, thickening of cervical mucus, body temperature ↑;
AE: acne, hepatic dysfunction, edema, weight gain, nausea, headache, dysmenorrhea;
CI: hepatic diseases, cholestasis, retained abort, vesicular mole

Levonorgestrel	EHL 11-45h, PRC X, Lact ?
Mirena *Intrauterine device (IUD) 52mg* **Norplant** *Implant 36mg* **Plan B** *Tab 0.75mg*	**Contraception:** implant complete system subdermal 8-10cm above the elbow crease within 7d after onset of menses (Implant) or fundal insertion of IUD; **postcoital contraception:** 1 Tab PO, rep in 12h, Tx within 24-72h after sexual intercourse
Medroxyprogesterone Acetate	EHL 38-46 h, PRC D, Lact +
ratio-MPA *Tab 2.5mg, 5mg, 10mg* **Depo-Provera** *Inj 50mg/ml, 150mg/ml* **Gen-Medroxy** *Tab 2.5mg, 5mg, 10mg* **Novo-Medrone** *Tab 2.5mg, 5mg, 10mg* **Provera** *Tab 2.5mg, 5mg, 10mg, 100mg*	**Contraception:** 150mg IM q13wk, inj only during first 5d after onset of menses or within 5d postpartum if not breastfeeding or, if breastfeeding, at 6wk postpartum; **secondary amenorrhea:** 5-10mg PO qd x 5-10d; **abnormal uterine bleeding:** 5-10mg PO qd x 5-10d beginning on the 16th or 21st day of the cycle (after estrogen priming); **hormone replacement Tx to prevent endometrial hyperplasia:** 10mg PO qd for the last 12d mo, or 2.5-5mg PO qd continuously; **endometrial hyperplasia:** 10-30mg PO qd (long-term) or 40-100mg PO qd (short-term) or 500mg IM biw
Megestrol	EHL 13-105h, PRC D (Tab), X (Susp) Lact ?
Megace *Tab 40mg, 160mg, Susp 40mg/ml* **Generics** *Tab 40mg, 160mg*	**AIDS anorexia:** 800mg Susp PO qd; **palliative Tx of advanced CA of the breast:** Tab 40mg PO qid; **endometrial CA:** Tab 40-320mg/d in div doses; **endometrial hyperplasia:** 40-160mg PO qd x 3-4mo; **CA-associated anorexia/cachexia:** 80-160mg PO qid

Norethindrone	EHL 4-13h, PRC X, Lact -
Micronor *Tab 0.35mg*	**contraception:** 1 Tab PO qd

Progesterone, micronized	EHL 16.8-18.3h, PRC X, Lact ?
Prometrium *Cap 100mg* **Generics** *Inj 50mg/ml*	**Hormone replacement Tx to prevent endometrial hyperplasia:** 200mg PO hs 12d/mo; **secondary amenorrhea:** 400mg PO hs x 10d; **hormone replacement Tx to prevent endometrial hyperplasia:** 100mg hs continuously

17.1.5 Hormone Replacement Combinations

Conjugated Estrogens + Medroxyprogesterone (MPA)	PRC X, Lact -
Premplus *Tab 0.625mg + Tab 2.5mg*	**Menopausal vasomotor symptoms, vulvar/ vaginal atrophy, and PRO of postmenopausal osteoporosis:** ini estrogen tab + 2.5mg MPA tab PO qd x 28 days, maint estrogen tab + 5.0 mg MPA PO qd x 28 days OR estrogen tab PO qd x 28 days + 10 mg MPA tab PO qd from day 15-28 of a 28-day cycle

Estradiol + Norethindrone	PRC X, Lact -
Estalis *Film (ext.rel, TD) (0.05mg + 0.14mg)/24h, (0.05mg + 0.25mg)/24h* **Estracomb** *Film (ext.rel, TD) (0.05mg + 0.25mg)/24h*	**Menopausal vasomotor symptoms, vulvar and vaginal atrophy, female hypogonadism, castration, primary ovarian failure, PRO of postmenopausal osteoporosis:** 2 patch/wk

Ethinyl Estradiol + Norethindrone	PRC X, Lact -
FemHRT *Tab 0.005mg + 1mg*	**Menopausal vasomotor symptoms, PRO of postmenopausal osteoporosis:** 1 Tab PO qd

17.2 Oral Contraceptives

17.2.1 Monophasics

MA (monophasics):administration of the same fixed amount of an estrogen-gestagen combination qd for 21d⇒antigonadotropic effects ⇒ suppression of ovulation;
AE/CI (monophasic): see triphasics →308

Desogestrel + Ethinyl Estradiol	PRC X, Lact -
Marvelon *Tab (21) 0.15mg + 0.03mg, Tab (21/7) 0.15mg + 0.03mg/plac* **Linessa 21, 28** *Tab (21) 0.1mg + 0.025mg, 0.125mg + 0.25mg, Tab (21/7) 0.15mg + 0.025mg/plac* **Ortho-Cept** *Tab (21) 0.15mg + 0.03mg Tab (21/7) 0.15mg + 0.03mg/plac*	**Contraception:** 1 Tab PO qd

Ethinyl Estradiol + Ethynodiol	PRC X, Lact -
Demulen 30 *Tab (21) 0.03mg+2mg, Tab (21/7) 0.03mg+2mg/plac*	**Contraception:** 1 Tab PO qd

Ethinyl Estradiol + Levonorgestrel	PRC X, Lact -
Alesse *Tab (21, 21/7) 0.02mg + 0.1mg/plac* **Min-Orval** *Tab(21,21/7) 0.03mg + 0.15mg/plac* **Portia** *Tab 0.03mg + 0.15mg/plac* **Seasonale** *Tab 0.03mg + 0.15mg/plac*	**Contraception:** 1 Tab PO qd; **postcoital contraception:** 0.1mg ethinyl estradiol + 0.5mg levonorgestrel or 5 Tab Alesse or 4 Tab Min-Orval, rep each in 12h within 72h after sexual intercourse

Ethinyl Estradiol + Norelgestromin	PRC X, Lact +
Evra *Film (ext.rel, TD) 0.75 + 6mg/d*	**Contraception**: apply 1 patch qd x 21 d then no patch for 7 d, repeat cycle

Ethinyl Estradiol + Norethindrone	PRC X, Lact -
Brevicon 0.5/35 *Tab 0.035mg + 0.5mg,* **Brevicon 1/35** *Tab 0.035mg + 1mg* **Loestrin 1.5/30** *Tab 0.03mg + 1.5mg* **Minestrin 1/20** *Tab 0.02mg + 1mg* **Ortho 1/35** *Tab 0.035mg + 1mg* **Ortho 0.5/35** *Tab 0.035mg + 0.5mg* **Select 1/35** *Tab 0.035mg + 1mg*	**Contraception:** 1 Tab PO qd

Ethinyl Estradiol + Norgestimate	PRC X, Lact -
Cyclen *Tab 0.035mg + 0.25mg*	**Contraception:** 1 Tab PO qd

Ethinyl Estradiol + Norgestrel	PRC X, Lact -
Ovral *Tab (21, 21/7) 0.05mg + 0.25mg/plac*	**Contraception:** 1 Tab PO qd; **postcoital contraception:** 2 Tab Ovral or 4 Tab Lo/ Ovral, rep each in 12h

17.2.2 Biphasics

MA (biphasic): first half of menstrual cycle: estrogen-only, or combination with low-dose gestagen; second half of menstrual cycle: regular estrogen-gestagen combination ⇒ inhibition of ovulation; **AE/CI** (biphasic): see triphasics →308

Ethinyl Estradiol + Norethindrone	PRC X, Lact -
Synphasic *Tab (10/11) 0.035mg+ 0.5mg/0.035mg + 1mg, Tab (10/ 11/7) 0.035mg + 0.5mg/0.035mg + 1mg/plac*	**Contraception:** 1 Tab PO qd

17.2.3 Triphasics

MA: 3 phases with different estrogen + gestagen combination ⇒ inhibition of ovulation
AE (estrogen-gestagen combinations): seborrhea, acne, dizziness, headache, N/V, breast tenderness, depression, vaginal candidiasis, thrombotic event;
CI (estrogen-gestagen combinations): hepatic dysfunction, cholestasis, hepatic tumors, hormone-dependent malignant tumors, past or present history of thrombosis

Ethinyl Estradiol + Levonorgestrel	PRC X, Lact -
Triphasil, Triquilar *Tab (6/5/10) 0.03mg + 0.05mg/0.04mg + 0.075mg/ 0.03mg+0.125mg, Tab(6/5/10/7) 0.03mg + 0.05mg/0.04mg + 0.075mg/ 0.03mg + 0.125mg/plac*	**Contraception:** 1 tab PO qd
Ethinyl Estradiol + Norethindrone	PRC X, Lact -
Ortho 7/7/7 *Tab (7/7/7) 0.035mg + 0.5mg/ 0.035mg + 0.75mg/0.035mg + 1mg*	**Contraception:** 1 Tab PO qd
Ethinyl Estradiol + Norgestimate	PRC X, Lact -
Tri-Cyclen *Tab (7/7/7) 0.035mg + 0.18mg/ 0.035mg + 0.215mg/0.035mg + 0.25mg*	**Contraception, adult acne** (tri-cyclen): 1 Tab PO qd

17.2.4 Progestin Only Contraceptives (Minipill)

MA: low-dose gestagen-only administration qd for 28 d ⇒ no inhibition (suppression) of ovulation, but cervical mucus viscosity↑; **AE:** irregular menstrual cycles, intracyclic menstrual bleeding; **CI:** serious hepatic dysfunction

Norethindrone	EHL 4-13h, PRC X, Lact -
Micronor *Tab 0.35mg*	**Contracept.:** 1 Tab PO qd

17.3 GnRH Agonists

MA/EF: high doses of gonadotropin releasing hormones ⇒ complete down regulation of pituitary receptors ⇒ production of sex hormones sinks to castration levels
AE (goserelin): bone pain, hot flashes, gynecomastia, impotence, breakthrough bleeding
AE (leuprolide): hot flashes, vaginal hemorrhage, bone pain, N/V, peripheral edema
AE (nafarelin): acne, hot flashes, irregular menstrual bleeding, breast enlargement
CI (goserelin): hypersensitivity to goserelin; **CI** (leuprolide): hypersensitivity to leuprolide / GnRH agonists; **CI** (nafarelin): undiagnosed vaginal bleeding, hypersensitivity to nafarelin

Ganirelix Acetate	EHL 12.8h (1x), 16.2h (multiple), PRC X, Lact -
Orgalutran *Inj 250mcg/0.5ml*	**Infertility:** 250mcg SC qd during early to mid follicular phase, continue Tx qd until day of hCG administration
Goserelin	EHL 2.3h (female), PRC X, Lact -
Zoladex *Implant System 3.6mg/syringe, 10.8mg/syringe*	**Endometriosis:** 3.6mg implant SC q28d x 6mo or 10.8mg implant SC q12wk x 6mo; **palliative Tx of breast CA:** 3.6mg implant SC q28d; **endometrial thinning prior to ablation for dysfunctional uterine bleeding:** 3.6mg SC 4wk preop or 3.6mg SC q4wk x 2, followed by surgery in 2–4wk
Leuprolide	EHL 3h, PRC X, Lact -
Lupron *Inj 5mg/ml* **Lupron Depot** *Inj 3.75mg/vial, 7.5mg/vial, 11.25mg/vial, 22.5mg/vial, 30mg/vial*	**Endometriosis/uterine leiomyomata (fibroids):** 3.75mg IM q mo or 11.25mg IM q3mo x6mo (endometriosis) or x3mo (fibroids) **central precocious puberty:** Inj: 50mcg/kg/d SC, incr by 10mcg/kg/d until total down regulation, Inj depot: 0.3mg/kg/4wk IM, incr by 3.75mg q4wk until adequate down regulation
Nafarelin	EHL 2.7 h, PRC X, Lact -
Synarel *Spray 2mg/ml*	**Endometriosis:** 200mcg spray into one nostril q am, the other nostril q pm x 6mo, incr prn to 4 x 200mcg/d; **central precocious puberty:** 2 sprays into each nostril q am + qpm, incr prn to 1,800mcg/d
Triptorelin	EHL 5.37 h, PRC X, Lact ?
Trelstar (Endometriosis) *Inj 3.75mg/vial*	**Endometriosis:** 3.75 mg IM q 28 days for no longer than 6 month

17.4 Fertility Drugs

17.4.1 Gonadotropins

AE (chorionic gonadotropin): headache, irritability, precocious puberty, gynecomastia, injection site pain;
AE (menotropins): adnexal torsion (with ovarian enlargement), ovarian cysts, flu-like symptoms, pulmonary/vascular complications;
CI (chorionic gonadotropin): precocious puberty, prostatic CA, other androgen dependent neoplasia, hypersens. to chorionic gonadotropin; epilepsy, migraine, asthma, cardiac/renal disease; **CI** (menotropins): vaginal/intracranial bleeding, adrenal/thyroid DO, ovarian cysts or enlargement, primary ovarian failure, pituitary tumor, primary testicular failure

Chorionic Gonadotropins, hCG EHL 5.6h, PRC X, Lact ?	**Induction of ovulation and pregnancy:** ini with menotropins 75U FSH/LH IM qd x 7-12d, then 5,000-10,000 U single shot of hCG IM the day after last menotropin dose, rep prn for 2 more cycles, if evidence for ovulation, incr mentropin dose prn to max 150U FSH/LH; **induction of spermatogenesis in male hypogonadotropic hypogonadism:** 75U FSH/LH IM 3x/wk, prior to administration of menotropins, hCG 5000 U IM 3x/wk until adequate serum testosterone levels and masculinization is achieved, then ini 75U FSH/LH IM 3x/ wk, reduce hCG to 2000 U 2 x/wk, continue for ≧ 4mo, incr prn to 150U FSH/LH
Profasi HP *Inj 10,000 U/vial* **Ovidrel** *Inj 250mcg/vial*	
Follitropins, FSH EHL 17-44h, PRC X, Lact ?	
Gonal-F *Inj 75 U, 150 U/vial, 300U/0.5ml, 450U/0.75ml, 900U/1.5ml, 1200 U/vial* **Puregon** *Inj 50, 100 U/vial* **Luveris** *Inj 75 U/vial*	
Menotropins, FSH/LH EHL 2.2-2.9h, PRC X, Lact ?	
Humegon *Inj 75+75 U/vial* **Menopur** *Inj 75+75 U/vial*	

17.4.2 Ovulatory Stimulants

AE (clomiphene): blurred vision, ovarian enlargement, vasomotor flushing, abdominal pain
CI (clomiphene): uncontrolledthyroid or adrenal dysfunction, liver disease, abnormal uterine bleeding, ovarian cysts, organic intracranial lesion

Clomiphene	EHL 5d, PRC D, Lact ?
Clomid *Tab 50mg* **Serophene** *Tab 50mg*	**Ovulation induction:** 50mg x 5d, ini at any time if no history of recent uterine bleeding, otherwise ini at 5th d of cycle, prn incr to 100mg x 5d in ≧ 30d, max 3 Tx
Gonadorelin	
Lutrepulse *Inj 3.2mg/10ml*	**Ovulation induction:** 1-20mcg SC/IV

17.5 Myometrial Relaxants

AE (indomethacin): headache, GI distress; **AE** (magnesium): flushing, hypotension, muscle weakness; **AE** (nifedipine): peripheral edema, headache, dizziness, tachycardia; **AE** (terbutaline): tremor, tachycardia, headache, nausea, palpitations; **CI** (indomethacin): hypersensitivity to the drug, asthma, history of recent rectal bleeding or proctitis, allergic reactions to ASA or other anti-inflammatories; **CI** (magnesium): 2hr preceding delivery, heart block; **CI** (nifedipine): hypersensitivity to nifedipine or other CCBs, symptomatic hypotension, persistent dermatologic reactions, CHF; **CI** (terbutaline): hypersensitivity to terbutaline products

Indomethacin	EHL 4.5h, PRC X, Lact -
Novo-Methacin *Cap 25mg, 50mg, Supp 50mg, 100mg* **Nu-Indo** *Cap 25mg, 50mg* **Generics** *Cap 25mg, 50mg, Supp 50mg, 100mg*	**Preterm labor** (2nd-3rd line): ini 50-100mg PO/PR, then 5mg PO/PR q6-12-48h; **primary dysmenorrhea:** 25mg PO tid-qid; **patent ductus arteriosus:** neonates <48h: 1st dose 0.2mg/kg, 2nd dose 0.1mg/kg, 3rd dose 0.1mg/ kg, 2-7d: 1st dose 0.2mg/kg, 2nd dose 0.2mg/kg, 3rd dose 0.2mg/kg, >7d: 1st dose 0.2mg/kg, 2nd dose 0.25mg/kg, 3rd dose 0.25mg/kg
Magnesium Sulfate	EHL no data, PRC A, Lact +
Generics *Inj 500mg/ml*	**Seizure prevention in preeclampsia or eclampsia:** 1-4g IV x 2-4min, 5g in 250ml D5W IV inf, max 3ml/min or 4-5g of 50% sol IM q4h prn; **premature labor:** 6g IV x 20min, then 2-3g/h titrated to decrease contractions; DARF: required, monitor serum level, maint urine output 100ml/4h
Nifedipine	EHL 49-137min (pregnancy), PRC C, Lact +
Adalat XL *Tab ext.rel 20mg, 30mg, 60mg* **Apo, Nu-Nifed** *Cap 5mg, 10mg* **Apo-Nifed PA** *Tab ext. rel. 10mg, 20mg* **Novo-Nifedin** *Cap 5mg, 10mg* **Generics** *Tab ext.rel 10mg, 20mg*	**Preterm labor:** ini 10mg PO/SL q20-30min, max 40mg in 1st h of Tx, if successful, maint 10-20mg PO q4-6h or 60-160mg ext.rel PO qd; DARF: not required
Terbutaline	EHL 11-26 h, PRC B, Lact +
Bricanyl Tablets *Tab 2.5mg, 5mg*	**Preterm labor:** 0.25mg SC q30min up to 1mg/4h or 2.5-10mcg/min IV, incr slowly to max 17.5-30mcg/min or 2.5-5mg PO q4-6h

17.6 Labor Induction, Cervical Ripening

MA (oxytocin): contraction of uterine smooth muscle, promotion of milk ejection by stimulation of smooth muscle contraction in the mammary gland
AE (dinoprostone): GI effects, back pain, fetal HR abnormality; **AE** (misoprostol): diarrhea, abdominal pain; **AE** (oxytocin): arrhythmias, subarachnoid hemorrhage, hypotension
CI (dinoprostone): cardiac/pulmonary/renal/hepatic disease, hypersensitivity to dinoprostone products, history cesarean section/ traumatic delivery , cephalopelvic disproportion, fetal distress
CI (misoprostol): hypersensitivity to misoprostol or prostaglandins
CI (oxytocin): significant cephalopelvic disproportion, unfavorable fetal positions, fetal distress, hypertonic uterus, when vaginal delivery is contraindicated, hypersensitivity to oxytocin, severe toxemia

Carbetocin	
Duratocin *Inj 100mcg/vial*	**Prevention of uterine atony:** 100mcg IV
Dinoprostone	EHL 2.5-5min, PRC X (C for cerv. ripen.), Lact ?
Cervidil *Insert ext.rel (vaginal) 10mg* **Prepidil** *Gel (endocervical) 0.5mg/syringe* **Prostin E2** *Tab 0.5mg, Gel (endocervical) 1mg/syringe, 2mg/syringe*	**Cervical ripening:** gel: 1 syringe via catheter placed into cervical canal below the internal os, rep prn q6h, max 3 doses. insert: 1 insert in the posterior fornix of the vagina
Ergonovine Maleate	
Generics *Inj 0.25mg/ml*	**Prevention of uterine atony:** 200mcg IV/IM
Misoprostol	EHL rapid, PRC X, Lact -
Generics *Tab 0.1mg, 0.2mg*	**Cervical ripening/labor induction:** 25-100mcg oral tablet intravaginally q3-4h, max 500mcg/24h or 50mcg PO q4h, max 6 doses or 200mcg PO q6-8h,max 2 doses
Oxytocin	EHL 3-5min, PRC X, Lact -, nasal spray +
Generics *Inj 10 U/ml*	**Induction/stimulation of Labor:** 10U in 1000ml NS, 1-2mU/min IV as continuous inf (6-12ml/h), incr by 1-2 mU/ min q30min until a contraction pattern is established, max 20mU/min; **promotion of milk ejection:** 1 spray in one nostril 2min prior to nursing during 1st wk of puerperium

17.7 Uterotonics

AE (carboprost): emesis/diarrhea, paresthesia, fever/chills, dystonia, breast tenderness
AE (methylergonovine): HTN, N/V, dizziness, palpitations, severe headache, hallucinations
CI (carboprost): hypersensitivity to prostaglandin, acute pelvic inflammatory disease
CI (methylergonovine): hypersensitivity to methylergonovine products, HTN/toxemia

Carboprost	EHL no data, PRC C, Lact ?
Hemabate *Inj 0.25mg/ml*	**Refractory post-partum uterine bleeding:** 250mcg IM, rep prn q15-90min, max 2mg

see Oxytocin →312

17.8 Vaginal Preparations

17.8.1 Antibacterials

Clindamycin Phosphate	EHL 1.5-5h, PRC B, Lact +
Dalacin *Crm (vag) 2%*	**Bacterialvaginosis:** 1 applicatorful (approx. 100mg clindamycin phosphate in 5g cream) intravaginally hs x 7d or one supp qhs x 3d

Metronidazole, local and systemic	EHL 6-11 h, PRC B/X (1st trimester), Lact ?
Flagyl *Cap 500mg, Crm (vag) 10%, Supp (vag) 500mg* **MetroCream** *Crm (top) 0.75%* **MetroGel** *Gel (top) 0.75%* **Nidagel** *Gel (vag) 7.5mg/g* **Noritate** *Crm (top) 1%* **Generics** *Tab 250mg, Inj 5mg/ml*	**Bacterial vaginosis** (local): 1 applicatorful (approx. 37.5mg metronidazole/5g) vag hs or bid x 5d; **bacterial vaginosis** (systemic): Flagyl ER: 750mg PO qd x 7d, other oral Tab: 500mg PO bid x 7d, in pregnancy (not 1st trimester): 250 mg PO tid x 7d; **trichomoniasis:** 2g PO single dose or 250mg PO tid x 1wk or 375-500mg PO bid x 1wk, treat sex partners, too; **Giardia:** 250 mg PO tid x 5-7d; **pelvic inflammatory disease:** 500mg PO bid + ofloxacin 400mg PO bid x 14d; DARF: GFR (ml/min) >10: 100%, <10: 50%

17.8.2 Antifungals

AE (clotrimazole, nystatin, terconazole, tioconazole; topical): vaginal irritation/pain
CI (butoconazole, clotrimazole, miconazole, nystatin, terconazole): hypersensitivity to product ingredients; **CI** (tioconazole): hypersensitivity to tioconazole or miconazole products

Clotrimazole	EHL 3.5–5h, PRC B, Lact ?
Canesten *Crm 1%, 2%, 10%* **Canesten Insert Combi-Pak** *Supp (vag) 200mg +Crm 1%, Supp (vag) 500mg +Crm 1%* **Canesten Cream Combi-Pak** *Crm appl. 500mg +Crm 1%* **Clotrimaderm** *Crm (vag) 1%, 2%*	**Local Tx of vulvovaginal candidiasis:** 1 applicatorful 1% cream hs x 7d or 1 applicatorful 2% cream hs x 3d, prn top cream for external symptoms bid x 7d
Econazole	PRC C, Lact ?
Ecostatin *Supp (vag) 150mg*	**Vaginal candidiasis:** 150mg vag qd x 3d
Fluconazole	EHL 30h, PRC C, Lact -
Diflucan *Tab 50mg,100mg, Cap 150mg, Susp 50mg/5ml, Inj 2mg/ml* **Generics** *Tab 50mg,100mg, Cap 150mg*	**vaginal candidiasis:** 150mg PO single dose
Miconazole	EHL 24 h, PRC C, Lact ?
Micatin *Crm 2%, Spray 2%* **Micazole** *Crm (vag) 2%* **Monistat** *Crm (vag) 2%, Supp (vag) 100mg, Supp (vag) 400mg, 1200mg* **Monistat 3** *Crm (vag) 4% applicators (total of 3)* **Monistat Derm** *Crm (top) 2%* **Monistat Dual-Pak** *Supp (vag) 100mg + Crm 2%, Supp (vag) 400mg + Crm 2%, Supp (vag) 1200mg + Crm 2%*	**Vulvovaginal candidiasis:** 1 applicatorful 2% cream vag hs x 7d or 100mg supp vag hs x7d or 200mg hs x 3d or 1200mg vag insert hs x 1, top cream for external symptoms bid x 7d
Nystatin	EHL not absorbed, PRC C, Lact ?
Candistatin *Crm 100,000 U/g* **Nilstat** *Powder 1 billion U/bottle, Crm 100,000 U/g, Oint 100,000U/g, Crm (vag) 100,000 U/g, Tab (vag) 100,000 U* **Nyaderm** *Crm 100,000 U/g, Oint 100,000 U/g, Crm (vag) 25,000 U/g*	**Local Tx of vulvovaginal candidiasis:** 100,000 U Tab vag hs x 2 wk, treat external lesions with cream

Terconazole	EHL 6.9 h, PRC C, Lact -
Terazol *Crm (vag) 0.4%, 0.8%, Supp (vag) 80mg* **Terazol Dual-Pack** *Supp (vag) 80mg + Crm (vag) 0.8%*	**Local Tx of vulvovaginal candidiasis:** 1 applicatorful 0.4% cream vag hs x 7d or 1 applicatorful 0.8% cream vag hs x 3d or 80mg supp vag hs x 3d

17.8.3 Postmenopausal Vaginal Preparations

Estradiol Vaginal Ring	EHL no data, PRC X, Lact -
Estring *Insert (ext.rel, vag) 0.0075mg/24h*	**Menopausal atrophic vaginitis:** insert into upper 1/3 of vaginal vault, replace after 90d
Estradiol Vaginal Tablet	EHL no data, PRC X, Lact -
Oestrilin *Supp (vag) 0.25mg* **Vagifem** *Tab (vag) 25 mcg*	**Menopausal atrophic vaginitis:** ini 1 Tab (vag) qd x 2wk, maint 1 Tab (vag) 2x/wk
Estrogen Gel/Cream	PRC X, Lact ?
Estrogel *Gel (vag) 0.06%* **Neo Estrone** *Crm (vag) 1mg/g* **Oestrilin** *Crm (vag) 1mg/g* **Premarin** *Crm (vag, conjugated estrogens) 0.625mg/g*	**Atrophic vaginitis/kraurosis vulvae:** Estrogel: 2.5g intravaginally qd cyclically, 3wk on and 1 wk off, Premarin: 0.5-2g intravaginally qd cyclically, 3wk on and 1 wk off

17.8.4 Other Vaginal Preparations

Progesterone Gel	EHL no data, PRC NR Lact ?
Crinone *Gel (vag) 8%*	**Progesterone supplementation in assisted reproduction technology:** 90mg progesterone (gel 8%) vag qd; **progesterone replacement in assisted reproduction technology:** 90mg progesterone (gel 8%) vag bid; **secondary amenorrhea:** progesterone (gel 4%) vag qod x 6 doses, prn gel 8% qod x 6 doses; **contraception:** fundal insertion of progestasert IUD

17.9 Other Gynecologic, Obstetric Drugs

AE (clonidine): CNS depression, orthostasis, localized reactions, dry mouth;
AE (danazol): hepatic dysfunction, weight gain, acne, menstrual disturbances;
AE (RHO Immune Globulin): chills, headache, intravascular hemolysis;
CI (clonidine): hypersensitivity to clonidine products, conduction defects, bleeding DO, injection site infection;
CI (danazol): undiagnosed abnormal vaginal bleeding, hepatic/renal/cardiac dysfunction;
CI (RHO Immune Globulin): hypersensitivity to human globulin B, Rho(D)/D(U) positive patients, Rho(D) negative patients sensitized to Rho(D)/D(U) antigens neonates, IgA deficiency

Clonidine	EHL 12-16 h, PRC C, Lact ?
Catapres *Tab 0.1mg, 0.2mg* **Dixarit** *Tab 0.025mg* **Generics** *Tab 0.1mg, 0.2mg*	**Menopausal flushing:** 0.1-0.4mg/d PO div bid-tid or TD 0.1mg/d (1 patch qwk)
Danazol	EHL 4.5h, PRC X, Lact ?
Cyclomen *Cap 50mg, 100mg, 200mg*	**Endometriosis:** ini 400mg PO bid, then decr to a dose sufficient to maintain amenorrhea x 3-6mo, max 9mo; **fibrocystic breast disease:** 100-200mg PO bid x 4-6mo; **menorrhagia:** 100-400mg PO qd x 3mo; DARF: contraind. in RF
Doxylamine + Pyridoxine	
Diclectin *Tab del. rel. 10mg + 10mg*	**Nausea of pregnancy:** 2 Tab PO qhs and 1 Tab PO bid PRN
Rho(D) Immune Globuline	PRC C, Lact ?
BayRho-D Full Dose *Inj 300mcg/vial* **WinRho SDF** *Inj 120mcg/vial, 300mcg/vial, 1000mcg/vial*	**PRO of isoimmunization in Rh-negative women following spontaneous or induced abortion or termination of ectopic pregnancy ≥12 wk gestation:** 50mcg (Microdose) **IM; PRO of maternal sensitization ot the Rh factor in pregnancy/after childbirth:** 300mcg IM if fetal packed RBC volume that entered mother's blood due to fetomaternal hemorrhage <15ml (30ml of whole blood), if >15ml, admin 600mcg IM

18 Toxicology

18.1 Drugs, Antidotes

Acetylcysteine	EHL 2.27h, PRC B, Lact ?
Mucomyst *Sol (inhal) 20%* **Parvolex** *Sol (inhal) 200mg/ml* **Generics** *Inj 200mg/ml*	**Acetaminophen toxicity:** loading dose 140mg/kg PO or NG as soon as possible, then 70mg/kg q4h x 17 doses, prn mix in water; IV use: pyrogen-free IV; acetylcysteine is available only through participating poison centers; **CH:** adult dose
Atropine	EHL 4h, PRC C, Lact ?
Generics *Inj 0.4, 0.6mg/ml*	**Organophosphate poisoning:** 2–5 mg IV, rep prn q10–30min; **CH:** 0.05mg/kg IV, rep prn q10–30min
Charcoal	PRC B, Lact +
Charcodote (in sorbitol) *Liquid (oral) 200mg/ml* **Charcodote aqueous (in water)** *Liquid (oral) 200mg/ml* **Charcodote TFS** *Liquid (oral) 200mg + 200mg (sorbitol)/ml*	**Gut decontamination:** 25–100g (0.5–1g/kg or 10 times the amount of poison ingested) PO or NG as soon as possible, rep prn q4h; **CH** >1y: adult dose
Deferasirox	EHL 8–16 h, PRC B, Lact ?
Exjade *Tab 125 mg, 250 mg, 500 mg*	**Chronic iron overload:** ini 20mg/kg PO qd, maint. 20–30mg/kg PO qd, max 30mg/kg/d; **CH** >2y: ini 20mg/kg PO qd, max 30mg/kg/d
Deferoxamine	EHL 3–6 h, PRC C, Lact ?
Desferal *Inj 500mg/vial, 2g/vial* **Desferrioxamine Mesilate** *Inj 500mg/vial* **Generics** *Inj 500mg/vial*	**Chronic iron overload:** 500mg–1,000mg IM qd and 2g IV inf (max 15mg/kg/h) with each unit of blood or 1–2g SC qd (20–40mg/kg/d) x 8–24h via contin. inf pump; **acute iron toxicity:** ini 1g IM, then 500mg IM q4h x 2 doses, rep prn 500mg IM q4–12h, max 6g/24h; IV route (only in patients with CVS collapse): ini 1g slowly IV (max 15mg/ kg/h), then 500mg x 4h for 2 doses at max rate of 125mg/ h, prn subsequent doses of 500mg x 4–12h at max rate of 125mg/h; DARF: contraind. unless undergoing dialysis

Digoxin Immune Fab	EHL 15-20h, PRC C, Lact ?
Digibind *Inj 38mg/vial*	**Digoxin intoxication:** single large dose intoxication: of vials= (total digital body load in mg/0.5) IV; based on steady-state concentrations: adult: of vials= ([serum digoxin in nmol/L x 0.781 x wt. in kg]/100) IV; **CH:** of vials = ([Serum digoxin in nmol/L x 0.765 x wt. in kg]/1000) IV
Dimercaprol	EHL very short (no exact data), PRC N, Lact ?
BAL in oil *Inj 100mg/ml*	**Arsenic/gold poisoning, mild:** 2.5mg/kg deeply IM 4x/d x 2d, bid on d3, then qd x 10d or until recovery; **arsenic/gold poisoning, severe:** 3mg/kg deeply IM q4h x 2d, qid on d3, bid x 10d or until recovery; **mercury poisoning:** ini 5mg/kg,then 2.5mg/kg qd-bid x 10d; **acute lead encephalopathy:** 4mg/kg q4h x 2-7d, after 1st dose, combined Tx with edetate calcium disodium at separate site; **lead poisoning, mild:** ini 4mg/kg, then 3mg/kg q4h x 2-7d; DARF: req
Edetate Calcium Disodium	EHL 1.4-3h, PRC C, Lact -
Calcium Disodium Versenate *Inj 200mg/ml*	**Lead poisoning:** rec dosage for blood lead level >20mcg/deciliter and <70mcg/deciliter: 1g/m^2/d IM x 8-12h x 5d, then interrupt Tx x 2-4d, then rep prn 5-day course of Tx, max 75mg/kg/d, mix for IM use 1ml of inj concentrate with 1ml lidocaine or procaine 1%; DARF: CrCl (mg/dl) 2-3: 50% q24h x 5d, rep prn qmo, 3-4: 50% q48h x 3 doses, rep prn qmo, >4: 50% qwk, rep prn qmo
Ethanol	EHL 0.232mg/(ml x h), PRC N, Lact -
Ethanol	**Methanol poisoning:** if acidosis, visual changes, blood MeOH level >25mg/deciliter, ini loading dose 10ml/kg of 10% ethanol in D5W x 20-30min, maint 1-2ml/kg/h, maint blood ethanol level 100-150mg/dl
Flumazenil	EHL 41-79min, PRC C, Lact ?
Anexate *Inj 0.1mg/ml* **Generics** *Inj 0.1mg/ml*	**Benzodiazepine sedation reversal:** 0.2mg IV x 15sec, after 30sec prn 0.2mg q1min, max 1mg total dose, usual dose 0.6-1mg; **benzodiazepine overdose reversal:** 0.2mg IV x 30sec, after 30sec prn 0.3mg, then prn 0.5mg q1min, max 3mg total dose; DARF: not required

Fomepizole	EHL 5h (oral), PRC C, Lact ?
Antizol *Inj 1g/ml*	**Methanol/Ethylene glycol toxicity:** ini loading dose 15mg/kg slowly IV x 30min, then 10mg/kg slowly IV q12h x 4 doses, then 15mg/kg slowly IV q12h, then until ethylene glycol concentrations <20mg/deciliter or ini 15mg/kg PO, in 12h 5mg/kg PO, then 10mg/kg PO q12h ethylene glycol plasma levels =0; DARF: consider additional dialysis
Ipecac Syrup	PRC C, Lact ?
Generics *Syr*	**Induction of emesis:** 15-30ml PO, then 3-4 glasses of water, rep if vomiting does not occur within 20-30min; **CH** 1-12y: 15ml, then 1-2 glasses of water, rep if vomiting does not occur within 20-30min
Methylene Blue	PRC C, Lact ?
Generics *Inj 50mg/5ml*	**Methemoglobinemia (drug induced):** 1-2mg/kg IV (0.1-0.2ml/kg of 1% sol) x 5min, do not use in cyanide poisoning; DARF: use with caution in severe RF
Penicillamine	EHL 1-7.5h, PRC D, Lact -
Cuprimine *Cap 125mg, 250mg* **Depen** *Tab 250mg*	**Wilson's disease:** 750mg-1.5g/d resulting incupriuresis of 2mg/d, adjust dosage based on urinary copper analysis and determination of free copper in the serum; **lead poisoning:** 1-1.5g/d x 1-2mo given 2h before or 3h after meals; DARF: GFR (ml/min) <50%: avoid drug
Sodium Thiosulfate	PRC C, Lact ?
Generics *Inj 2.5g/10ml*	**Cyanide poisoning:** 12.5g IV at a rate of 0.625-1.25g/min; **CH:** 412.5mg/kg or 7g/square meter body surface area IV at a rate of 0.625-1.25 g/min
Sorbitol	PRC N, Lact +
Generics *Sol (oral) 70%*	**Laxative:** 30-150ml (70% sol) PO or 120ml (25-30% sol) PR; **CH** 2-11y: 2ml/kg (70% sol) PO or 30-60 ml (25-30% sol) PR

18.2 Poison Control Centers

ALBERTA
Poison and Drug Information Services,
Foothills General Hospital,
1403-29th St. N.W.
Calgary, AB. T2N 2T9
1-800-332-1414;
(403) 670-1414 local;
(403) 670-1472 (fax)

BRITISH COLUMBIA
B.C. Drug and Poison Information Centre,
St. Paul's Hospital,
1081 Burrard St.,
Vancouver, BC V6Z 1Y6
1-800-567-8911
Tel: 604-682-5050 (Lower Mainland)
Tel: 1-800-567-8911 (remainder of Province)
Fax: 604-806-8262
E-mail: daws@dpk.bc ca

MANITOBA
Provincial Poison Information Centre,
Children's Hospital
840 Sherbrook St.,
Winnipeg, MB R3A 1S1
(204) 787-2591 emergency inquiries
(204) 787-4807 (fax)

NEW BRUNSWICK
Poison Control Centre,
774 Main St 6th floor
Moncton NB E1C 9Y3
Tel: Call 911 in New Brunswick for poison information.
Fax: 506-867-3259

NEWFOUNDLAND
Poison Information Centre,
The Janeway Child Health Centre
300 Prince Philip Dr
St. John's NL A1B 3V6

NORTHWEST TERRITORIES
Emergency Department,
Stanton Territorial Hospital
550 Byrne Rd
PO Box 10
Yellowknife NT X1A 2N1
Tel: 867-669-4100
Tel: 1-800-268-9017
Fax: 867-669-4171

NOVA SCOTIA
Poison Control Centre,
The Izaak Walton Killam Children's Hospital,
P.O.Box 3070,
Halifax, NS B3J 3G9
Tel: 902-470-8161
Tel: 1-800-565-8161 (Nova Scotia and Prince Edward Island)
Tel: 1-902-470-8161 (remainder of Provinces)
Fax: 902-470-7213

ONTARIO
Ontario Regional Poison Information Centre
The Hospital for Sick Children
555 University Ave
Toronto ON M5G 1X8
Tel: 416-813-5900
Tel: 1-800-268-9017
Fax: 416-813-7489

PRINCE EDWARD ISLAND
Poison Control Centre,
The Izaak Walton Killam Children's Hospital,
P.O.Box 3070,
Halifax, NS B3J 3G9
1-800-565-8161

QUÉBEC
Centre anti-poison du Québec,
1050 ch Ste-Foy
"L" wing 1st Floor
Quebec QC G1S 4L8
Tel: 418-656-8090
Tel: 1-800-463-5060
Fax: 418-654-2747

SASKATCHEWAN
Poison and Drug Information Service
Foothills Hospital
1403-29th St NW
Calgary AB T2N 2T9
Tel: 1-866-454-1212

YUKON TERRITORY
Emergency Department,
Whitehorse General Hospital,
5 Hospital Road,
Whitehorse, YT Y1A 3H7
Tel: 867-393-8700
Fax: 867-393-8762

Bibliography

1. Arana GW, Hyman SE, Rosebaum JF, ed: Handbook of Psychiatric Drug Therapy, edn 4. Philadelphia: Lippincott Williams & Wilkins, 2000.

2. Bartlett JD, Jaanus SD, ed: Clinical Ocular Pharmacology, edn 4. Woburn: Butterworth-Heinemann, 2001.

3. Bauer LA, ed: Applied Clinical Pharmacokinetics, edn 1. New York: McGraw-Hill, 2001.

4. Bezchlibnyk-Butler KZ, ed: Clinical Handbook of Psychotropic Drugs, edn 11. Seattle, Hogrefe and Huber, 2001.

5. Billups NF, Billups SM, ed: American Drug Index 2001, edn 45. Philadelphia: Facts & Comparisons, 2001.

6. Braunwald E, Fauci AS, Kasper DL, Hauser SL, Longo DL, Jameson JL, ed: Harrison's Principles of Internal Medicine, edn 15. New York: Lippincott Williams & Wilkins, 2001.

7. Canadian Immunization Guide. Sixth Edition, http://www.hc-sc.gc.ca/, Health Canada, 2002.

8. Colbert BJ, Mason BJ, ed: Integrated Cardiopulmonary Pharmacology, edn 1. Upper Saddle River: Prentice Hall, 2001.

9. Compendium of Pharmaceuticals and Specialties, Thirty-sixth Edition. Canadian Pharmacists Association, 2001.

10. Compendium of Pharmaceuticals and Specialties. Thirty-seventh Edition. Canadian Pharmacists Association, 2002.

11. Compendium of Pharmaceuticals and Specialties. Thirty-eight Edition. Canadian Pharmacists Association, 2003.

12. Compendium of Pharmaceuticals and Specialties. Thirty-nine Edition. Canadian Pharmacists Association, 2004.

13. Compendium of Pharmaceuticals and Specialties. Fortieth Edition. Canadian Pharmacists Association, 2005.
14. Drug Product Database, http://www.hc-sc.gc.ca/hpb/drugs-dpd/, Health Canada.
15. Electronic Orange Book, http://www.fda.gov/cder/ob/, FDA, 2001.
16. Gibaldi M, ed: Drug Therapy, 2000: A Critical Review of Therapeutics, edn 1. New York: McGraw-Hill, 2000.
17. Joel G, Hardman LE, ed: Goodman & Gilman's The Pharmacological Basis of Therapeutics, edn 10. New York: McGraw-Hill, 2001.
18. Russ A, Nudo CG, Canadian Drug Pocket, first edition: Borm Bruckmeier Publishing, 2004.
19. Mycek MJ, Harvey RA, Champe PC, ed: Lippincott's Illustrated Reviews: Pharmacology: Special Millennium Update, edn 2. Philadelphia: Lippincott Williams & Wilkins, 2000.
20. Physician's Desk Reference 2001 (Library Edition), edn 55. Oradell: Physician's Desk Reference, 2001.
21. Reese RE, Betts RF, Gumustop B, ed: Handbook of Antibiotics, edn 3. Philadelphia: Lippincott Williams & Wilkins, 2000.
22. Skolnick P, ed: Antidepressants: New Pharmacological Strategies; edn 1. Totowa: Humana Press, 1997.
23. Wolverton SE, ed: Comprehensive Dermatologic Drug Therapy, edn 1. London: Saunders, 2001

Important Formulas

A-a O_2 gradient
= $(Fi_{O2}\% / 100) \times (P_{atm} - 47\,mmHg) - (Pa_{CO2} / 0.8) - Pa_{O2}$
(all units in mmHg)

Anion gap
= $(Na^+ + K^+) - (Cl^- + [HCO_3^-]$
(all units mmol/L)

BSA (m^2)
= $\sqrt{}$height(cm) x weight(kg)/60
(Mosteller. NEJM 1987; 317:109)

Lean Body Weight (men)
= (1.10 x weight(kg)) - 128 (weight^2 / (100 x height(m))^2)
Lean Body Weight (women)
= (1.07 x weight(kg)) - 148 (weight^2 / (100 x height(m))^2)

Ideal Body Weight (men)
= 50 + 2.3 (height(in) - 60)
Ideal Body Weight (women)
= 45.5 + 2.3 (height(in) - 60

Body Mass Index
= Weight(kg) / Height(m)^2

Estimated Creatinine Clearance (CrCl ml/min)
= [[140 - age(yr)] x weight(kg)] / [72 x serum Cr(mg/dL)]
(multiply by 0.85 for women); Cr: µmol/l = 88.4 x mg/dl

Fractional Excretion of Sodium (FE_{Na})
= $(U_{Na} \times P_{Cr}) / (P_{Na} \times U_{Cr}) \times 100$

Serum Osmolality
= $(2 \times (Na^+ + K^+))$ + (BUN) + (glucose)
(all units mmol/L)

Numerics

A

C

D

E

F

G

H

I

J

K

L

M

N

O

Q

R

S

T

U

V

W

X

Y

Z

Notes

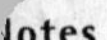

Notes

Notes

Note

Notes

Notes

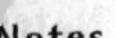

Notes

Notes

Medical Spanish pocketcard Set

Vital communication tool for anyone working with Spanish-speaking patients!

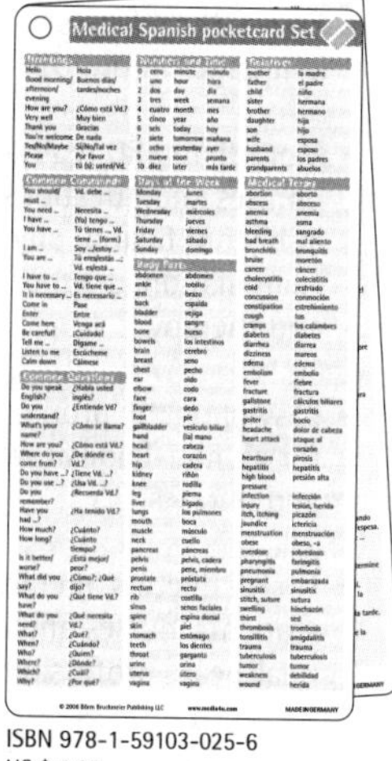

ISBN 978-1-59103-025-6
US $ 6.95

- Numerous ready-to-use words and phrases including greetings, common commands and questions, body parts, medical terms, physical exam terms, and much more
- With its clearly organized structure, the Medical Spanish pocketcard set is an ideal companion in the doctor's office, on hospital rounds, and during consultations
- With these pocketcards, language should never be a barrier to communicating with Spanish-speaking patients
- Perfect supplement to our Medical Spanish pocket.

Table of Contents, Text Samples, PDA Demo Files... www.media4u.com

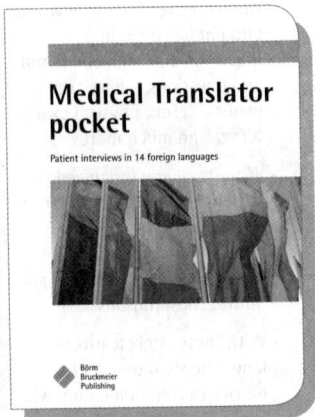

Börm Bruckmeier Products

pockets

Acupuncture pocket	ISBN 978-1-59103-248-9	US $ 12.95
Anatomy pocket	ISBN 978-1-59103-219-9	US $ 16.95
Canadian Drug pocket 2009	ISBN 978-1-59103-238-0	US $ 14.95
Differential Diagnosis pocket	ISBN 978-1-59103-216-8	US $ 14.95
Drug pocket 2008	ISBN 978-1-59103-240-3	US $ 12.95
Drug pocket plus 2008	ISBN 978-1-59103-241-0	US $ 19.95
ECG pocket	ISBN 978-1-59103-230-4	US $ 16.95
ECG Cases pocket	ISBN 978-1-59103-229-8	US $ 16.95
Homeopathy pocket	ISBN 978-1-59103-250-2	US $ 14.95
Medical Abbreviations pocket	ISBN 978-1-59103-221-2	US $ 16.95
Medical Classifications pocket	ISBN 978-1-59103-223-6	US $ 16.95
Medical Spanish pocket	ISBN 978-1-59103-232-8	US $ 16.95
Medical Spanish Dictionary pocket	ISBN 978-1-59103-231-1	US $ 16.95
Medical Spanish pocket plus	ISBN 978-1-59103-239-7	US $ 22.95
Medical Translator pocket	ISBN 978-1-59103-235-9	US $ 16.95
Normal Values pocket	ISBN 978-1-59103-205-2	US $ 12.95
Nursing Dictionary pocket	ISBN 978-1-59103-237-3	US $ 12.95
Respiratory pocket	ISBN 978-1-59103-228-1	US $ 16.95
Wards 101 pocket	ISBN 978-1-59103-236-6	US $ 19.95

pocketcards

Alcohol Withdrawal pocketcard	ISBN 978-1-59103-031-7	US $ 3.95
Anesthesiology pocketcard Set (3)	ISBN 978-1-59703-050-8	US $ 9.95
Antibiotics pocketcard 2008	ISBN 978-1-59103-041-6	US $ 3.95
Antifungals pocketcard	ISBN 978-1-59103-013-3	US $ 3.95
Asthma pocketcard Set (2)	ISBN 978-1-59103-046-1	US $ 6.95
COPD pocketcard Set (2)	ISBN 978-1-59103-047-8	US $ 6.95
Dementia pocketcard Set (3)	ISBN 978-1-59103-053-9	US $ 9.95
Diabetes pocketcard Set (3)	ISBN 978-1-59103-054-6	US $ 9.95
Dyslipidemia pocketcard Set (2)	ISBN 978-1-59103-055-3	US $ 6.95
ECG pocketcard	ISBN 978-1-59103-028-7	US $ 3.95
ECG Ruler pocketcard	ISBN 978-1-59103-002-7	US $ 3.95
ECG pocketcard Set (3)	ISBN 978-1-59103-003-4	US $ 9.95
Echocardiography pocketcard Set (2)	ISBN 978-1-59103-024-9	US $ 6.95

Börm Bruckmeier Products

pocketcards

Epilepsy pocketcard Set (2)	ISBN 978-1-59103-034-8	US $ 6.95
Geriatrics pocketcard Set (3)	ISBN 978-1-59103-037-9	US $ 9.95
History & Physical Exam pocketcard	ISBN 978-1-59103-022-5	US $ 3.95
Hypertension pocketcard	ISBN 978-1-59103-042-3	US $ 6.95
Immunization pocketcard	ISBN 978-1-59103-044-7	US $ 6.95
Medical Abbreviations pc Set (2)	ISBN 978-1-59103-010-2	US $ 6.95
Medical Spanish pocketcard	ISBN 978-1-59103-027-0	US $ 3.95
Medical Spanish pocketcard Set (2)	ISBN 978-1-59103-025-6	US $ 6.95
Neurology pocketcard (2)	ISBN 978-1-59103-021-8	US $ 6.95
Normal Values pocketcard	ISBN 978-1-59103-023-2	US $ 3.95
Parkinson pocketcard Set (2)	ISBN 978-1-59103-043-0	US $ 6.95
Periodic Table pocketcard	ISBN 978-1-59103-014-0	US $ 9.95
Psychiatry pocketcard Set (2)	ISBN 978-1-59103-033-1	US $ 6.95
Vision pocketcard	ISBN 978-1-59103-032-4	US $ 3.95
Wound Ruler pocketcard	ISBN 978-1-59103-051-5	US $ 3.95

pockettools

Asthma pockettool	ISBN 978-1-59103-802-3	US $ 9.95
DARF pockettool	ISBN 978-1-59103-803-0	US $ 9.95
ECG pockettool	ISBN 978-1-59103-800-9	US $ 9.95
ECG Ruler pockettool	ISBN 978-1-59103-805-4	US $ 9.95
Medical Spanish pockettool	ISBN 978-1-59103-804-7	US $ 9.95
Normal Values pockettool	ISBN 978-1-59103-801-6	US $ 9.95

PDA software

Differential Diagnosis pocket for PDA	ISBN 978-1-59103-600-5	US $ 16.95
Drug Therapy pocket for PDA	ISBN 978-1-59103-605-0	US $ 16.95
ECG pocket for PDA	ISBN 978-1-59103-601-2	US $ 16.95
Homeopathy pocket for PDA	ISBN 978-1-59103-650-0	US $ 16.95
ICD-9-CM 2005 for PDA	ISBN 978-1-59103-606-7	US $ 24.95
Medical Abbreviations pocket for PDA	ISBN 978-1-59103-603-6	US $ 16.95
Medical Calculator pocket for PDA	ISBN 978-1-59103-616-6	US $ 16.95
Medical Spanish pocket for PDA	ISBN 978-1-59103-602-9	US $ 16.95
Medical Spanish Dic. pocket for PDA	ISBN 978-1-59103-607-4	US $ 16.95
Medical Spanish pocket plus for PDA	ISBN 978-1-59103-608-1	US $ 24.95